MODERN CONCEPTS IN PSYCHIATRIC SURGERY

DEVELOPMENTS IN PSYCHIATRY

MODERN CONCEPTS IN PSYCHIATRIC SURGERY

Proceedings of the 5th World Congress of Psychiatric Surgery
held in Boston MA, U.S.A. on August 21-25, 1978

Editors

E.R. Hitchcock

H.T. Ballantine, Jr.

and

B.A. Meyerson

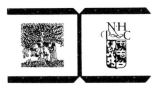

1979

ELSEVIER/NORTH-HOLLAND BIOMEDICAL PRESS
AMSTERDAM · NEW YORK · OXFORD

ISBN for this volume: 0-444-80108-1
ISBN for the series: 0-444-80107-3

Published by:
Elsevier/North-Holland Biomedical Press
335 Jan van Galenstraat, P.O. Box 211
Amsterdam, The Netherlands

Sole distributors for the USA and Canada:
Elsevier North-Holland Inc.
52 Vanderbilt Avenue
New York, N.Y. 10017

PRINTED IN THE NETHERLANDS

PREFACE

These papers represent some of the contributions held at Pine Manor College in Brooklyn, Massachusetts, in August, 1978.

Although we were saddened by the recent death of the President, Sixto Obrador, we were steered through a successful meeting by the President of the Congress, Tom Ballantine.

The papers presented here represent the most modern concepts of psychiatric surgery and reveal the increasing awareness of the relationship between biogenic amines and ablative and stimulation surgery. Many of these papers present the findings of teams of neurosurgeons, psychiatrists, psychologists and biochemists - a trend strongly supported by the society.

The use of photo offset reproduction has meant that most authors have been responsible for their own manuscript editing. The Editors hope that for the rapidly changing field of Psychiatric Surgery the early publication made possible by this method will excuse any minor inaccuracies.

E.R.H.

CONTENTS

viii

SOCIETY AND PSYCHIATRIC SURGERY

BIOCHEMICAL AND STIMULATION STUDIES

© 1979 Elsevier/North-Holland Biomedical Press
Modern Concepts in Psychiatric Surgery
E.R. Hitchcock, H.T. Ballantine, Jr. and B.A. Meyerson, eds.

NEUROTRANSMITTER MECHANISMS UNDERLYING PSYCHIATRIC SURGERY,

ELECTROCONVULSIVE THERAPY AND ANTIDEPRESSIVE DRUG THERAPY

HOFSTATTER, L. and GIRGIS, M.

University of Missouri-Columbia, School of Medicine, Department
of Psychiatry, Missouri Institute of Psychiatry, U.S.A.; &
University of Sydney, Australia and University of Missouri-
Columbia, same as above.

Involvement of Neurotransmitters (NT) in all treatment modalities, including Psychiatric Surgery, for psychiatric illness,
particularly depressive states is implied in the title. Therefore
we shall proceed to point out the essential part of the NT
system in mental health and illness, the significance of NT
equilibrium and disequilibrium for mental health and mental
illness respectively, the equal and equalizing role of aminergic
and cholinergic NTs in the maintenance of NT balance, and the
paramount importance of restoration of NT balance for the therapeutic effectiveness of the three treatment modalities, particularly in depression.

Their clinically and experimentally established foundation
is in sharp contrast to the originators' conception of their
ingeniously conceived treatment methods, i.e. disruption of a
vicious cycle of fixed cell connections in the brain by Egas
Moniz (1936)[1], antagonism of epilepsy and schizophrenia by
L.V. Meduna (1938)[2], and the origin of non-hypnotic ataractic
psychotropic drugs from a study of histamines (1952).

Our data was derived from neuro-histochemical neuro-physio-
logical and neuro-pharmacological investigations at the Missouri
Institute of Psychiatry, U.S.A., and the University of Sydney,
Australia and will enable the psychologically and biologically
oriented neuro-scientist to better understand the workings of
the components of his/her armamentarium.

The present investigation attempts to establish plausible
and heuristic evidence of an abnormal NT imbalance with a relative
predominance of acetylcholine (ACh) in some limbic structures
as one of the biochemical substrates of depressive states; they

have so far commonly been attributed to underactivity or deficiency of aminergic NT according to the pioneering catecholamine hypothesis of affective disorders (Schildkraut 1965)[3]. The effective reduction of ACh and/or elevation of aminergic NT levels in these areas to reestablish normal NT equilibrium will be shown to be the common denominator, basic principle and central goal of all treatment modalities, surgical axotomy, pharmacological or electroconvulsive therapy (ECT) and available tricyclic antidepressants, responsible and essential for their success in treating depressive states.

The maintenance of a delicate self-regulating and self-correcting balance of opposing NTs within a narrow range of safety is based on their synergistic reciprocal relationship and is the condition essential for adaptive, i.e. normal emotional behavior.

This concept can be traced back to the time honored principles of constancy of the internal environment by Claude Bernard (1872), to W.B. Cannon's natural tendency toward homeostasis of bodily processes in the service of self-preservation and survival (1932), and to W.R. Hess' (1924)[4] and E. Gellhorn's (1953)[5] critical balance and synergism between ergotropic and trophotropic elements of the autonomous nervous system. They apply not only to the realm of physiology but also to that of psychiatry and were elaborated in L.V. Bertalanffy's Open System Theory of Living Systems (1966)[6] with its dynamic steady state of balanced tension and reciprocal interaction of opposing forces. Perez-Cruet, et al (1971)[7] have first presented experimental evidence of a reciprocal relationship between central cholinergic and adrenergic NTs. Marrazzi (1966)[8] stressed the relationship of excessive and nonadaptive emotional responses in mental illness and a dynamic imbalance or distorted homeostasis between excitatory and inhibitory NTs, chemical compounds that convey information between adjacent nerve cells. Janowsky (1972)[9] has laid the foundation for a bivariate cholinergic-adrenergic hypothesis of Mania and Depression, and indicated that a given affective state may represent a balance between central cholinergic and adrenergic NT activity in those areas of the brain which regulate affect. Balance among the central NT has been the subject of some recent reviews (Pradhan 1978)[10].

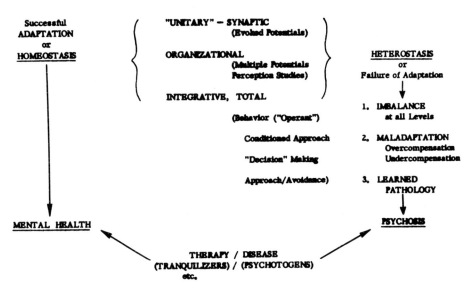

Fig. 1. Cerebral Adaptive System.
(Reproduced with permission of Dr. A. Marrazzi[8])

There is further evidence that points to specific limbic
structures of the medio-orbito-temporal region and to malfunc-
tioning neural mechanisms in that area, normally subject to
cholinergic mediation as a source of disturbed behavior and a
target for therapeutic intervention in psychotic depression.

Histochemical light microscopic studies with a modified
Koelle's thiocholine technique (Girgis, 1967)[11] brought out a
strikingly high, though uneven, concentration of acetyl-
cholinesterase (AChE) in all relays in the "Cortical Circuits
of Emotion" of Papez (1937)[12]. The limbic system ranks highest
among cerebral structures in AChE content and activity throughout the animal kingdom, from rodents to primates with variation
from nucleus to nucleus and from animal to animal. Invariably,
however, the magno-cellular part of the amygaloid nucleus
stains intensely in all mammalian brains, including the brain
of man.

AChE concentration is only slight in neocortical areas,
excepting moderate concentrations in the posterior orbito-frontal
cortex (area 13) and the cingulate gyrus.

6

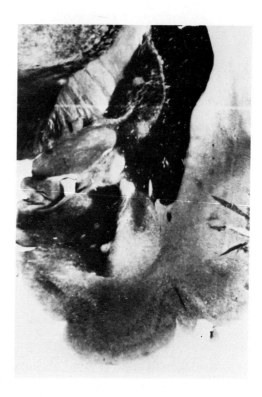

Fig. 2. Distribution of AChE in rabbit amygdala and other
limbic structures.

   The high concentration of readily available AChE in the limbic
system may serve an important stabilizing and protective function in the maintenance of a more or less steady level of ACh
within narrow limits of safety; it may be operative by safeguarding the physiological threshold of sensitivity of ACh and
by preventing the development of pathological cholinergic hyper-
reactivity or hypersensitivity in susceptible neurons of the
limbic system, (Hofstatter and Girgis, 1973)[12a].
   Electron Histochemistry, has allowed more exact cytological
localization of AChE than the light microscope (Shute and Lewis,

1965)[13].

The electron microscopic study with a modified Koelle technique (Tsuji, 1974)[14] showed AChE in the cisternae of rough endoplasmic reticulum of the perikarya of cholinergic neurons and in their nuclear envelope, with which the cisternae often communicate. Occasionally, as in the septum (The source of the cholinergic supply to the hippocampus) AChE is also present in the plasma membrane.

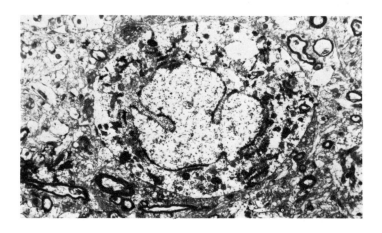

Fig. 3. Ultrastructural localization of AChE in cell bodies of Amygdala.

The Electronmicrogram of the above mentioned magno-cellular part of the basal amygdaloid nucleus shows also numerous positive synaptic endings around these cholinergic cells, suggesting both the cholinergic as well as cholinoceptive nature of a large number of its neurons.

Ultrastructural studies indicate that the enzymes needed for both synthesis and hydrolysis of the neurotransmitter are manufactured in the perikarya of the cholinergic neurons and transported in neurotubular structures in a slow but constant flow down in the axoplasm of the axon at a rate of about 20 to 400 mm/day, to be released at its terminals, the active synaptic sites, (Lewis and Hughes, 1957[15]; Haggendal, et al,

1971[16]; Lubinska, 1975[17]). There ACh is synthesized from
Choline and acetate with the help of the enzyme choline-acetyl-
transferase.

That transport system becomes blocked when a cholinergic nerve
or axon is ligated or transected. Transitory accumulation of
enzyme proximal to the lesion and disappearance of AChE distal
to the lesion was demonstrated (Hughes and Lewis, 1961[18];
Eccles, 1961[19]; Pradham and Dutta, 1970[20]); the axoplasmic
flow that carries the synthesizing system no longer reaches
the terminals, where it is required for the generation of ACh.

This mechanism becomes readily applicable to the effect of
psychiatric surgery. Any surgical procedure from the antiquated
lobotomy to the modern stereotactic techniques in various topo-
graphical areas of the brain, e.g. in the medio-orbito-frontal
area for the treatment of depressive states, results in sever-
ance of fiber structures in the brain, i.e. in axotomy, and
thus in disruption of the axoplasmic flow. The supply of the
raw materials necessary for the synthesis of ACh, is prevented
from reaching the terminals at some distance from the surgical
target. Thus synthesis and storage of excessive ACh in the
area responsible for abnormal behavior is reduced. Absence of
regeneration in the central nervous system renders the discon-
tinuation of the transected fibers permanent. The resulting
cessation of axoplasmic flow and enzyme transport with the consequent reduction of excessive ACh synthesis and store contri-
butes to the enduring effect of axotomy, i.e. psychiatric surgery
through restoration of NT balance.

Electroconvulsive therapy for psychotic depression has been
accepted for its therapeutic efficacy, rapidity, and superiority
of outcome. It is brought about in a small series of bilateral
or unilateral non-dominant application of alternating electric
current at the temples. It is administered 2-3 times per week
with precautionary measures, such as positioning of the patient
in hyperextension of the spine, i.v. thiopental or methohexital
anesthesia, blockade of the inconsequential motor component of
the convulsions by muscle relaxants like succinyl-choline
(Anectine), and by hyperoxygenation. It exerts its effect
through the cerebral component, however, i.e. a multitude of
wide spread biochemical concomitants, among them the chemical
processes induced on the neuroregulatory system, stirring both
the biogenic amines and the cholinergic and ACh system in an

apparent effort to re-establish equilibrium and restore the
situation toward normal. The mobilization of the ACh system
by ECT is reflected in the immediate, though not persistent
effect of single seizures on the ACh content of the brain and
its depletion into the cerebrospinal fluid (CSF). The levels
of bound and free ACh in the brain increase significantly during
the seizure itself, postictally, particularly after a series of
seizures, however, both, more so the free ACh, decrease gradually because of the increased synthesis and turnover (Karczmar,
1974[21]), saturation and blockage of cholinergic receptors
(Goldberg, et al, 1976)[22], and the appearance of considerable
amounts of cholin and ACh in the cerebrospinal fluid (CSF)
(Fink, 1966[23]; Essman, 1972[24]). Increased release of ACh from
many cortical and subcortical areas of the brain into extracellular space, cerebral ventricle, and the cerebrospinal fluid
is a general, non persisting corollary of convulsions whether
induced by head trauma, epilepsy, ECS, or chemical agents like
the inhalant flurothyl (indoklone), or I.V. pentylenetetrazole,
i.e. metrazole (Bornstein, 1946[25]; Tower and MacEachern, 1948[26];
Fink, 1966[23]). ACh was also collected from the CSF of persons
who had died after generalized convulsions (Hitchcock, 1968)[27].

The prompt adaptive responsiveness of the ACh system to
repeated ECT is shared by the biogenic amines, with their persistent alteration of metabolism, in the direction of increased
synthesis, release, turnover, and concentration of serotonin
(Kety, et al, 1967[28]), dopamine (Engel, et al, 1968[29]; Billiet,
et al, 1970[30]), and nor-ephedrine (Kety, et al, 1967[28]; Ladisch,
Steinhauff, & Matussek, 1969[31]; Schildkraut & Draskoczy, 1974[32]).
They participate effectively in the destabilization of the
neurotransmitter disequilibrium with their newly elevated level
of availability and functioning; they seem to contribute to the
establishment of a new neurotransmitter balance that may vary
in different people (Barchas, et al, 1978)[33]. The reestablished
physiological synergism of cholinergic and aminergic neurotransmitters may account for the restoration of normal emotional
life by ECT in the previously severely and/or suicidal depressed
patient.

TRICYCLIC ANTIDEPRESSANTS.

The psychopharmacology of depression, including biochemical
subtypes, of the past has ever since 1957 focussed mainly on

functional underactivity or deficiency of biogenic amines and
adhered to the univariate catecholamine or norepinephrine and
serotonine hypothesis (Bunney, 1978)[34]. Therefore, antidepressive drugs, thymoleptics, capable of elevating the level
of available biogenic amine concentration in the synaptic gap
at the receptor came into general use. Some, like mono-amine-
oxydase inhibitors would counteract their metabolic breakdown,
others like the more effective tricyclics, would block their
re-uptake into the presynaptic neuron that released them into
the synaptic cleft. The beneficial effect of administering
tryptophane, a precursor of the aminergic neurotransmitter
serotonin, to patients with depression support the generally
accepted hypothesis.

On the other hand, the anti-depressant activity of certain
anticholinergic drugs (Feldberg & Sherwood, 1955)[35] and the
anticholinergic "side" effects of the important antidepressant
tricyclic drugs suggest some role of the ACh system in clinical
depression and in the beneficial effects of antidepressant
drugs (Kety, 1974)[36]. The precipitation of depression by CHE
inhibitors that increase the available level of ACh in the
brain, be it by accidental poisoning with cholinesterase inhibitor insecticides and poisoning with nerve gasses, or by experimental administration of physostigmine to manic patients
(Janowsky, et al, 1972)[9] are compelling evidence for the important part of an elevated ACh level in the biochemistry of
depression.

Both the aminergic and the cholinergic system seem to have
their share in producing the neurotransmitter disequilibrium,
necessary and responsible for emotional dysfunction in depression; the pathological shift in the physiological balance of
opposing though normally synergistic neurotransmitter systems
represents a tipping of the scale--in favor of ACh, to which
both systems apparently may contribute by overfunction or under-
function, respectively.

Restoration of neurotransmitter balance and recovery from
emotional depression requires either considerable alteration
of one or the other, or both mutually reinforcing transmitter
system, i.e. diminution or increase respectively, or a simul-
taneous moderation of both systems as well exemplified in
Parkinson's Disease. The presently available antidepressant

drugs, the tricyclics with their norepinephine-potentiating and ACh blocking properties appear to fulfill the latter requirement. Although their peripheral anticholinergic side effects are unpleasant and undesirable, the central anticholinergic action of tricyclics appears to contribute to the establishment of a new neurotransmitter equilibrium, and to their therapeutic effect in depression.

SUMMARY AND CONCLUSION.

Evidence was presented for the significance of the pathological disequilibrium of the ordinarily balancing and reciprocal cholinergic-aminergic neurotransmitter systems due to a relative ACh preponderance in the visceral brain of emotions, responsible for depression.

Destabilization of the abnormal disequilibrium of cholinergic-aminergic neurotransmitters by reducing the relative ACh predominance and establishment of a new neurotransmitter balance was established as the principle purpose and goal of all (three) treatment modalities available in the treatment of psychotic depression.

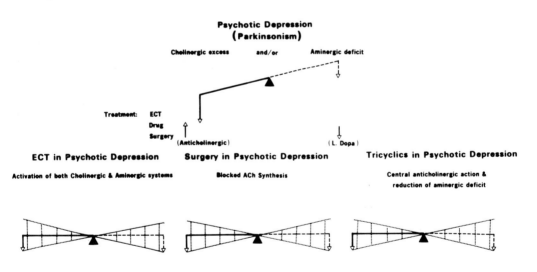

Fig. 4. Neurotransmitter Mechanisms and Restoration of Neurotransmitter balance underlying the effectiveness of Psychiatric Surgery, Electroconvulsive Treatment, and Tricyclic Drug Therapy in Psychotic Depression.

The effectiveness of tricyclic antidepressive drugs consists in balancing ACh preponderance through both aminergic receptor blocking and central anticholinergic action. Successful electro convulsive treatment results in temporary clearing of super-abundant central ACh into the cerebro-spinal fluid and simul-taneous elevation of aminergic activity levels in the limbic system.

Psychiatric surgery for depression owes its success to cutting off the supply routes, the axoplasmic flow of building materials for the synthesis of excessive ACh in the limbic system, remote from the surgical target area.

REFERENCES

1. Moniz, E., and Lima, A.: (1936) Premiers essais de psycho-chirurgie; technique et resultats, Lisboa med. 13:152.

2. Meduna, L. von (1938) General discussion of the cardiazol therapy. Am. J. Psychiat. 94(Supp.):40.

3. Schildkraut, J.J. (1965) The Catecholamine Hypothesis of Affective Disorders: A Review of Supporting Evidence. Am. J. Psychiat. 122: 509-522.

4. Hess, W.R. (1924) Ueber die Wechselbeziehungen zwischen psychischen und vegetativen Funktionen. Schweiz. Arch. Neurol. 15, 260.

5. Gellhorn, E. (1953) Psychiological Foundations of Neurology and Psychiatry, Minneapolis, University of Minnesota Press.

6. Bertalanffy, L. von (1966) General System Theory and Psy-chiatry in American Hankbook of Psychiatry. (ed. Arieti, G.), Basic Books, New York, 3:705.

7. Perez-Cruet, J., Gesse, G.L., Tagliamonte, A., and Taglia-monte, P. (1971) Evidence of a balance in the basal ganglia between cholinergic and dopaminergic activity. Annual Meeting of Federation of American Societies for Experimental Biology, Chicago, Illinois. April 12-17.

8. Marrazzi, A.S. (1966) An Experimentalist Looks at Psychiatry, in Recent Advances in Biological Psychiatry, Ed., J. Wortis, Plenum Press, New York, 9:143.

9. Janowsky, D.S.; El-Yousef, M.D.; Davies, J.M.; & Sekerke, H.J. (1972) A cholinergic-adrenergic hypothesis of mania and depression. Lancet (i),632.

10. Pradhan, N.S., and Bose, S. (1978)Interactions among Central Neurotransmitters, In Psychopharmacology: A Generation of Progress, Ed. Lipton, M.A., DiMascio,A., Killam, K. Raven

Press, New York.

11. Girgis, M. (1967) Distribution of cholinesterase in the basal rhinencephalic structures of the Coypu (Myocaster Coypus). J. Comp. Neurol., 129, 85.

12. Papez, J.W. (1937) A proposed mechanism of emotion. Arch. Neurol. Psychiat. 38, 725.

12a. Hofstatter, L. & Girgis, M. (1973) Depth electrode investigations of the limbic system of the brain by radiostimulation, electrolytic lesions and histochemical studies. I: Surgical Approaches in Psychiatry (ed. Laitinen & Livingston) Baltimore, University Park Press.

13. Shute, C.C.D., & Lewis, P.R. (1965) The fine localization of cholinesterase in the hippocampal formation. J. Anat. (Lond) 99, 938.

14. Tsuji, S. (1974). On the chemical basis of thiocholine methods for demonstration of cholinesterase activities. Histochemie, 42, 99.

15. Lewis, P.R. & Hughes, A.F.W. (1957) The cholinesterase of developing neurones in Xenopus larvae. In: Metabolism of the Nervous System. London: Pergamon Press.

16. Haggendal, C.J., Saunders, N.R., & Dahlstrom, A.B. (1971) A rapid accumulation of acetylcholine in nerve above a crush. J. Pharm. Pharmacol., 23, 552.

17. Lubinska, L.: (1975) On Acoplasmic Flow, In: International Review of Neurobiology. Vol. 17. Ed. by Pfeiffer & Smythles. Academic Press, New York, San Francisco, London.

18. Hughes, A.F.W. & Lewis, P.R. (1961). Effect of limb ablation on neurones in Xenopus larvae. Nature, 189:333.

19. Eccles, J.C. (1961). Mechanism of synaptic transmission. Ergebnisse der Physiologie, 51:299.

20. Pradhan, S.N. & Dutta, S.N. (1970) Central cholinergic mechanism and behavior. Int. Rev. Neurobiol. 13:173.

21. Karczmar, A.G. (1974). Brain acetylcholine and seizures. in: Psychobiology of Convulsive Therapy. Ed. by Fink, Kety, McGaugh & Williams. Winston & sons, Washington, D.C.

22. Goldberg, A.M. and Hanin, I. (1976) Biology of Cholinergic Function. Raven Press, New York.

23. Fink, M.,(1966) Cholinergic Aspects of Convulsive Therapy. J. Nervous and Mental Disease, 24:475-484.

24. Essman, W.B. (1972) Neurochemical Changes in ECS and ECT. Seminars in Psychiatry, 4:67-79.

25. Bornstein, M. (1946) Presence and action of ACh in experimental brain trauma. J. Neurophysiol. 9:349.

26. Tower, D.B. & McEachern, D. (1948). Acetylcholine and neuronal activity in craniocerebral trauma. J. Clin. Invest., 27, 558.

27. Hitchcock, E.R. and Forrester, J.M. (1968) The structure and functions of the nervous system. in: A Companion to Medical Studies. 1, 24.88. Blackwell Scientific Publications, Oxford and Edinburgh.

28. Kety, S.S., Javoy, F., Thierry, S.M., Julou, L., and Glowinski, J. (1967) A sustained effect of electroconvulsive shock on the Turnover of norepinephrine in the central nervous system of the rat. Proceedings of the National Academy of Sciences, United States of America. 58, 1249-1254.

29. Engel, J., Hanson, L.C.F., Roos, B.E., and Strombergsson, L.E. (1968) Effect of electroshock on dopamine metabolism in rat brain. Psychopharmacologia, B, 140-144.

30. Billiet, M., Bernard, P., Delaunois, A., and DeSchaepdryver, A (1970) Electroshock and nucleus dopamine. Archives Internationales de Pharmacodynamie et de Therapie, 186,179-181.

31. Ladisich, W., Steinhauff, N., and Matussek, N. (1969) Chronic administration of electroconvulsive shock and Norephedrine metabolism in the rat brain, Psychopharmacol. 15, 296-304.

32. Schildkraut, J.J. and Draskoczy, P.R. (1974) Effects of Electroconvulsive Shock on Norepinephrine Turnover and Metabolism: Basic and Clinical Studies: in Psychobiology of Convulsive Therapy. Ed. by Fink, Kety, McGaugh & Williams. Winston & Sons, Washington, D.C..

33. Barchas, J.D., Akil, H., Elliot, G.R., Holman, R.B., Watson, S. (1978) Behavioral Neurochemistry: Neuroregulators and Behavioral States. Science 200, 964-974.

34. Bunney, E.Jr. (1978) Drug Therapy and Psychobiological Research Advances in the Psychoses in the Past Decade. Am. J. Psychiatry 135, July, Supplement.

35. Feldberg, W.C. and Sherwood, S.L. (1955). Intraventricular administration of drugs. Lancet

36. Kety, S.S. (1974) Biochemical and Neurochemical Effects of Electroconvulsive shock, in Psychobiology of Convulsive Therapy. Ed. Fink, Kety, McGaugh & Williams, Winston & Sons, Washington, D.C.

© 1979 Elsevier/North-Holland Biomedical Press
Modern Concepts in Psychiatric Surgery
E.R. Hitchcock, H.T. Ballantine, Jr. and B.A. Meyerson, eds.

ESTIMATION OF CSF AND URINARY BIOGENIC AMINES
IN FUNCTIONAL BRAIN DISORDERS

by

S. SUBRAHMANYAM and B. RAMAMURTHI

MADRAS - INDIA

INTRODUCTION

The role of biogenic amines in functional disorders of the brain is becoming

more obvious. An upset in the delicate balance between the different amines in

the brain may cause behavioural changes. Schieldkraut et al (1964)[1] studied

the effect of antidepressant drugs on the urinary excretion of VMA and suggested

a mechanism of action for imipramine. Rosenblatt et al (1969)[2] first suggested

that changes in noradrenaline in the brain may be involved in depression. The

changes in brain chemistry are being studied extensively by analysing the bio-

chemical deviations in blood, CSF and urine in patients with functional dis-

orders.

The important biogenic amines are the Indole (5-hydroxy tryptamine or

serotonin) and catechol amines (noradrenaline and dopamine). They are con-

centrated in brain areas concerned with behaviour. Catechol and Indole amines

are produced both centrally and peripherally. Only small amounts of circulating

hormones can enter the brain because of the blood brain barrier.

Noradrenaline is synthesised in the brain from the amino acid tyrosine

through the intermediates, Dopa and Dopamine and stored in the intraneuronal

granules. MHPG (3-methoxy 4-hydroxy phenyl glycol) is the major metabolite

of noradrenaline in the brain, whereas VMA is the major metabolite in the urine

and is derived mainly from peripheral tissues.

The dopa gets converted into dopamine which is metabolised into homovanillic acid (HVA). In areas where dopamine is in high concentration, dopamine beta oxidase which converts it into noradrenaline is absent.

An attempt has been made in this study to correlate the change in the CSF and urinary end products of biogenic amines with the clinical state of patients with functional disorders.

MATERIALS AND METHODS

The patients were selected from the Institute of Neurology and the Govt. Mental Hospital, Madras. Consent was obtained from the patients before including them in the study. The following groups of cases were selected:

Group	No	Nature of treatment	
		Medical	Surgical
1. Normal subjects	12		
2. Acute Schizophrenia	36	24	12 Basofrontal leucotomy
3. Depression	36	20	10 Basofrontal leucotomy
4. Aggressive hyper-kinetic behaviour	20		14 Bilateral amygdalotomy
5. Temporal lobe epilepsy	20	9	11 Bilateral amygdalotomy
6. Drug Addiction			
a) Alcohol	10		6 Bilateral cingulumotomy
b) Morphine	6		4 Bilateral cingulumotomy
c) Multiple drugs	8		6 Cingulumotomy - 4 Sequential Surgery - 2

As many patients underwent surgery under anaesthesia, a study was made about the effect of anaesthesia on the levels of biogenic amines in the urine and in the CSF. All the patients were on a standard restricted diet and no drug was administered for 24-hours prior to the collection of specimens. Premedication was standardized in the patients who underwent surgery.

The diagnosis of the various groups of cases was made by the concerned specialists after a careful study of the patients. The patients with schizophrenia and depression were chosen for surgery by two experienced psychiatric colleagues. All the cases of aggressive hyperkinetic behaviour who underwent surgery have had extensive medical therapy with no benefit. In temporal lobe epilepsy only those patients who had no relief from adequate medication and who showed a demonstrable focus of disturbance in the temporal lobe were chosen for stereotaxic excision of the discharging focus in the amygdala and the periamygdaloid region. The patients with drug addiction varied from highly intellectual personnel to the illiterate. In all these cases when repeated attempts at curing the patients of the addiction had failed, stereotaxic bilateral cingulumotomy was carried out.

Estimations of biogenic amines and their metabolites were done for the past $3\frac{1}{2}$ years and the cases have been followed for a period of 24 months.

Methods

The metabolites of biogenic amines were estimated in the lumbar CSF and urine. The metabolites assayed in the CSF were 5-HIAA, MHPG and HVA and in the 24-hour sample of urine, 5-HIAA, MHPG, VMA and HVA. In the CSF, 5-HIAA was estimated by the method of Ashcroft and Sharman (1962)[3], MHPG by the method of Schanberg et all (1968)[4] and HVA by the method of Curzon et al (1970)[5]. In the urine VMA was estimated by the method of Armstrong et al (1957)[6], MHPG by the method of Mass and Faucet (1968)[7], HVA by the method of Mellinger (1968)[8] and 5-HIAA by the method of Subrahmanyam and Narayanan (1973)[9]. Patients were examined every 6 months.

RESULTS

Anaesthesia did not have any significant effect on the levels of metabolites of noradrenaline and 5-HT in the CSF.

Schizophrenia

In acute schizophrenia, (Tables 1 & 2) both 5-HIAA and MHPG were reduced in the CSF and in the urine. There was no apparent change in HVA. With medical treatment the levels tended to increase. The same was the result with surgical treatment also. In a few cases that were followed for 12-24 months, it was found that the amine levels were almost restored to normal. Medical treatment especially with chlorpromazine tended to increase the HVA level.

Depression

36 Cases of depression were studied (Tables 3 & 4). They were not categorised as endogenous and exogenous. Medical treatment was administered in 20 of them and in 10 cases basofrontal leucotomy was performed. In all cases, 5-HIAA, MHPG and HVA were reduced considerably. After medical treatment for a period of about 12 months, there was an improvement in the amine levels which were maintained even after 24 months of treatment, and clinically the patients appeared to be normal. Immediately after surgery there was an elevation in the amine levels. After 12-24 months it was found that almost normal levels were attained.

Hyperkinetic & aggressive behavioural disorder

In this group there were 20 cases, 16 of them were children (Tables 5 & 6). There was no significant change in the 5-HIAA level in the CSF, but HVA and MHPG were increased. Bilateral amygdalotomy was performed in 14 cases and this served to reduce the levels of HVA and MHPG immediately after the operation and the levels were maintained during the observation period of 24 months.

TABLE 1 - SCHIZOPHRENIA
Lumbar C.S.F. (ng/ml)

GROUP	No	5-HIAA	MHPG	HVA
Normal	12	40.6+4.2	20.6+2.4	40.2+4.0
Control (with no neurological morbidity	12	40.2+3.8	21.4+3.2	42.4+3.6
Acute Schizophrenia	36	19.8+1.8	11.2+1.7	41.2+3.6
Medical treatment(3-12 months)	24	25.6+3.2	15.6+1.8	46.2+4.4
Medical treatment(12-24 months)	12	32.6+3.6	18.4+1.0	48.6+3.6
Basofrontal leucotomy	12	30.2+4.8	18.6+3.2	40.4+6.2
3-12 months later	6	32.4+3.6	17.5+2.4	44.0+5.6
12-24 months later	4	38.6+3.2	18.5+3.2	42.2+4.2

TABLE 2 - SCHIZOPHRENIA
Urine (mg/day)

GROUP	No	5-HIAA	MHPG	HVA	VMA
Normal	12	4.36+0.9	2.09+.3	8.2+1.2	4.8+.8
Control (no neurological morbidity)	12	4.00+0.4	2.09+.2	7.8+8.8	4.4+.6
Acute schizophrenia	36	2.6 +0.4	1.4 +.4	8.2+0.8	3.6+.4
Medical treatment (3-12 months)	24	3.8 +0.8	1.4 +.3	12.2+1.1	3.8+.3
Medical treatment (12-24 months)	12	4.0 +0.08	1.8 +.2	12.6+0.8	4.2+.6
Basofrontal Leucotomy	12	3.8 +0.4	1.6 +.2	9.0+1.2	3.8+.4
3-12 months later	6	4.2 +1.0	1.5 +.3	9.6+1.3	4.0+.6
12-24 months later	4	4.4 +0.8	1.8 +.8	9.2+1.2	4.2+.8

TABLE 3 - DEPRESSION
Lumbar C.S.F. (ng/day)

GROUP	No.	5-HIAA	MHPG	HVA
Normal	12	40.6±4.2	20.6±2.4	40.2±4.0
Depression	36	18.0±2.6	14.2±2.6	22.2±3.8
Medical Treatment	20	28.2±4.8	16.6±3.4	38.6±3.6
Basofrontal leucotomy	10	30.2±4.2	18.6±2.2	34.4±4.2
12 Months later	8	32.4±4.8	16.2±4.2	36.4±3.8
24 Months later	4	36.2±3.4	20.2±3.0	39.2±4.0

TABLE 4 - DEPRESSION
Urine (mg/day)

GROUP	No.	5-HIAA	MHPG	HVA	VMA
Normal	12	4.36±.9	2.09±.3	8.2±1.2	4.8±.8
Depression	36	3.6 ±.6	1.0 ±.4	5.6±0.4	3.2±.4
Medical treatment(24 months)	20	3.6 ±.4	1.6 ±.2	7.2±1.2	3.6±.2
Basofrontal leucotomy	10	4.0 ±.2	1.8 ±.4	7.6±0.8	4.4±.4
12 Months later	8	4.1 ±.6	1.6 ±.4	7.9±1.0	4.2±.4
24 Months later	4	4.2 ±.4	1.8 ±.6	7.8±0.8	4.2±.5

TABLE 5 - AGGRESSIVE HYPERKINETIC BEHAVIOUR
Lumbar C.S.F. (ng/day)

GROUP	No.	5-HIAA	MHPG	HVA
Normal	12	40.6±4.2	20.6±2.4	40.2±4
Aggressive behaviour	20	43.4±4.2	36.4±3.2	56.0±2.6
After amygdalotomy	14	41.2±5.6	26.2±3.8	44.8±5.2
12 Months later	6	40.6±4.2	25.2±4.4	46.4±4.2
24 Months later	3	41.6±3.8	24.8±2.6	47.4±3.6

TABLE 6 – AGGRESSIVE HYPERKINETIC BEHAVIOUR
Urine (mg/day)

GROUP	No.	5-HIAA	MHPG	HVA	VMA
Normal	12	4.36+0.9	2.09+.3	8.2+1.2	4.8+.8
Aggressive behaviour	20	4.6 +1.0	3.2 +.8	10.6+1.4	5.6+.6
Amygdalotomy	14	5.0 +0.8	2.8 +.4	9.2+0.8	5.8+.8
12 Months later	6	4.8 +0.6	3.0 +.4	9.0+0.8	4.8+.6
24 Months later	3	4.6 +0.4	2.8 +.6	9.0+0.6	4.9+.4

TABLE 7 – TEMPORAL LOBE EPILEPSY
Lumbar C.S.F. (ng/ml)

GROUP	No.	5-HIAA	MHPG	HVA
Normal	12	40.6+4.2	20.6+2.4	40.2+4
Temp. Lobe epilepsy	20	22.4+3.2	24.6+3.8	42.8+4.5
Medical treatment – 12 months	9	28.6+4.0	20.2+2.8	43.6+3.0
After amygdalotomy	11	30.2+3.6	23.2+3.6	45.1+4.8
12 Months after	6	28.4+2.2	22.4+2.8	42.6+5.2
12-24 Months after	4	32.6+3.2	21.6+1.8	41.2+4.2

TABLE 8 – TEMPORAL LOBE EPILEPSY
Urine (mg/day)

GROUP	No.	5-HIAA	MHPG	HVA	VMA
Normal	12	4.36+.9	2.09+.3	8.2+1.2	4.8+.8
Temp. lobe epilepsy	20	2.2 +.2	2.0 +.6	8.2+1.0	5.2+.6
Medical treatment – 12months	9	3.6 +.04	2.0 +.03	8.0+0.08	4.6+.4
Amygdalotomy	11	4.0 +.4	1.8 +.8	7.8+0.6	4.0+.6
12 Months later	11	4.2 +.6	1.6 +.6	8.0+0.6	4.2+.4
12-24 Months after	5	4.0 +.4	1.8 +.4	8.4+0.6	4.8+.6

The normal levels were not reached at any time during the study. There was no alteration in 5-HIAA levels in the urine and no change was noticed after surgery. But the MHPG, HVA and VMA levels were increased in them. After amygdalotomy there was a steady decline and the levels reached almost normal by the end of 24 months. Clinically also the few patients that turned up for the follow-up studies were apparently normal; although they had become unusually calm. The parents had nothing much to complain about them. Mild recurrence of symptoms was noticed in 2 cases and the amine levels showed the original pattern. They were controlled by tranquilisers.

Temporal lobe epilepsy

There are 20 cases in the series studied (Tables 7 & 8). 5-HIAA levels were low (roughly about half of the normal value). MHPG and HVA were slightly increased in CSF. The same was the case with urine. In 11 cases bilateral amygdalotomy was performed and from 6 cases CSF could be collected after 12 months and from 4 cases after 24 months whereas urine could be collected from 11 cases and 5 cases at the end of 12 months and 24 months respectively. Stereotaxic surgery improved the 5-HIAA levels but not restored to normal especially in CSF even after 24 months. Medical treatment also had the same effect.

Drug Addiction (Tables 9 & 10)

In alcohol addicts, 5-HIAA was low in CSF, HVA was normal and MHPG was raised. In the urine the metabolites of catechol amines, namely VMA and MHPG were increased and HVA was normal and 5-HIAA reduced. In morphine addicts, 5-HIAA was low in both CSF and urine and the others were within the normal range. In multiple addiction 5-HIAA was reduced in CSF and urine and MHPG and VMA were high in the urine. After cingulumotomy there was a tendancy

TABLE 9 - DRUG ADDICTION
Lumbar C.S.F.(ng/day)

GROUP	No.	5-HIAA	MHPG	HVA
Normal	12	40.6+4.2	20.6+2.4	40.2+4.0
Drug Addiction				
a) Alcohol	10	20.6+1.2	26.2+2.6	40.4+3.6
After cingulumotomy	6	30.2+2.6	17.2+2.4	38.2+2.8
3-18 Months after	3	32.4+3.2	18.6+2.6	40.0+2.2
b) Morphine	12	28.6+4.2	20.8+2.4	38.6+2.6
After cingulumotomy	10	32.6+3.8	20.2+1.6	38.6+3.2
3-18 Months after	4	36.2+6.6	21.2+1.8	36.8+3.8
c) Multiple	8	25.6+2.6	30.4+1.8	40.6+3.8
After cingulumotomy	6	32.8+4.2	19.2+1.4	38.6+1.8
3-18 Months after	3	36.6+5.4	18.6+1.2	38.0+3.2

TABLE 10 - DRUG ADDICTION
Urine (mg/day)

GROUP	No.	5-HIAA	MHPG	HVA	VMA
Normal	12	4.36+0.9	2.09+.3	8.2+1.2	4.8+0.8
Drug Addiction					
a) Alcohol	10	3.6 +0.8	3.2 +.06	8.2+1.2	5.4+0.8
Cingulumotomy	6	3.8 +0.6	1.8 +.2	7.0+0.6	4.6+0.6
3-18 Months after	3	3.9 +0.8	1.7 +.3	7.2+0.4	4.8+0.8
b) Morphine	12	3.6 +1.2	2.0 +.04	8.0+1.8	4.6+1.0
Cingulumotomy	10	4.8 +1.2	1.8 +.06	7.6+0.8	4.2+0.6
3-18 Months after	4	4.3 +0.8	1.6 +.1	7.8 +0.8	4.4 +0.6
c) Multiple	8	3.8 +0.6	3.6 +.04	7.6+0.8	5.9+0.8
Cingulumotomy	6	4.0 +0.4	2.7 +.08	7.6+0.8	3.6+0.6
3-18 Months after	3	4.2 +0.6	1.9 +.1	8.0+0.6	4.5+0.5

for restoration of normal levels. There was definite clinical improvement and in most of them there was no craving for drugs and the patients have been followed up for about 18 months. In two patients sequential surgery had to be performed.

Summary of the results is given in Table 11.

DISCUSSION

In schizophrenia the metabolites of noradrenaline and 5-HT were low in CSF and urine suggestive of either decreased synthesis or metabolism of the amines in the brain. HVA was normal. Our findings are in accordance with those of Ashcroft et al (1966)[10], Greenspan et al (1970)[11], Dencker et al (1966)[12] and of the earlier studies of Subrahmanyam (1975)[13]. The amine levels improve both by medical and surgical therapy but not restored to normal in most of the cases. Copin (1971)[14] observed that clinical recovery was not accompanied by total correction of the abnormality of the amine levels. Hence changes in amine metabolism may form only part of the chemical pathology and perhaps other factors are involved to produce the clinical picture.

Antun et al (1971)[15] suggested that schizophrenia may be due to inhibition of the enzyme converting dopamine into noradrenaline, thus raising the brain dopamine level. In the present study dopamine could not be estimated in the brain tissue. There was no change in the HVA level initially in the CSF but continued treatment with Chlorpromazine had a tendency to increase the HVA in CSF and urine.

Depression in this series of studies was characterised by a decrease in the levels of MHPG, HVA and 5-HIAA in CSF and urine. Functional deficiency of noradrenaline or 5-HT may occur at receptors in brain in depression as evinced

TABLE 11 - SUMMARY OF THE RESULTS

	C.S.F.			URINE			
	MHPG	HVA	5-HIAA	MHPG	VMA	HVA	5-HIAA
Acute Schizophrenia	↓	↔	↓	↓	↓	↔	↓
Medical Chlorpromazine	↑	↑	↑	↑	↑	↑	↑
Surgical	↑	↔	↑	↑	↑	↑	↑
Depression	↓	↓	↓	↓	↓	↓	↓
Medical	↑	↑	↑	↑	↑	↑	↔
Surgical	↑	↑	↑	↑	↑	↑	↑
Hyperkinetic behaviour	↑	↑	↔	↑	↑	↑	↔
Surgical	↓	↓	↔	↓	↓	↓	↔
Temp. lobe epilepsy	↑	↑	↓	↔	↑	↔	↓
Medical	↓	↑	↑	↔	↓	↔	↑
Surgical	↓	↔	↑	↔	↓	↔	↑
Drug addiction							
Alcohol	↑	↔	↓	↑	↑	↔	↓
Surgery	↔	↔	↑	↓	↓	↓	↑
Morphine	↔	↔	↓	↔	↔	↔	↓
Surgery	↔	↓	↑	↓	↔	↔	↑
Multiple drugs	↑	↔	↓	↑	↑	↓	↓
Surgery	↑	↔	↑	↓	↓	↔	↑

by a fall in their levels in the CSF. Similar observations were made by Schild-kraut in 1970[16]. In 1965[17] he suggested that depression is associated with deficiency of catechol amines at functionally important adrenergic sites in the brain and mania with excess of these amines. Hence drugs which increase catechol amines in appropriate neurones should alleviate depression or produce mania and agents which cause decrease in amine levels at receptor sites should worsen depression. Functional deficiency of NA and 5-HT at receptors is evidenced by the low level of their metabolites in the CSF and urine.

Electroconvulsive therapy, an effective somatic treatment for severe depressive reactions, produces sustained increase in synthesis, utilisation and turnover of the amines in the brain. Antidepressant drugs increase free amines either by decreasing the metabolism of amines (MAO inhibition) or by interfering with the cellular binding. The effect of tricyclic antidepressants, electroconvulsive therapy and other drugs on the turn over and metabolism correlates well with their clinical effects seen in active states. The present findings are in agreement with that of Schildkraut (1970)[18] and Bunny and Davies (1965)[19]. Papeschi and McCluere (1971)[20] found lower concentration of HVA and 5-HIAA in CSF. Shaw (1966)[21] claimed that one of the causes of affective disorders can be alteration of brain excitability caused by abnormal distribution of NA and K ions across the cell membranes of the neurones. Abnormal CSF findings can result not only from deranged brain metabolism but also from defective transport of metabolites from CSF or brain to blood.

Aggressive hyperkinetic behaviour is associated with an increase in the metabolites of catechol amines. Segal and Mandell (1970)[22] infused noradrenaline into the cerebral ventricles of a rat and noticed increase in the exploratory behaviour and locomotor activity. Post et al (1973)[23] found that depressed patients when stimulated to manic hyperactivity for a few hours had higher

5-HIAA, HVA and MHPG in CSF than at rest. 5-HIAA and HVA are correlated

with motor activity and they were least in depression and highest in mania and

aggressive behaviour. Medical and surgical therapy lowered the MHPG and

HVA levels. It can be postulated that aggressive behaviour may be due to in-

creased synthesis of catechol amines. Stereotaxic amygdalotomy brings down

the amine levels resulting in improvement.

The symptoms in temporal lobe epilepsy are diverse. The EEG records in

the patients studied were positive according to the criteria of Mani (1973)[24]

and showed definite seizure discharges with well defined spikes, sharp waves

or spike and waves, focal or generalised. In them low levels of 5-HIAA with

raised MHPG were found. Low ventricular and lumbar concentration of HVA have

been reported by Burnheimer et al (1966)[25] and Barolin et al (1967)[26] in

epileptic patients. Papeschi et al (1972)[27] noticed low 5-HIAA levels in ventri-

cular fluid in epilepsy. Shaywitz et al (1973)[28] observed accumulation of

5-HIAA after probenecid. Garelis and Sourker (1974)[29] found low levels of

5-HIAA in CSF in epileptic patients with no change in HVA, similar to the find-

ings in this   study. Stereotactic ablation of the medial temporal structures

increased the 5-HIAA levels.

In alcohol and in multiple drug addicts 5-HIAA was low in CSF, HVA was

normal and MHPG was raised. In the urine VMA and MHPG were increased and

HVA and 5-HIAA were normal. In morphine addicts, 5-HIAA was low in CSF and

urine and the others were within the normal range. The results are different

for different drugs.

It has been postulated that there are receptors for morphine like drugs in the

central and peripheral nervous system. They play an important role in drug tolerance, dependance and withdrawal symptoms. Opium receptors are scattered throughout the brain, the highest density being in the limbic system.

Kianmaa et al (1975)[30] found that a lesion in the dorsal NA bundle which innnervates the cortex increases alcohol intake and alcohol preference. Euphoric state of alcoholics may be due to release of catechol amines from the cortical, subcortical and hypothalamic NA neurones. Reduced forebrain NA activity may lead to compensatory increase in alcohol preference. In the present study in alcohol and multiple addiction, 5-HIAA was low, HVA was normal and MHPG and VMA were raised. After cingulumotomy the levels were restored almost to normal. Increased NA turnover after alcohol intake shows that alcohol may further augment amine release from the remaining nerve terminals. Cingulumotomy perhaps inhibits these neurones thereby reducing either the synthesis or the release of CA from the monoaminergic neurones.

In morphine addiction, 5-HIAA was low in CSF and urine without any significant change in MHPG and HVA in human subjects. Tolerance to morphine may involve increased synthesis of catecholamines and 5-HT (Way et al 1968)[31]. 5-HT is implicated in opium tolerance and physical dependance. No reference in literature could be obtained regarding the effect of surgery on the amine levels in drug addiction for comparing the results.

SUMMARY

1. The levels of metabolites of biogenic amines namely, MHPG, VMA, HVA and 5-HIAA were studied in the CSF and urine in normal subjects and in patients suffering from different types of behavioural disorders.

2. The cases studied were schizophrenia, depression, temporal lobe epilepsy, aggressive hyperkinetic behaviour and drug addiction. The

patients were from the Institute of Neurology, and the Govt.Mental Hospital, Madras.

3. The estimations were done before and after medical and surgical therapy.

4. There is definite alteration in the levels of the metabolites of the biogenic amines in different types of behavioural disorders.

5. Other factors may also perhaps be concerned in the production of behavioural disorders but the biogenic amines definitely play an important role in the etiology of these conditions.

6. The defect may be in the synthesis, metabolism, turnover or utilisation of the amines. This aspect needs further study.

ACKNOWLEDGEMENT

Our thanks are due to the Indian Council of Medical Research, New Delhi for the financial assistance rendered for this project.

REFERENCES

1. Schildkraut, J.J., Klerman, G.L., Hammond, R. and Friend, D.G.(1964) Excretion of 3-methoxy 4-hydroxy mandelic acid (VMA) in depressed patients treated with antidepressant drugs, J.Psychiat. Res, 2, p.257.

2. Rosenblatt, S., Charley, J.D. and Leighton, W.P. (1969 A) Temporal change in the distribution of urinary tritiated metabolites in affective disorders, J.Psyhciat. Res, 6, p.321.

3. Ashcroft, G.W. and Sharman, D.F. (1962) Changes in the concentration of 5-OH indolyl compounds in cerebrospinal fluid and caudate nucleus, Brit. J.Pharmacol, 19, p.153.

4. Schanberg, S.M., Breese, G.R., Schildkraut, J.J., Gorden, E.K. and Kopin, I.J. (1968 A) MHPG sulphate in brain C.S.F., Biochem.Pharmacol, 17, p.2006.

5. Curzon, G. and Bridges, P.K. (1970) Tryptophan metabolism in depression, J.Neurol.Neurosurg.Psychiat, 33, p.698.

6. Armstrong, M.D., McMillan, A. and Shaw, D.M. (1957) VMA in the body

fluids, Acta-Biochem-Biophys, 25, p. 422.

7. Mass, J.H., Fawcet, J. and Dekirminjain, H. (1968) MHPG excretion in depressed subjects : A pilot study, Arch.Gen.Psychiat, 18, p.129.

8. Mellinger, T.J. (1968) Spectroflourimetric determination of HVA in urine, Am.J.Cl.Path, 49(No.2) p.200.

9. Subrahmanyam, S. and Narayanan, S. (1973) A quick colorimetric method of estimation of 5-HIAA in urine, Curr.Med.Pr., 17, p.46.

10. Ashcroft, G.W., Growford, T.B.B., Eccleston, D., Sharman, D.F., MacDougall, E.J., Stanton, J.B. and Binns, J.K. (1966) 5-Hydroxy indole compounds in the cerebrospinal fluid of patients treated for psychiatric or neurological diseases, Lancet, 2, p.1049.

11. Greenspan, K., Schildkraut, J.J., Gordon, E.K., Baei, L., Annog, M.S. and Dwell, J. (1970) Catecholamine metabolites in patients treated with lithium carbonate, J.Psychiat. Res, 7, p.171.

12. Dencker, S.J., Malm. M. and Roose, B.E. (1966) Acid monoamine metabolites of CSF in mental depression and mania, J. Neurochem, 13, p.1545.

13. Subrahmanyam, S. (1975) Role of biogenic amines in certain pathological conditions, Brain Res, 87, p.355.

14. Copin, A.J. (1971) Biogenic amines in affective disorders, Brain Chemistry & Mental Disease. Plenum Press, New York.

15. Antun, F., Eccleston, D. and Smythies, R. (1971) Transmethylation process in schizophrenia, Brain Chemistry and Mental Diseases, Plenum Press, New York.

16. Schildkraut, J.J. (1970) Neuropsychopharmacology and the affective disorders, Boston, Little Brown.

17. Schildkraut, J.J. (1965) The catecholamine hypothesis of affective disorders. A review of supporting evidence, Amer.J.Psychiat., 122, p.509.

18. Schildkraut, J.J., Winokur, A. and Applegate, W (1970) Norepnephrine turnover and metabolism in rat brain after long term administration of imipramine, Science, 168, p.867.

19. Bunny, W.E. Jr. and Davies, J.M. (1965) Norepinephrine in depressive reactions, Arch.Gen.Psychiat., 13, p.483.

20. Papeschi, R. and McClure, D.J. (1971) Homovanillic acid and 5-hydroxy-indole acetic acid in cerebrospinal fluid in depressed patients, Arch.Gen.Psychiat., 25, p.354.

21. Shaw, D.M.(1966) Mineral metabolism, Mania and Malancholia, Brit.

Med.J, 2, p.262.

22. Segal, D.S. and Mandell, A.J. (1970) Infusion or norepinephrine into the ventricles in rat, Proc.Acad.Sc, 66, p.289.

23. Post, R.M., Kopin, I.J., Goodwin, K. and Gorden, E.K. (1973) Psychomotor activity and CSF amine metabolites in affective illness, Amer.J. Psychiat, 130 (No.1) p.67.

24. Mani, K.S. (1973 b) Interictal EEG in epilepsy - Possible factors associated with definite seizure discharges, Neurology ʻIndia) 21, p.51.

25. Bunheimer, H., Birkmayer, W. and Hornyjiewicz, O (1966) Homovanillins in Liquor cerebrospinalis : Untersuchugen bein Parkinson-Syndrom and anderen Erkrankungen Des. ZNS, Wiener Klinische Wochenschrift, 78, p.417.

26. Barolin, G.S. and Hornykewicz, O. (1967) Zur diagnostischen Wertigkeit der Homovanillinsaure in Liquor cerebrospinalis, Wiener Klinische Wochenschrift, 79, p.815.

27. Papeschi, R., Moline, Negro, P., Sourker, T.L. and Erba, C. (1972) The concentration of homovanillic acid and 5-hydroxy-indole acetic acid in ventricular and lumbar CSF., Neurology (Minneap), 22, p.1151.

28. Shaywitz, B.A., Cohen, D.J. and Bowers, M.B.Jr. (1973) Brain monoamine turnover in children, preliminary results in epilepsy, Minimal brain dysfunction, Neurology, 23, p.428.

29. Garelis, E. and Sourker, T.L. (1974) Use of CSF drawn at pneumoencephalography in the study of monoamine metabolism in man, J.Neurol. Neurosurg. & Psychiat, 37, p.704.

30. Kianmaa, K., Fuxe, K., Johnson, G. and Ahtee, L. (1975) Evidence for involvement of central NA neurons in alcohol intake : Increased alcohol consumption after degeneration of NA pathway to the cortex cerebri. Neuroscience Letters, 1, p.41.

31. Way. E.L., Loh, H.H. and Shen, Γ.H. (1968) Morphine tolerance, physical dependence and synthesis of brain 5-HT, Science, 162, (3859), p.1290.

© 1979 Elsevier/North-Holland Biomedical Press
Modern Concepts in Psychiatric Surgery
E.R. Hitchcock, H.T. Ballantine, Jr. and B.A. Meyerson, eds.

ALTERATION IN MONOAMINERGIC FUNCTIONS IN HYPERKINETIC SYNDROMES: SOME
NEUROCHEMICAL AND PHARMACOLOGICAL DETERMINANTS

SABIT GABAY

Biochemical Research Laboratory, Veterans Administration Medical Center,
Brockton, Massachusetts 02401 U.S.A. and Section of Psychiatry and Human
Behavior, Brown University, Providence, Rhode Island

ABSTRACT

   A permanent hyperkinetic syndrome, characterized by excitation, choreiform head and neck movement and circling, which had led to it being called
collectively the "ECC-Syndrome" is induced in rats by 7-day IP administration of β-β´-iminodipropionitrile. Findings from regional neurochemical studies (measurement of monoamine levels in five regions of the rat
brain and uptake of [^{3}H]-biogenic amines into midbrain and striatal synaptosomal preparations) and, particularly, responses to various neuropsycho-
pharmacologic agents closely resemble those observed in human dyskinesias.

INTRODUCTION

   The significance of monoaminergic nervous transmission in the regulation of the central nervous system has been most clearly demonstrated in
the nigrostriatal dopaminergic pathway of the basal ganglia. While there
is no doubt that this pathway plays an important role in controlling the
activity of the caudate-putamen and globus pallidus, the contribution of
other neuronal pathways within the basal ganglia to the overall activity
and functioning of this complex system remains unclear. Oftentimes the
nature of such widespread connections and their functional interrelationships become evident only when their delicate balance is disturbed.

Considerable effort, therefore, has been expended in inducing extrapyramidal motor disturbances in laboratory animals in the hope that an examination of the accompanying biochemical and pathological changes would provide useful information concerning the role of the various areas and pathways of the basal ganglia in the maintenance of normal motor control.

Presently available models involve selective lesions of the basal
ganglia area of the experimental animals in which, among other altered
monoamine levels, abnormal striatal dopamine metabolism has been suggested
as a possible explanation for hyperkinetic motor activity.

The work carried out in our laboratories has been concerned with the
elucidation of monoaminergic mechanisms of a very complex syndrome. Following daily intraperitoneal injection of purified β-β´-iminodipropio-
nitrile·HCl (IDPN·HCl), 300 mg/1000 g body weight for seven days, rats
display a permanent abnormal behavior on the seventh day without fail and
with virtually no mortality nor changes in the syndrome during the entire
life span. This hyperkinetic syndrome is characterized by excitation,
choreiform head and neck movement, circling behavior which has led to it
being called collectively the "ECC-Syndrome". This paper summarizes a
series of (a) regional neurochemical studies[1-3], namely endogeneous levels
of the biogenic amines norepinephrine (NE), dopamine (DA), serotonin
(5-HT) and its metabolite, 5-hydroxyindoleacetic acid (5-HIAA) in five
regions of the rat brain as well as the uptake of [^{3}H]-biogenic amines
into midbrain and striatal synaptosomal preparations[1-3], and (b) extensive behavioral pharmacologic manipulations[4,5]. These studies have
demonstrated the possible involvement of monoaminergic functions in the
pathogenesis of this chemically-induced "ECC-Syndrome" without any evidence of cellular loss and is, therefore, a non-lesioned, noninvaded
(implanted connulae, intracerebral infusion, etc.) animal model in which

hyperactivity (choreiform movements and circling) can be consistently produced and studied separately or cooperatively.

CHEMICALS AND DRUGS

IDPN·HCl was purified in our laboratory by saturating an ethanolic solution of the free base (Eastman Kodak) with dry HCl and recrystallizing the resultant product twice in ethanol (m.p. 152-153°C).

The drugs used throughout these studies were donated by the companies. d-Amphetamine-sulfate (Benzedrin), Chlorpromazine·HCl (Thorazine), and Phenoxybenzamine·HCl (Dibenzylene), Smith, Kline and French, Philadelphia, Pennsylvania; Promethazine·HCl (Phenergan), Wyeth Laboratories, Philadelphia, Pennsylvania; Amantadine·HCl (Symmetrel), Endo Labs, Garden City, New York; 1-(3,4-methylene-dioxybenzyl)4-(2-pyrimidyl)piperazine mono-methane sulfonate (ET-495), Servier Labs, Orleans, France; Clonidine·HCl (Catapres), Boehringer Ingelheim, Ltd., Elmsford, New York; Quipazine maleate, Miles Laboratories, Inc., Elkart, Indiana; Methysergide maleate, Sandoz Pharmaceuticals, East Hanover, New Jersey; and 2-chlorocinanserin· HCl (SQ10,631), Squibb Institute of Medical Research, Princeton, New Jersey were dissolved in distilled water just prior to injection. Haloperidol (Haldol) injectable solution, McNeil Laboratories, Inc., Ft. Washington, Pennsylvania, bis-(4-methyl-1-homopiperazinyl thiocarbonyl)disulfite (FLA-63), Regis Chemical Co., Morton Grove, Illinois, and Pimozide (ORAP), McNeil Labs, were obtained commercially. FLA-63 along with an equal weight of ascorbic acid was dissolved in water and adjusted to pH 6.0. Pimozide (2.5 mg free base) was dissolved in 50 µl glacial acetic acid, diluted to 5.0 ml with boiling water and allowed to cool to room temperature before injecting. All doses given are those of the salt forms and were administered intraperitoneally, except for quipazine which was given subcutaneously.

METHODS

Neurochemical Assays. Control and IDPN-treated rats (125-150 g) were guillotinized between 0800-0900 hr. On day-7 (24 hr after induction) because on this day the syndrome is fully expressed and on day-14 (a week after the syndrome appeared) because this time interval permitted the animal to regain fully their weight loss and to stabilize their behavior. Brains were quickly removed and placed on a cold plate, -4°C and then were dissected into five regions[6]. NE, DA, 5-HT and 5-HIAA were extracted in ice-cold 0.4N perchloric acid containing 0.02% ascorbic acid and 0.5% EDTA. Centrifugation, neutralization of the supernatant ($26,000xg_{max}$), column separation and elution procedure are described in great detail in Ref. 3. Once eluted from the column, the amines and amino acid were immediately measured spectrofluorometrically and quantitated against an internal standard. Native fluorescence was used to determine 5-HIAA[7] and 5-HT[8]. Trihydroxyindole derivative techniques were employed in the measurement of NE[9] and DA[10]. Known quantities of each of the biogenic amines and amino acid, in amounts similar to those expected in the sample, were added directly to tissue homogenates and used in calculating recovery rates. The average percent recovery values were as follows: 5-HT, 74%; 5-HIAA, 75%; NE, 88%; and DA, 95%. All results reported are uncorrected values. Measurement of [^{3}H]-amine uptake in the striatal and midbrain synaptosomal preparations were also performed[3]. The molar concentration that produced 50% inhibition of the uptake were determined graphically.

Behavioral Pharmacologic Experiments. Measurement of the circling behavior and choreiform movements and the effects of numerous neuropsycho-pharmacologic agents, administered systemically, were carried out. The circling behavior was achieved by manually counting the number of turns (continuous, complete 360° rotations) made by the rat in an enclosed circular arena (40 cm dia). To avoid complications from stimulation caused by being handled, injected and placed in observational arena, measurements were not begun until 15 min after rats were placed in arena. At least three separate measurements of the spontaneous rotational rate of the IDPN-treated rats were made just prior to drug administration. Rotations and choreiform movements were observed as described previously[4,5].

RESULTS AND DISCUSSION

Effect of IDPN on Regional Biogenic Amine Levels. The levels of the biogenic amines, NE, DA, 5-HT and its metabolite 5-HIAA, were measured in the striatum, midbrain, medulla, cortex, and cerebellum on the day the syndrome appeared (day 7) and one week later (day 14). The biogenic amine most affected by IDPN administration was 5-HT. On day 7, striatal 5-HT levels increased and 5-HIAA levels decreased while in the medulla and midbrain, 5-HIAA levels increased. On day 14, significant reductions in both 5-HT, in the midbrain, striatum, and cortex, and 5-HIAA in all regions except the cortex, were observed. NE was markedly increased in the medulla, midbrain, and striatum on day 7, whereas on day 14 it was found to be within the normal range in these same regions. With the exception of a slight, but significant, increase in the cortex on day 7, DA levels in all regions were found to be relatively unaffected by IDPN administration on both day 7 and day 14[3].

Uptake of Labelled Biogenic Amines. In an attempt to detect degenerative changes which might be taking place in the brain and which might provide an explanation for the permanency of the behavioral disturbances, the uptake of [^{3}H]-labelled NE, DA, and 5-HT into synaptosomal-rich preparations of striatum and the uptake of NE and 5-HT into the midbrain area were compared between normal and syndromized rats on both day 7 and day 14. Small changes were observed but they were not statistically significant.

Another method for examining synaptosomal membrane systems, other than direct measurement of the transport of the naturally occurring amines, is by measuring the degree of inhibition of uptake which has been demonstrated to be produced by several classes of compounds. CPZ was more potent in inhibiting the uptake of DA than 5-HT into the striatum. The IC_{50} values for the 5-HT uptake were very similar for both normal and IDPN-treated rats, while small differences in the DA uptake were observed.

The alterations of 5-HT and 5-HIAA levels in several regions of the brain under the conditions examined may indicate that IDPN's neurotoxicity primarily affects 5-HT-containing neurones. The active membrane transporting system of the nerve endings studied, however, remained relatively intact. This latter finding eliminates the possibility that neuronal degeneration in these areas is responsible for the decreased 5-HT and 5-HIAA levels or is the pathology underlying the permanency of the syndrome. These results were evaluated in terms of a possible model for hyperkinetic disorders[3].

Effect of Neuropharmacologic Agents. The possibility of an involvement of brain dopaminergic mechanisms in the choreiform movements and circling behavior induced by IDPN was investigated from a behavioral pharmacologic approach[4]. Concretely, the effect of neuroleptic drugs with DA receptor blocking properties, i.e., CPZ, haloperidol and pimozide and the noradrenergic receptor antagonist, phenoxybenzamine, was tested on the potentiation of these hyperkinesias by amphetamine (2.0 mg/kg, i.p.). It was found that very low doses of the neuroleptics, haloperidol (0.1 mg/kg), pimozide (0.1 mg/kg) and CPZ (1.0 mg/kg) produce complete inhibition of the amphetamine potentiation, whereas the non-neuroleptic phenothiazine, promethazine (1, 5 and 10 mg/kg), had no effect. High dose of the central noradrenergic antagonist, phenoxybenzamine (20 mg/kg), produced only a slight reduction in response to amphetamine. The exacerbation of choreiform movements and circling by amphetamine was completely blocked by α-methyl-para-tyrosine induced depletion of brain NE and DA, while depletion of only NE by FLA-63 resulted in only a partial antagonism. This antagonism of hyperkinesia by neuroleptics could not be attributed to their sedative properties, for neither chlordiazepoxide (50 mg/kg) nor sodium pentobarbital (10 mg/kg) produced any significant inhibition of the effects of amphetamine.

The central DA stimulators, i.e., amantadine, apomorphine and ET-495 and the direct noradrenergic receptor agonist, clonidine, were also tested for their ability to exacerbate these hyperkinetic movements. Amantadine, 50 and 80 mg/kg, produced a biphasic response characterized by an initial inhibition during the first 30 mins followed by a marked increase in both circling and choreiform movements which lasted for 120 mins. Apomorphine, at varying doses from 0.05 to 5.0 mg/kg, as well as ET-495 from 1.0 to 5.0 mg/kg, produced a similar exacerbation of the choreiform head and neck movements. Unlike amphetamine and amantadine, these two direct DA-receptor stimulants, showed no consistent potentiation of the IDPN-induced circling. Clonidine, 1.0 and 5.0 mg/kg, had no effect on either form of hyperkinesia[4].

The 5-HT agonist, Quipazine (2-(1-piperazinyl) quinone maleate), reportedly increases brain 5-HT activity by directly stimulating 5-HT receptor[11-14] and by inhibiting the neuronal uptake of 5-HT[15,16]. Thus, by observing the behavioral effects resulting from pharmacological stimulation of brain 5-HT mechanisms, a study was carried out in order to determine if the reduction in brain 5-HT was directly related to the

"ECC-Syndrome". A number of IDPN-treated animals were pretreated with
5-HT antagonists, methysergide and SQ10,631. Several animals were also
pretreated with haloperidol, the DA receptor blocker, since dopaminergic
mechanisms have also been implicated in quipazine behavioral action[17].

Rather than alleviating the IDPN-induced "ECC-Syndrome", quipazine
(5-25 mg/kg) administration resulted in a marked exacerbation of circling
behavior. Increasing the dose of quipazine lengthened the duration of
increased circling or the severity of choreiform movements seen with a
threshold dose of 5 mg/kg (15 mg/kg produced the most consistent increase
in circling: 10-fold during 5-15 min period). Circling and choreiform
movements were never observed in normal rats treated with this or any other
dose of quipazine[5]. Pretreatment with SQ10,631 (25 mg/kg; 30 min) and
methysergide (5 mg/kg; 30 min) completely blocked the increased circling
and the exacerbatory effect on choreiform movements induced by quipazine.

These findings suggest that the previously observed reductions in brain
5-HT and 5-HIAA levels may not be causally related to the motor disturbances. Instead, this apparent reduction in 5-HT biosynthesis and turnover may be the result of a compensatory feedback inhibition caused by
the toxic action of IDPN on some other cell population. Therefore, increasing serotonergic activity by quipazine administration counteracts
this adaptive feedback inhibition and results in further behavioral disturbances. On the other hand, reducing serotonergic activity with methysergide or SQ10,631 not only blocks quipazine exacerbation of circling and
choreiform movements but also reduces or eliminates these disturbances
present in unmedicated hyperkinetic rats.

An interesting finding was haloperidol antagonism of quipazine action
on this syndrome. At low dose used (0.5 mg/kg, i.p.), haloperidol selectively blocks DA receptors. Hence, it is unlikely that the antagonism of

quipazine actions by haloperidol is due to its direct interference with quipazine action on 5-HT neurons. A more plausible explanation is that an intact dopaminergic pathway is necessary for the behavioral expression of 5-HT receptor stimulation by quipazine. Haloperidol antagonism of the quipazine effect on the "ECC-Syndrome" may be the result of its blockade of a DA receptor which is serially 1 synapse higher than the 5-HT receptor stimulated by quipazine. A functional dependence of 5-HT pathways on intact DA neurons has been suggested to explain the ability of brain DA depletion to inhibit a hyperactive syndrome produced by tranylcypromine and L-tryptophan administration[18]. It may be that rather than being mutually antagonistic, brain DA- and 5-HT-mediated neuronal pathways may, in fact, interact synergistically to control certain body movements and behaviors. The serotonergic raphe-striatal and dopaminergic nigro-striatal pathways have been proposed to display such a relationship[19] and possibly could be involved in the circling and choreiform movements induced by IDPN.

The various behavioral pharmacologic studies described above are interpreted as evidence that dopaminergic mechanisms are involved in the hyperkinetic components of the "ECC-Syndrome". The role of DA, however, remains to be elucidated. The effect of IDPN on midbrain and striatal 5-HT levels points to a possible decreased serotonergic innervation of striatal neurons. Thus, the involvement of dopaminergic mechanisms might be secondary; the primary disturbance induced by IDPN being an impairment of the ascending raphe-striatal 5-HT system. It would, therefore, be of interest to investigate this possibility through an enzyme approach, i.e., to examine the activity of the enzymes responsible for the biosynthesis and metabolism of both 5-HT in the raphe system and DA in the nigrostriatal areas of IDPN-treated rat brain.

Before an experimentally-induced motor disturbance in the rat can be proposed as a suitable model for human motor disorders, it should, among other criteria, display similar responses to the same neuropsychopharmacological agents. The striking similarity in the pharmacological profile of the hyperkinetic movements of both the "ECC-Syndrome" and human dyskinesias seems to fulfill this requirement.

For example, there are several close parallels between the "ECC-Syndrome" and Huntington's Chorea. First, normal or near normal striatal DA levels are found in both the "ECC-Syndrome"[3] and Huntington's Chorea[20]. DA antagonists (neuroleptics) ameliorate while certain DA agonists exacerbate the abnormal involuntary movements of Huntington's Chorea[21] and the "ECC-Syndrome". On this point, it should be noted that similar to its effect on the "ECC-Syndrome", apomorphine has been observed to ameliorate the choreic movements of Huntington's disease[22]. Treatment with α-methyl-p-tyrosine produces a definite improvement in patients with Huntington's Chorea[23]. Thus, there is a similarity between the drug responses of the hyperkinetic movements induced by IDPN and those of Huntington's Chorea and its consequences.

SUMMARY

A permanent syndrome is induced in rats by seven daily injections of IDPN (300 mg/kg, i.p.) and is characterized by marked locomotor and behavioral excitation, choreiform head and neck movement and circling; "ECC-Syndrome". The "ECC-Syndrome", by the very nature of its motor disturbances and symptomatology, appears to be a useful model for human dyskinetic disorders.

A series of regional neurochemical studies and behavioral pharmacologic manipulations have demonstrated the possible underlying involvement of dopaminergic mechanisms in the pathogenesis of this chemically-induced "ECC-Syndrome" without any evidence of cellular loss and is, therefore, a non-lesioned, noninvaded (implanted connulae, intracerebral infusion, etc) animal model in which hyperactivity (choreiform movements and circling) can be consistently produced and studied separately or cooperatively.

The levels of the biogenic amines, NE, DA, 5-HT and its metabolite 5-HIAA were measured in the striatum, midbrain, medulla, cortex and cerebellum on the day the syndrome appeared (day 7) and one week later (day 14). The biogenic amine most affected by IDPN administration was 5-HT. On day 7, striatal 5-HT levels increased and 5-HIAA levels decreased while in the medulla and midbrain, 5-HIAA levels increased. On day 14, significant reductions in both 5-HT, in the midbrain, striatum and cortex, and 5-HIAA, in all regions except the cortex, were observed. NE was markedly increased in the medulla, midbrain, and striatum on day 7, whereas on day 14 it was found to be within the normal range in these same regions. With the exception of a slight, but significant, increase in the cortex on day 7, DA levels in all regions were found to be relatively unaffected by IDPN administration on both day 7 and day 14.

In an attempt to detect degenerative changes which might be taking place in the brain and which might provide an explanation for the permanency of the behavioral disturbances, the uptake of [^{3}H]-labelled NE, DA and 5-HT into synaptosomal-rich preparations of striatum and the uptake of NE and 5-HT into the midbrain area were compared between normal and syndromized rats on both day 7 and day 14. The data did not reveal changes. Neither the reduced levels of 5-HT and 5-HIAA nor the permanency of the syndrome, therefore, can be explained by gross cellular degenerative lesions in these areas.

Behavioral pharmacological studies[4] have demonstrated the possible underlying involvement of dopaminergic mechanisms in the pathogenesis of these movements. Neuroleptic drugs (CPZ, haloperidol and pimozide) are quite effective in abolishing the choreoathetoid movements, circling behavior and hyperactivity induced by IDPN. Administration of amphetamine (2.0 mg/kg, i.p.) produces a profound exacerbation of this syndrome, an effect which can be completely blocked by pretreatment with neuroleptics. Reduction in brain DA and NE levels by inhibition of tyrosine hydroxylase with α-methyl-p-tyrosine, completely antagonizes the exacerbating effect of amphetamine. However, depletion of only NE levels by inhibition of DA-β-hydroxylase with FLA-63 produces only a slight reduction in the effect of amphetamine. The importance of dopaminergic rather than noradrenergic mechanisms in amphetamine's action is supported by the inability of phenoxybenzamine, a central noradrenergic receptor antagonist, to block the effect of amphetamine. Similarly, clonidine, a central noradrenergic receptor agonist, has no effect on the "ECC-Syndrome".

Two direct DA receptor stimulants, apomorphine and ET-495 (Piribedil) have some unusual effects on the choreoathetoid head and neck movements and circling behavior. At low doses of apomorphine (0.01-2.0 mg/kg, i.p.) and ET-495 (0.1-5.0 mg/kg), rather than stimulating circling behavior, as is seen in the unilateral nigro-striatal lesion model, both of these drugs reduce or completely abolish the IDPN-induced circling behavior. Following these treatments most animals appear to be in a semi-stuporous state, hunching motionless with their eyes partially closed. Lower doses of apomorphine and ET-495 also produce either no change or an amelioration of the choreoathetoid movements. Larger doses produce no consistent effect on the circling behavior while definitely exacerbating the choreoathetoid movements. The results of these pharmacological experiments provide evidence that some alteration of dopaminergic systems exists in this syndrome.

Following the administration of quipazine, the 5-HT agonist, which reportedly increases 5-HT activity by directly stimulating the neuronal uptake of 5-HT was found to exacerbate the "ECC-Syndrome". Quipazine potentiation of circling and choreiform movement was effectively inhibited by pretreatment with the 5-HT antagonists, SQ10,631 and methysergide, as well as the DA receptor antagonist, haloperidol (500 µg/kg). These observations are discussed with respect to our previously observed reductions in brain 5-HT and 5-HIAA as well as the nature of the involvement of brain serotonergic and dopaminergic systems.

While it is hazardous to draw analogies between an animal syndrome and a human disorder, the neurochemical findings and the response of circling and choreiform movements in these animals to various pharmacological agents closely resembles those responses seen in human hyperkinesias. It is thus felt that the "ECC-Syndrome" seems to represent a useful model for screening drugs potentially effective in the treatment of Huntington's disease and its consequences. It is suggested that more thorough biochemical, pharmacological, physiological and morphological studies be conducted on this syndrome. The results of such studies should contribute greatly to our understanding of the chemistry and physiology of the complex networks which regulate involuntary movements and the types of disturbances in these systems which result in hyperkinesia.

ACKNOWLEDGMENT

The author is greatly indebted to Mr. Philip J. Langlais for his very valuable collaboration from 1972-1976. This work is supported by the Medical Service of the Veterans Administration.

REFERENCES

1. Gabay, S. (1966) Rec. Adv. Biol. Psychiat 8, 73-85.

2. Gabay, S., Langlais, P. J. and Huang, P. C. (1974) The Pharmacologist 8, 308.

3. Langlais, P.J., Huang, P.C. and Gabay, S. (1975) J. Neurosci. Res. 1, 419-435.

4. Langlais, P.J., Huang, P.C. and Gabay, S. (1977) Int. J. Neurol. 12, 97-112.

5. Langlais, P.J., Huang, P.C. and Gabay, S. (1977) J. Neurosci. Res. 3, 135-141.

6. Iversen, L.L. (1970) Adv. Biochem. Pharmac. II, 109-132.

7. Lindqvist, M. (1971) Acta Pharmac. (Kbh.) 29, 303-313.

8. Anden, N.-E. and Magnusson, T. (1967) Acta Physiol. Scand. 69, 87-94.

9. Bertler, A., Carlsson, A. and Rosengren, E. (1958) Acta Physiol. Scand. 44, 273-292.

10. Shellenberger, M.K. and Gordon, J.H. (1971) Anal. Biochem. 39, 356-372.

11. Hong, E. and Pardo, E.G. (1966) J. Pharmac. Exp. Ther. 153, 259-265.

12. Hong, E., Sancilio, L.F., Vargas, R. and Pardo, E.G. (1969) Eur. J. Pharmac. 6, 274-280.

13. Rodriguez, R., Rojas-Ramirez, J.A. and Drucker-Colin, R.R. (1973) Eur. J. Pharmac. 24, 164-171.

14. Costall, B. and Naylor, R.J. (1975) J. Pharm. Pharmac. 27, 368-371.

15. Medon, P.J., Lelling, J.L. and Phillips, B.M. (1973) Life Sci. 13, 685-691.

16. Fuller, R.W., Snoddy, H.D., Perry, K.W., Roush, B.W., Molloy, B.B., Bymaster, F.P. and Wong, D.T. (1976) Life Sci. 18, 925-934.

17. Grabowska, M., Antkiewicz, L. and Michaluk, J. (1974) J. Pharm. Pharmac. 26, 74-76.

18. Green, A.R. and Grahame-Smith, D.G. (1974) Neuropharmacology 13, 949-959.

19. Cools, A.R. and Hanssen, H.-J. (1974) Eur. J. Pharmac. 28, 266-275.

20. Barbeau, A. (1973) The Psychiat. Forum 4, 8-15.

21. Klawans, H.L. (1970) Eur. J. Neurol. 4, 148-163.

22. Tolosa, E.S. and Sparber, S.B. (1974) Life Sci. 15, 1371-1380.

23. Birkmayer, W. (1969) Wein. Klin. Wschr. 81, 10-12.

© 1979 Elsevier/North-Holland Biomedical Press
Modern Concepts in Psychiatric Surgery
E.R. Hitchcock, H.T. Ballantine, Jr. and B.A. Meyerson, eds.

THERAPEUTICAL ELECTRICAL STIMULATION OF THE BRAIN. BIOCHEMICAL
CHANGES INDUCED IN THE VENTRICULAR CEREBRO SPINAL FLUID WITH
REGARD TO OPIATE-LIKE SUBSTANCES.

J.G. MARTIN-RODRIGUEZ and S. OBRADOR.
Department "Sixto Obrador" of Neurosurgery. Centro Especial
"Ramón y Cajal" of the Spanish Social Security. Madrid, Spain.

What we believe was the first case reported in the literature of therapeutic electrical stimulation of the brain (TESB)
by means of a chronically fully implanted subdermal stimulator
was presented by our group at the III World Congress of Psychiatric Surgery in Cambridge on 1972. Since then, a total
of 10 patients have been treated in two consecutive series of
5 cases each. All the patients suffered from chronic intractable pain of different ethiologies and as the first group had
been previously reported (Delgado et al.[1], 1973; Obrador et
al.[2], 1973; Obrador et al.[3],1974; Obrador et al.[4], 1975;
Martín-Rodriguez et al.[5], 1977) we shall only refer in this
presentation to the second group of 5 patients in 3 of whom
we had the opportunity of measuring variations of endorphin -
like substances in the ventricular cerebro spinal fluid
(V-CSF) before and after cerebral stimulation.

MATERIAL and METHODS.- A group of 5 patients, 3 males and
2 females, were studied in detail at our "pain clinic". Age
ranged from 48-65 years old. Facial anaesthesia dolorosa was
the cause of illness in two of the patients while phantom limb
pain, thalamic syndrome and cancer pain accounted for each one
of the remaining 3 patients. Overall duration of the pain
syndrome ranged from 1 to 40 years.

A trial of psychopharmacological therapy, was given following our recommendations presented at the IV World Congress
of Psychiatric Surgery in Madrid on 1975 before they were selected for Surgery (Martín-Rodriguez et al.[5], 1977). The only

exception to this rule was the patient suffering from cancer pain. Their pre-surgical evaluation included detailed neurological history, social history, clinical examination, pain chart,blood and urine analysis, EEG, ECG, skull and chest x-ray, CT scanner and psychiatric-psychological examination.

Details of the surgical technique will be given in extension at our second presentation today (pag.95). We shall only mention now, that a four contacts deep brain Medtronic electrode was implanted stereotaxically from a coronal burr-hole into the Posterior Commisure-periventricular-Parafascicular-Centre Median area contralateral to the side of the pain. Later it was coupled to a subdermal bipolar Medtronic stimulator. An Ommaya reservoir was implanted at the beginning of the operation in a opposite coronal burr-hole. This was a modification from our previous technique, being the rational behind it, the possibility of later performing serial ventriculography with safety and minimum disturbance to the patient, in any of those cases in whom electrode displacement could be suspected as the cause of sudden failure during the course of a successfully running treatment. Advantage was taken from this modification to draw CSF samples from the III Ventricle under full sterile conditions using the Ommaya reservoir.

The first sample used for tracing a basal measurement, was taken at the time of surgery, while the other basal specimens were withdrawn at a later date so that at least two of the basal samples were taken on different times. All the remaining CSF samples were taken at random from each patient with regards to post-stimulation periods. After withdrawl, the samples were immediately frozen down to -20°C and sent to Dr. Agneta Wahlstrom in Sweden who performed the analysis for endorphin-like substances. A total of 22 V-CSF specimen were withdrawn from 3 patients and sent for analysis: 3 of them were lost during processing because of the small amount supplied and 2 further ones were discarded as they were taken following a Naloxone test and this substance does interfere with the analysis technique.

The samples of V-CSF were tenfold concentrated and ultrafiltered through an AMICON PM 10. Chemical separation and partial desalting was obtained by running the concentrated ultrafiltered samples through a G 10 SEPHADEX column. Ultrafiltration removed high-molecular weight components such as enzymes of blood origin if present. This procedure also preserved endorphin activity in the sample as well as protected the column. Two fractions called Fractions I and II were isolated and tested for opiate receptor affinity in a radioreceptor-assay method that measures receptor-active material with no other restrictions regarding their chemical composition.[6, 7,8,9]

RESULTS.- The principal active molecular species in Fractions I and II are yet to be chemically characterized. It seems clear that they do not represent any of the previously known endorphins (Wahlstrom et al.[10]; Terenius and Wahlstrom [11]) and with all probability they are not enkephalines as both fractions appear to be more basic in character. On the other hand, they probably have a lower molecular weight than β-endorphin since they differ from that substance in not being excluded from SEPHADEX C 10 gels. However, in lumbar CSF, Terenius and Wahlstrom[11], using a radio-immuno-assay, have found a slight crossreaction of Fraction II endorphin with leucine-enkephaline directed antiserum, indicating its genetic relationship. It is likely that al least in part, it could derived from the Central Nervous System, as a fraction with similar properties to Fraction II could also be isolated from the human brain as demonstrated by the group of Terenius.[11]

Values of endorphins contents in lumbar-CSF of normal subjects[7] are presented in Table 1 as supplied by Drs. Wahlstrom and Meyerson.[14] However, as far as we know, there are no data available of endorphin values in V-CSF of normal subjects.

TABLE 1

NORMAL VALUES OF ENDORPHIN IN CSF

Fraction I	=	1.0 pmole/ml CSF	$\pm$ 0.8 SEM
Fraction II	=	2.5 pmole/ml CSF	$\pm$ 0.3 SEM
n = 19			

CASE 1: (Patient S.G.C.) This 60 years old male patient with
a left limb phantom pain of 40 years duration, does achieve full
pain relief following stimulation sessions lasting between 15-30
minutes. Analgesia does begin within 30 minutes of ending TESB
and reaches its maximum 2 hours later. At the last follow-up
in July 78, it did last between 3-6 days, a change from the 2-4
days pain relief previously reported. The parameters of stimulation used since the beginning are 50 Hz. of frequency with a
pulse width (PW) of 0.4 ms. Current intensities cannot be measured with the implanted devices available at present because
being the values of electrode impedance unknown, the voltage
range applied to the stimulator do lack any reality. A Naloxone test was performed in two different occasions with a very
positive result following an intravenous (IV) injection of 1 and
0.5 mg. respectively. Naloxone reversal with full recurrence of
pain occurred within 5-15 minutes of initiating the IV injection.

TABLE 2

CASE 1: V-CSF ENDORFHINS CONTENT AFTER TESB

Samples	Fraction I [*]	Fraction II [*]
Basal V-CSF	0.6	0.5
" "	0.7	$\leqslant$0.4
" -- "	0.4	0.5
30 min. after stim.[a]	0.7	0.5
4 h. " " [a]	1.7	2.5
72 h. " " [b]	<0.4	<0.4
96 h. " " [b]	0.4	2.0

[*] Concentration expressed in pmole/ml V-CSF
[a] Following the same stim. session
[b] Following another stim. session

As may be seen in Table 2, following stimulation, there are no
significant increments in concentration of either Fractions I or

II in V-CSF when compared to the normal values of lumbar-CSF. However, if they are compared with the values of the 3 basal V-CSF samples taken from the same patient on different days and times, it is clearly apparent the increments of both Fractions I and II 4 hours after stimulation, as well as Fraction II 96 hours since stimulation. On the contrary, the low values of both Fractions 72 hours after stimulation should be noted. The patient was pain-free at the time when all the post-stimulation samples were taken.

CASE 2: (Patient C.M.P.) This 52 years old female suffered for 2 years a left facial anesthesia dolorosa following a Frazier operation for a trigeminal neuralgia involving the II and III divisions. Good analgesia lasting between 4-48 hours could be achieved with 15-30 minutes TESB at 30 Hz and a PW of 0.6. A Naloxone reversal test has been considered doubtful as a slow IV injection of 0.5 mg of N-alil-morphine induced some degree of mental confusion lasting 15-20 minutes, after which she complained of varying degrees of pain affecting her in a wave like pattern. The test was not repeated.

TABLE 3

CASE 2: V-CSF ENDORPHINS CONTENT AFTER TESB

Samples	Fraction I *	Fraction II *
Basal CSF	1.3	0.8
" "	1.8	1.5
" "	1.1	5.3
1 h. after stim.[a]	0.8	2.7
4 h. " " [a]	4.0	0.4
8 h. " " [a]	4.0	<0.4
12 h. " " [a]	1.1	2.8

* Concentration expressed in pmole/ml V-CSF
[a] Samples taken in different days and following different stim. session.

The results presented in Table 3 reveal a significant

increment of the concentration of Fraction I in the V-CSF when
compared to both the normal lumbar and to her own basal V-CSF
samples, at 4 and 8 hours following two different TESB sessions
and being the patient pain-free. On the other hand, concentration
values for Fraction II endorphins remained rather low in all specimens and however, the high concentration found in one of the basal samples taken while she was in pain, should be noted. To further complicate the picture we shall report that this is the only
case in the whole series that has had up to date 3 different episodes of addiction to stimulation requiring TESB interruption for
at least 5 days before pain control could be regained. A check
ventriculogram was performed on the second occasion to discard
electrode displacement and we have plotted the electrode points
in the atlas of Van Buren and Borke[12] being the stimulation points
1 (cathode) versus 2 (anode) well within the Parafascicularis and
Centre Median nucleus, respectively, as the electrode runs upward,
forward and laterally from the wall of the III Ventricle where its
tip was located 1 mm lateral to it and at the border of the posterior commisure.

CASE 3: (Patient L.L.A.) This 48 years old male patient presented
a thalamic syndrome affecting the right hemibody with umbearable
pain during one year. Psychopharmacological therapy failed to
control the pain. TESB sessions not longer than 10 minutes duration at 30 Hz with a PW of 0.2 ms, produced immediate analgesia
with subjective values ranging between 50-80% and lasting from
6-14 hours. Any attempt to prolong TESB over 10 minutes produced
a contrary effect worsenning his original pain. In fact, TESB had
to be disconnected as soon as a feeling of muscle tone relaxation
in the right limbs was reported by the patient, analgesia following immediately afterwards. Otherwise he will get a sensation of
tightness in the right hemibody, mainly at the upper limb, that
will be followed by excruciating pain. Objective evidence of these muscle tone changes were obtained by direct measurements of active and passive contraction during stimulation. This pattern had
somewhat changed at the last follow-up when he reported tolerating
TESB sessions of up to 15 minutes with a lasting analgesia of 8-14
hours. Whatever degree of analgesia was produced by TESB it would

be mantained without important variations. A Naloxone reversal
test was not performed.

TABLE 4
CASE 3: V-CSF ENDORPHINS CONTENT AFTER TESB

Samples	Fraction I *	Fraction II *
Basal CSF	0.8	0.7
" "	0.5	3.4
1 h. after stim.	1.1	1.2

* Concentration expressed in pmole/ml V-CSF

Table 4 shows that there are not variations of significant value
in the V-CSF endorphin content of the only sample taken in this
case at 1 hour after TESB.

DISCUSSION.- The actual relation between CNS endorphin activity and CSF levels is not yet known. From a hypothetical basis it
may be accepted that endorphin levels in CSF do reflect CNS endorphin activity since the CSF is very similar in its composition to
that of the extracellular fluid of the CNS. However, it cannot
be said with certainty, at least in our cases, that the endorphins
being analysed in the V-CSF did originate from the periventricular
gray and medial thalamus itself, as their origin may had been the
pituitary gland.
 As has been said, the nature of endorphins analysed in the CSF
is not yet known and above all, normal values in V-CSF together
with natural variation along the day or under different emotional
conditions, are factors that need to be known before the possible
role played by TESB with relation to endorphin variation in V-CSF
could be analysed with certainty. The same may be said for the
mechanisms played by endorphins with regards to analgesia in response to TESB. Three points may be appraised from this presentation that may bear some relevance when relating TESB and endorphin

mechanisms in analgesia: a) the pattern of building-up analgesia following the end of TESB, b) the episodes of addiction to stimulation and c) the effects of the Naloxone reversal test, seems to suggest a positive biochemical role played by neurotransmitters following electrical stimulation of the brain.

However, if those mechanisms should be related to increase production of neurotransmitters, to changes induced in the functional situation of the specific binding receptors, to both or to none is hard to say at present. As was stressed in Cases 1 and 2, there were both positive and negative correlation between the V-CSF endorphin contents and analgesia induced by TESB, depending on the time when the samples were taken. The results were conflicting as well with regards to the values of the different Fractions when the patients were or were not in pain as was stressed for Fraction II in the second case.

It is evident that the benefitial effects following TESB could not be accounted only on biochemical mechanisms and there are no doubts of a direct and immediate relationship between TESB and analgesia that must be caused by a straight forward disruption of the afferent pain message. That is the case in our third patient as well as in several others of our series and in a good number of reports from the literature.

The area of the brain subjected to TESB, mainly the CM-Pf complex, has been stereotactically destroyed as a mean of successfully treating chronic pain as may be seen in the postmortem specimen from one of our cases with cancer pain presented in Figs. 1 and 2. Full control of pain was obtained until death three months after operation without any need of the morphine treatment she was receiving before surgery. This is again a conflicting finding, as Pert et al.[13] have demonstrated in animal studies that the medial intralaminar thalamus with its major implications in the mediation of affective components of pain, is a region highly enriched in opiate receptor binding sites.

ACKNOWLEDGEMENT.- We are deeply indebted to Dr. Agneta Wahlstrom from Sweden for the analysis of the V-CSF samples and to Dr. Bjorn Meyerson for his help and critical discussion of this presentation.

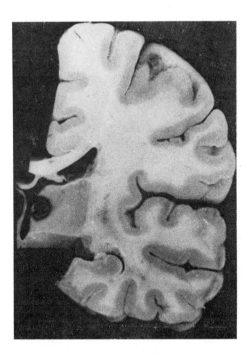

Fig.1. Post-mortem specimen showing the destruction of the CM-Pf nucleus by a cryogenic lesion stereotaxically placed. The outer edge of the lesion only encroaches up to the medial part of CM remaining the lateral half of the nucleus undestructed. A similar lesion was placed in the contralateral thalamus in the same surgical session without any untoward effect.

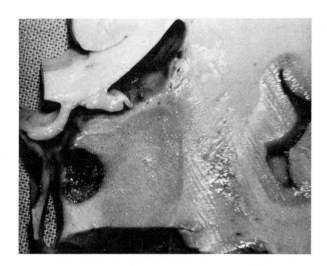

Fig. 2. Close-up view of the cryogenic lession in fig. 1.

REFERENCES

1. Delgado, J.M.R., Obrador, S. and Martín-Rodriguez, J.G. (1973) in Surgical Approaches in Psychiatry, Laitinen, L.V. and Livingstone, K.E. eds., MTP, Lancaster, pp.215-223.

2. Obrador, S., Delgado, J.M.R., Martín-Rodriguez, J.G., Santo-Domingo, J. and Alonso, A. (1973) Arch. Neurobiol., 36, 181-186.

3. Obrador, S., Delgado, J.M.R. and Martín-Rodriguez, J.G. (1974) in Progress in Neurological Surgery, Sano, K. and Ishii, S. eds., Elsevier, New York, pp. 265-269.

4. Obrador, S., Delgado, J.M.R. and Martín-Rodriguez, J.G. (1975) in Cerebral Localization, Zulch, K.J., Creutzfeldt, O. and Galbraith, G.C. eds., Springer-Verlag, Berlin, Heidelberg, New York, pp. 171-183.

5. Martín-Rodriguez, J.G., Delgado, J.M.R., Obrador, S., Santo-Domingo, J. and Alonso, A. (1977) in Neurosurgical Treatment in Psychiatry, Pain and Epilepsy, Sweet, W.H., Obrador, S. and Martín-Rodriguez, J.G. eds., University Park Press, Baltimore, London, Tokyo, pp. 639-649.

6. Almay, B.G.L., Johansson, F., Von Knorring, L., Terenius, L. and Wahlstrom, A. (1978) Pain 5, 153-162.

7. Lindstrom, L.H., Widerlov, E., Gunne, L.-M., Wahlstrom, A. and Terenius, L. (1978) Acta Psychiat. Scand., 57, 153-164.

8. Terenius, L. and Wahlstrom, A. (1975) Life Sci., 16, 1759-1764.

9. Terenius, L., Wahlstrom, A., Lindstrom, L. and Widerlov, E. (1976) Neurosci. Lett., 3, 157-162.

10. Wahlstrom, A., Johansson, L. and Terenius, L. (1976) in Opiates and Endogenons Opioid Peptides, Kosterlitz, H.W., ed., North-Holland, Amsterdam, pp. 49-56.

11. Terenius, L. and Wahlstrom, A. (1978) in Centrally Acting Peptides, Hughes, G. ed., McMillan, London.

12. Van Buren, J.M. and Borke, R.C. (1972) Variations and Connections of the Human Thalamus: Vol 2, Variations of the Human Diencephalon, Springer-Verlag, Berlin, Heidelberg, New York.

13. Pert, A. and Yaksh, T. (1974) Brain Research, 80, 135-140.

© 1979 Elsevier/North-Holland Biomedical Press
Modern Concepts in Psychiatric Surgery
E.R. Hitchcock, H.T. Ballantine, Jr. and B.A. Meyerson, eds.

ELEVATION OF B-ENDORPHIN-LIKE SUBSTANCES AND PRO-OPIOCORTIN (31K ACTH) BY PERIAQUEDUCTAL GRAY STIMULATION (PAGS) IN HUMANS

YOSHIO HOSOBUCHI

Department of Neurological Surgery, University of California School
of Medicine, San Francisco, San Francisco, California 94143 (USA)

INTRODUCTION

Hosobuchi, et al.[1] and Richardson and Akil[2] reported that permanent clinical pain states, as well as normal pain perception, can be blocked by electrical stimulation of the periventricular and periaqueductal gray matter in humans. Since the initial isolation of endogenous opiate-like substances from mammalian brain, it has been speculated that stimulation-produced analgesia (SPA) in animals is mediated by the release of endogenous, opiate-like substances or polypeptides, the endorphins. More recently, we have found that intraventricular administration of human B-endorphin in humans produces a prolonged state of analgesia[3].

In collaboration with Drs. Rossier, Bloom, and Guillemin of the Salk Institute, I conducted a study to determine whether or not the analgesia produced by periaqueductal gray stimulation (PAGS) is accompanied by an elevation of B-endorphin levels in the ventricular cerebrospinal fluid (CSF)[4].

We selected two groups of patients. One group obtained pain relief by PAGS or by opiates; the other suffered from deafferentation pains, and obtained pain relief by neither opiates nor PAGS, but rather by electrical stimulation of the posterior limb of the internal capsule[5]. We expected that PAGS of patients in the first group should increase the B-endorphin levels in the ventricular CSF, but that internal capsule stimulation of patients in the second group should not produce that effect.

MATERIALS AND METHODS

Ventricular fluid was collected from six patients undergoing stereotactic implantation of chronic brain electrodes for pain control. Three patients suffering from deafferentation pain received electrode implantation in the posterior limb of the internal capsule contralateral to their pain[5]. The other group had pain of peripheral origin, and had electrodes implanted bilaterally in the rostral position of the periaqueductal gray matter (Table 1).

Table 1
CLINICAL SUMMARY OF PATIENTS

Patient	Age	Sex	Etiology of Pain	Location of Pain
A	47	M	Postcordotomy dysesthesia	Bilateral, lower extremities
B	54	M	Postcordotomy dysesthesia	Right lower extremity
C	63	M	Thalamic syndrome	Right arm and leg
D	51	F	Lumbosacral arachnoiditis	Low back and both legs
E	57	F	Carcinoma of rectum	Abdomen and perineum
F	66	F	Carcinoma of colon	Abdomen

All six patients obtained significant or complete pain relief from stimulation of either the internal capsule or the periaqueductal gray matter. Ventricular fluids were collected from these patients, and radioimmunoassays for B-endorphin were performed according to the method of Guillemin and colleagues[6].

RESULTS

Control levels of immunoreactive B-endorphin $\int$ (ir) B-endorphin $\rceil$ in the patients' ventricular fluid ranged from 140 to 210 pg/ml. In three patients, stimulation of the internal capsule did not effect any increase of (ir) B-endorphin above the control levels; however, after stimulation of the periaqueductal area, there was a twofold to sevenfold increase in their (ir) B-endorphin levels (Table 2).

In two of these patients (B and F), radioimmunoassays for Leu[5]-enkephalin also were performed as described previously[6]. The assay is highly selective for Leu[5]-enkephalin, as it does not read alpha-, beta-, gamma-, or delta-endorphin, but does show a 3% cross-reactivity with Met[5]-enkephalin. The sensitivity of this assay is such that it could have detected as little as 25 pg/ml of Leu[5]-enkephalin per milliliter of original ventricular fluid. No Leu[5]-enkephalin immunoreactive material could be detected in the ventricular fluid of either patients E or F before or after stimulation of the periaqueductal gray matter.

Table 2

(ir) B-ENDORPHIN (pg/ml) IN VENTRICULAR FLUID

Patient	Baseline	End of 15 min stimulation	15 min after cessation of stimulation	30 min after cessation of stimulation
A	180	190	190	170
B	140	140	140	Not collected
C	160	160	Not collected	Not collected
D	170	230	270	Not collected
E	210	650	720	640
F	200	14010	720	980

Ventricular CSF samples were collected from a ventricular catheter inserted to perform intraoperative ventriculography. The tip of the catheter was usually located just at the foramen of Monro, but not in the third ventricle. Two cc of ventricular fluid were collected 1) at the onset of the surgery prior to ventriculography, insertion of the electrode, and stimulation (baseline); 2) just at the end of stimulation; 3) 15 min after the cessation of the stimulation; and 4) 30 min after cessation. Further collection of the fluid would have prolonged the usual time required for the closure of the surgical wound; it was thus not attempted. Tubes containing the collected ventricular fluids were immediately immersed in boiling water for 10 min to halt possible peptide degradation and then frozen.

COMMENT

In the rat brain, B-endorphin immunoreactive fibers are highly concentrated in the anterior periaqueductal gray matter. These fibers are part of the long projections of the B-endorphin immunoreactive cell bodies located in the basal tuberal hypothalamus[7]. Fibers of this pathway are rather dense around the wall of the third ventricle, especially in the anterior part of the ventricle. Futhermore, the anterior part of the rat hypothalamus exhibits the highest concentration of (ir) B-endorphin[8]. It seems possible that the (ir) B-endorphin observed here in samples of the third ventricular CSF could come from these B-endorphin-containing fibers packed in the anterior hypothalamus, and that electrical stimulation of the periaqueductal gray matter might induce antidromic stimulation of the anterior hypothalamic B-endorphin fibers, thereby causing the subsequent release of B-endorphin into the third ventricle. The stimulation of the B-endorphin-containing cell bodies in anterior hypothalamus could be orthodronic from the periaqueductal gray matter through the rostral projection system. Once B-endorphin is released into the third ventricle, it initiates its analgesic activity by binding with the many opiate receptors located in the periaqueductal area.

Neither opiates nor PAGS is effective in producing pain relief in cases of deafferentation dysesthesia [9]. In these cases, pain can be relieved by chronic stimulation of the somatosensory system, presumably mediated by an activation of the inhibitory corticofugall fibers[5]. This relief is not reversed by naloxone[1], nor is stimulation acompanied by increased (ir) B-endorphin levels in the CSF, as it was in the other patients who underwent PAGS.

It has been shown that naloxone reverses the pain relief obtained from both PAGS[1,10] and intraventricularly injected B-endorphin[3] in humans. Therefore, the mechanisms underlying the pain relief obtained by PAGS and endorphins may well be similar. The only other known endogenous opioid peptides in the periaquecductal gray, the enkephalin pentapeptides, are known to produce only transient analgesia in experimental animals[11,12], and are less likely to be the source of the longer-lasting analgesia observed in humans after PAGS. In a recent study based on a radioreceptor assay, Akil et al.[13] reported that PAGS produced a moderate increase (50%) of an uncharacterized enkephalin-like compound in the third ventricle. We found no such increase of Leu-enkephalin immunoreactivity in our study. Meyerson et al. also reported that PAGS caused an elevation of the "endorphin" level in lumbar CSF, but that dorsal column stimulation did not. However, since their method of "endorphin" measurement is based on the radioreceptor assay, one cannot be certain about what substance is actually being determined[14].

Our findings of a severalfold increase in levels of (ir) B-endorphin in the ventricular CSF demonstrate that the pain relief produced by PAGS has considerable anatomical and pharmacological specificity, inasmuch as the internal capsule stimulation resulted in no changes of (ir) B-endorphin levels in the CSF. Naturally, more data are needed to determine how much the "basal" levels measured in these patients differ from levels in unstressed patients who are not undergoing neurosurgical procedures, and whether or not the site of CSF collection is critical to the increments of changes in endorphins observed. Clearly, additional research is also required to define the precise mechanisms mediating the changes in endogenous opioid peptides detected in CSF and the pain relief resulting from PAGS.

COROLLARY EXPERIMENTATION

Release of a Large Molecular-Weight Adrenocorticotropic Hormone, Pro-opiocortin (31K-ACTH) by PAGS in Humans: Preliminary Result

High molecular-weight forms of adrenocorticotropic hormone (ACTH) have been observed in pituitary extracts and pituitary tumor extracts from several different species[15]. It has been confirmed by Mains and Eipper[15] that these high molecular-weight ACTH molecules are glycoproteins, and that the compound has molecular weight of 31,00 dalton. The entity it is now called 31K-ACTH or pro-opiocortin.

Figure 1 illustrates the many interesting fragments contained in 31K-ACTH[16]. Near the N-terminal, there is a 16K fragment with a carbohydrate attached. The amino acid sequence of this fragment has not been thoroughly defined, but it appears that calcitonin is a part of the molecule. After the 16K fragment, there is a molecule of 4.5K-ACTH, a commonly known form of ACTH: in certain species, a carbohydrate is attached. Finally, there is B-lipotropin. B-lipotropin degradation from 31K-ACTH has been demonstrated in both the pituitary gland and the hypothalamus. Their interdependence has not been clearly elucidated.

After confirming the release of B-endorphin by PAGS, I collaborated with Mains and Eipper's laboratory to determine if the common precursor hormone 31K-ACTH was released into the CSF by PAGS. Because the antibody for the human 16K fragment is not yet available, the mouse 16K-fragment antibody was used for the radioimmunoassay. Despite this technical difficulty, the initial result is highly encouraging. PAGS-induced

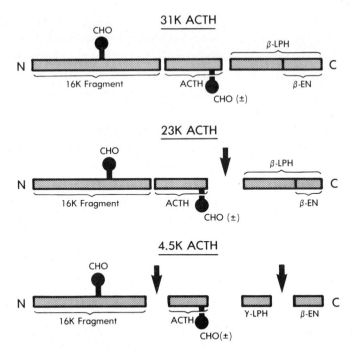

Fig. 1. Schematic representation of the degradation process from the common precursor hormone 31K-ACTH to each active component.

elevations of (ir) B-endorphin, 4.5K-ACTH, and the 16K fragment are shown in Table 3. The evidence suggests strongly that PAGS releases the precursor hormone 31K-ACTH. It is not clear whether the precursor arises from the pituitary gland or from the hypothalamus.

Table 3

31K-ACTH DETERMINATION (fmole/ml)

	B-Endorphin	4.5K-ACTH	16K Fragment
Prestimulation	18	170	72
Poststimulation	150	570	150

The ventricular fluid specimen was obtained during sterotactic implantation of PAGS electrode. (48-year-old female with carcinoma of the colon with sacral pain.)

Rose et al. demonstrated that PAGS induced a delayed elevation of blood ACTH levels in dogs[17] and, interestingly, that stress-induced ACTH release was inhibited by the electrical stimulation of the locus ceruleus and the N. sublocus ceruleus[18].

A concomitant rise of B-endorphin and ACTH levels in response to stress has been demonstrated by Guillemin, et al.[19]. Clearly, additional studies are necessary; however, one may speculate that the analgesia induced by PAGS is, in part, due to the activation of the organism's stress response.

REFERENCES

1. Hosobuchi, Y., Adams, J.E. and Linchitz, R. (1977) Science, 197, 183.

2. Richardson, D.E. and Akil, H. (1977) J. Neurosurgery, 47, 178.

3. Hosobuchi, Y. and Li, C.H. (1978) Commun. Psychopharmacology, 2, 33.

4. Hosobuchi, Y., Rossier, J., Bloom, F. and Guillemin, R. (in press) Science.

5. Adams, J.E., Hosobuchi, Y. and Fields, H.C. (1974) J. Neurosurgery, 41, 740.

6. Guillemin, R., Ling, N. and Vargo, T. (1977) Biochem. Biophys. Research Communications, 77, 361.

7. Bloom, F., Battenberg, E., Rossier, J., Ling, N. and Guillemin, R. (1978) Proc. National Academy of Science, USA, 75, 1591.

8. Rossier, J., Vargo, T.M., Minick, S., Ling, N., Bloom F.E. and Guillemin, R. (1977) Proc. National Academy of Science, USA, 74, 5162.

9. Garcin, R. (1968) in: Pain, Soulairac, A., Chan, J. and Charpentier, J.M., eds., Academic Press, New York, p. 521.

10. Adams, J.E. (1976) Pain, 22, 161.

11. Belluzi, J.D., Grant, N., Garsky, V., Sarantakis, R., Wise, C.D. and Steil, L. (1976) Nature, 260, 625.

12. Hosobuchi, Y., Adams, J.E. and Rutkin, B. (1973) Arch. Neurology, 29, 158.

13. Akil, H., Richardson, D.E., Hughes, J. and Barchas, J.D. (1978) Science, 201, 463.

14. Meyerson, B.A., Boethius, J., Trenius, L. and Wahlstrom A. (in press) J. Applied Neurophysiology.

15. Mains, R.E. and Eipper, B.A. (1976) J. Biological Chemistry, 251, 4115.

16. Mains, R.E., Eipper, B.E and Ling, N. (1977): Proc. National Academy of Science, USA, 74, 3014.

17. Rose, J.C., Goldsmith, P.C. and Ganong, W.F. (1976) Fed. Proc., 35, 1172.

18. Rose, J.C., Goldsmith, P.C., Lovinger, R., Aubert, M.L., Kaplan, S.L. and Ganong, W.F. (1977) Neuroendocrinology, 23, 223.

19. Guillemin, R., Vargo, T., Rossier, J., Minick, S., Ling, N., Rivier, C., Vale, W. and Bloom, F. (1977) Science, 197, 1367.

© 1979 Elsevier/North-Holland Biomedical Press
Modern Concepts in Psychiatric Surgery
E.R. Hitchcock, H.T. Ballantine, Jr. and B.A. Meyerson, eds.

HOMOVANILLIC ACID CONCENTRATION OF THE THIRD VENTRICULAR CSF
BEFORE AND AFTER ELECTRICAL STIMULATION OF THE MIDBRAIN
CENTRAL GRAY AND THE PERIVENTRICULAR GRAY IN HUMAN

KEIICHI AMANO, MASAO NOTANI, HIROSHI ISEKI, HIROKO KAWABATAKE,
TATSUYA TANIKAWA, HIROTSUNE KAWAMURA and KOITI KITAMURA
Department of Neurosurgery, Neurological Institute, Tokyo
Women's Medical College, Toyko, Japan

ABSTRACT

During stereotactic rostral mesencephalic reticulotomy (RMR)
and posteromedial hypothalamotomy for pain relief, homovanillic acid (HVA) concentration was measured in the
third ventricular cerebrospinal fluid (CSF) before and
after the electrical stimulation of the midbrain central gray
matter and the periventricular gray matter of the third
ventricle in human. Electrical stimulation of the periventricular gray matter of the third ventricle produced
marked increase of HVA in the third ventricular CSF. In case
of RMR, increase of HVA of the third ventricle was observed
when the stimulating electrode was in the midbrain central
gray matter. When the stimulating electrode was lateral to
the central gray matter, namely in the midbrain reticular
formation, increase of HVA was not noticed. Either periventricular gray or central gray stimulation evoked profound
autonomic response and fear response but no sensory response
such as pain. Sensory phenomenon such as burning sensation or
pain was reproduced only when the electrical stimulation was
delivered not to the central gray or periventricular gray but
to the reticular formation of the midbrain. Although the
authors have been aware of the possibility that humoral
factors such as monoamines or endorphins may play an important
role in perception of pain, the authors emphasize, based on
the above clinical observation, that pain relief by electrical
stimulation of the central gray or the periventricular gray
of the third ventricle, recently reported by other investigators[1], should remain unwarranted.

INTRODUCTION

Past several years we have been in the process of investigating humoral factors which may influence the interpretation of pain perception. By means of ventricular catheter which is inserted into the third ventricle during our stereotactic procedure, we are able to perform chemical analysis of the ventricular CSF. Because of the fact that there exist a number of monoamine-containing neurons in the periventricular gray matter, we started to investigate homovanillic acid (HVA) concentration in the third ventricular CSF during posteromedial hypothalamotomy(PMH) for pain relief[2,3]. As reported already in the previous publication, motivational pain or pain as suffering is relieved by PMH[3]. The target of PMH is 2 mm behind the midpoint of the AC-PC line, 2 mm below the AC-PC line and 2 mm lateral to the wall of the third ventricle. The target is included in the ergotropic triangle designated by Sano[4]. But this area in human is not really " hypothalamus " and it should be more appropriate if we call it rostral extension of the periaqueductal gray matter. On the Schaltenbrand-Bailey's atlas, the target area of the so-called PMH is identical to the rostral extension of the mesencephalic central gray matter[5]. During rostral mesencephalic reticulotomy (RMR) to alleviate motivational as well as discriminative pain[2,6], HVA in the third ventricular CSF was measured before and after electrical stimulation of the central gray matter.

MATERIALS AND METHODS

PMH was performed in 23 patients to alleviate intractable pain. These 23 patients were composed of 14 males and 9 females in the range of 28 to 66 years old. Primary diseases which caused intractable pain in these 23 patients were malignant neoplasm (16 cases), neuralgia (4 cases), causalgia (2 cases) and thalamic syndrome secondary to cerebral thrombosis (1 case). The stereotactic target of PMH for pain relief was 2 mm posterior to the midpoint of the AC-PC line, 2 mm below the AC-PC line and 2 mm lateral to the wall of the third ventricle[2].

RMR was done for relief of intractable pain in 13 patients
(10 males and 3 females) in the range of 47 to 65 years old.
The patients were composed of 11 cases of thalamic syndrome
secondary to cerebral thrombosis and 2 cases of malignant
neoplasm. The stereotactic target of RMR for pain relief was
14 mm posterior to the midpoint of the AC-PC line, 5 mm below
the AC-PC line and 5 mm lateral to the center of the aqueduct
[2,6]. In both PMH and RMR, a small plastic indwelling catheter
was inserted into the third ventricle to measure intraoperative
HVA change in the CSF. In our study HVA was measured by
oxidative coupling and fluorescein quantitative analysis
based on modified Nils-Erik's method. High frequency electrical stimulation (60 Hz) was delivered to these targets with
a bipolar concentric electrode (2 mm in outer diameter),
stimulation strength being 1 to 10 V. in intensity with 1.0
msec pulse width. The third ventricular CSF (10 ml) was
obtained before and after the stimulation of these targets
for HVA analysis. Single neuron discharge from these targets
were recorded with tungsten microelectrode and observed for
both spontaneous firing and evoked firing by peripheral pin-
prick stimulation.

RESULTS
    1) PMH for pain relief
    In the previous publication[2], we reported the nociceptive
neurons in the human periventricular gray matter during PMH
for pain relief. The top and middle recordings of Figure 1
clearly show the firing of nociceptive neurons responding to
contralateral face stimulation by pin-prick. The bottom tracing shows the firing of the neurons evoked by pin-prick stimulation of ipsilateral face. After recording the neuronal
activity with microelectrode, the microelectrode was removed
and replaced with conventional bipolar concentric electrode
for electrical stimulation study. The location of electrical
stimulation was confirmed postoperatively by demonstrating
radiofrequency lesion on computed tomograms[7] and/or at
autopsy. High frequency electrical stimulation of the human
periventricular gray matter during PMH produced marked
increase in HVA as shown in Figure 2. Inspite of the dilution

UNITARY RESPONSE IN HUMAN POSTERIOR HYPOTHALAMUS
TO PIN PRICK STIMULATION

Response Patterns of Hypothalamic Neurons to Contralateral and
Ipsilateral Face Stimulation

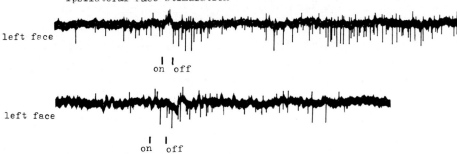

Patient F.T. 40 years old female, intractable pain in the left
Fig. 1   leg due to fibrosarcoma of the lumbar spines

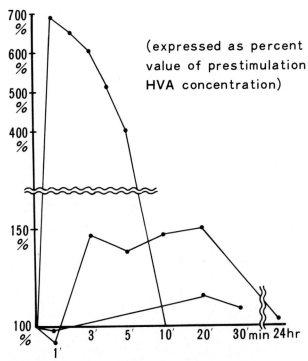

Fig. 2. Chronological alteration in the third ventricular
HVA value after stimulation of the periventricular gray.

HVA Concentration in Human 3rd Ventricular CSF
before and after Stimulation of Periventricular Gray Matter

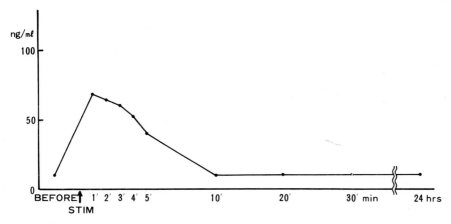

Fig. 3

effect in the third ventricular CSF, elevation of HVA occurs
within 20 minutes after the stimulation. In Figure 2, post-
stimulation value of HVA is expressed as percent value of
prestimulation concentration. Figure 3 shows a typical case
of periventricular electrical stimulation demonstrating chronological change of HVA in the ventricular CSF. Electrical
stimulation of the human posterior hypothalamus produced
signs of elevated sympathetic function characterized by
pupillary dilatation, tachycardia, rise in blood pressure
and medioinferior eye ball deviation. EEG changes were either
cortical desynchronization or high voltage slow waves[4]. The
patient noticed unpleasant sensation or fear or horror during
stimulation of the periventricular gray matter[2,4].

2) RMR for pain relief
Based on our concept that there are two different projections of nociceptive impulse, one projection reaching to the
posterior thalamus from the midbrain, the other taking a
route to the limbic system from the midbrain, we have performed 13 cases of rostral mesencephalic reticulotomy (RMR)

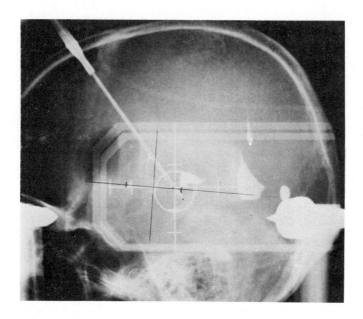

Fig. 4

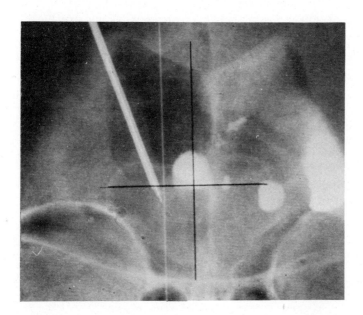

Fig. 5.

for pain relief trying to abolish these two different pain by
making a small lesion in the rostral midbrain reticular formation near the periaqueductal gray matter. The area has been
considered to be the dividing zone of these two different
projections of ascending extra-lemniscal fine-fibered system
[2,6]. The target for RMR is 14 mm posterior to the midpoint of
the AC-PC line, 5 mm below the AC-PC line and 5 mm lateral to
the center of the aqueduct. Figure 4 shows the lateral view
and Figure 5 is a close-up view of the AP projection. Since
our trajectory to the midbrain with small-diameter electrode
was determined to be considerably slunted to the AC-PC line
(approximately 55 to 60 degrees to the AC-PC line on the
lateral view and 60 to 70 degrees to the AC-PC line on AP
view), penetration with the electrode into the superior
colliculus and pretectal area was avoided. Untoward complications reported by Nashold[8], such as Parinaud's sign, were not
noticed postoperatively in our cases. The electrode path goes
through the nucleus ventrocaudalis portae and part of the
nucleus limitance portae of the thalamus, thus entering MRF
without penetrating the pretectal area. The trajectory to the
midbrain, therefore, has to be carefully selected to preserve
postoperative function of extraocular movement. Single neuron
analysis of MRF, investigated in 4 patients with intractable
pain during RMR, revealed characteristics of neuronal firing
as follows; 1) abrupt change of background noise on entering
the reticular formation 2) firing of neurons mostly composed
of small cells and 3) bilateral projection from the periphery with wide receptive fields. Another characteristic of
MRF neurons is the predominance of delayed firing in response
to peripheral pin-prick stimulation. The unit latency of
these nociceptive neurons is classified into early response
type, intermediate type and delayed response type[6]. Figure 6
shows the projection from ipsilateral arm. High frequency
electrical stimulation of MRF produced pain sensation mainly
in the face but also in the trunk and extremities contralateral to the side of stimulation. This sensory phenomenon
by electrical stimulation was seen when the electrode was in
the reticular formation, more than 5 mm from the midline of
the aqueduct. When the stimulating electrode was more medial

ROSTRAL MESENCEPHALIC RETICULOTOMY   No. 510630

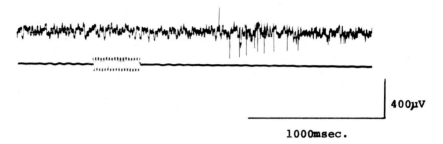

MRF UNIT IN RESPONSE TO PIN-PRICK STIMULATION OF IPSILATERAL ARM

Fig. 6

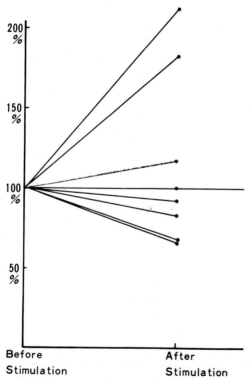

Fig. 7. HVA concentration of the third ventricular CSF after midbrain stimulation (expressed as percent value of pre-stimulation HVA).

in the central gray matter, the patient expressed fear
sensation and also noticed burning sensation of the entire
body rather than pain. In one case, at the time of central
gray stimulation, the patient said, " Somebody is now chasing
me, I am trying to escape from him. ". Another patient stated
on central gray stimulation that he had an abrupt feeling of
uncertainty just like entering into a long, dark tunnel.
Other patient said, on central gray stimulation, " I am standing at seashore and surf is coming from all directions ".
Figure 7 shows HVA concentration of the third ventricular CSF
after midbrain stimulation. Poststimulation HVA is expressed
as percent value of prestimulation HVA concentration. Figure 8
is a schematic diagram of HVA response pattern on electrical
stimulation of the human midbrain. When the stimulating
electrode is located within the central gray, marked increase
of HVA and fear sensation are seen as shown on the left of
Figure 8. If the stimulating electrode is off the central
gray and within the reticular formation, decrease of HVA
occurs as shown on the right of Figure 8. Intermediate type
of HVA response is seen if the electrode is located around
the border between the central gray and the reticular formation.

Loci of Midbrain Stimulation and Response Pattern of 3rd Ventricular HVA

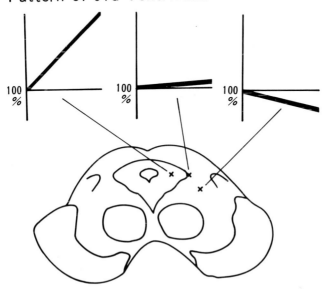

Fig. 8

DISCUSSION

   Homovanillic acid (HVA), namely 4-hydroxy-3-methoxy-
phenyl acetic acid, is a DOPA metabolite. It has been considered that monoamine metabolism is reflected in the level of
HVA. The target of PMH for pain relief is in the posterior
part of the periventricular gray matter around the third
ventricle. Since this target is considered to be the rostral
extension of the mesencephalic central gray[5], the rise in HVA
after electrical stimulation of the periventricular gray
matter during PMH can be regarded as essentially the same as
the increase in HVA after electrical stimulation of the midbrain central gray matter. Although either periventricular
gray or central gray stimulation evoked profound autonomic
response and fear response, no sensory response, neither pain
nor feeling of pain relief was observed during the electrical
stimulation in our patients. Inspite of the possibility that
humoral factors such as monoamines or endorphins may play a
significant role in perception of pain, we emphasize, based
on our clinical observation, that pain relief by electrical
stimulation of the central gray or the periventricular gray
of the third ventricle, recently reported by other investigators[1], should remain unwarranted. Since the increase of HVA
after electrical stimulation of the periventricular gray or
the central gray is accompanied by autonomic response and
fear response, alteration of HVA may reflect psycho-emotional
aspect of pain perception. The periventricular gray and the
central gray contain nociceptive neurons as well as monoaminergic neurons[2]. These areas are also known to receive C fiber
projection from the periphery. In view of the fact that serotonergic system has been studied in relation to nociception,
humoral factors such as monoamines may be related to perception of pain or threshold of nociception, whereas neural
mechanism may be more or less restricted to conduction and
transmission of nociception.

   Benzodiazepines (such as diazepam and clonazepam) are
known to suppress HVA in the striatum and the limbic forebrain produced by administration of chlorpromazine or haloperidol[9]. The mechanism of HVA suppression by benzodiazepines
is explained by the fact that benzodiazepines increase the

function of GABAnergic strio-nigral system, which leads to decreased activity of mesencephalic dopamine neuron and then reduces feedback activation of dopamine neuron by neuroleptics. Our result of HVA decrease by electrical stimulation of the mesencephalic reticular formation (scheme on the right of Figure 8) may be similar to the effect of benzodiazepines on HVA in that the electrical stimulation increase the inhibit ory action of striatonigral GABA system on mesencephalic dopamine neuron.

Many aspects of pain perception still remain as unsolved problems. Although the other investigators[1] showed evidence of analgesia by stimulation of the central gray and peri- ventricular gray matter, the background of electrical stimu- lation for pain relief has to be further investigated. Endorphins in the central gray matter are certainly a possibi- lity of humoral factor for pain relief as well as monoamines. Although alteration of HVA after central gray stimulation is a tantalizing phenomenon in regard to the direct solution of the problem, the present study may stimulate further progress of investigation in this field.

ACKNOWLEDGEMENTS

The authors gratefully acknowledge Sankyo Company Product Development Laboratory, Tokyo, Japan   for its technical assistance of the study on monoamines.

REFERENCES

1. Richardson, D. E. and Akil, H. (1978) J. Neurosurg, 47, 178-194.
2. Amano, K., Kitamura, K., Sano, K. and Sekino, H. (1976) Neurol. medico-chirur, 16 (part 1), 141-153.
3. Sano, K., Sekino, H., Hashimoto, I., Amano, K. and Sugiyama, H. (1975) Confin. neurol, 37, 285-290.
4. Sano, K. (1962) Neurol. medico-chirur, 4, 112-142.
5. Schaltenbrand, G. and Bailey, P. (1959) Introduction to stereotaxis with an atlas of the human brain, Vol. 2, Thieme, Stuttgart.
6. Amano, K., Tanikawa, T., Iseki, H., Kawabatake, H., Notani, M., Kawamura, H. and Kitamura, K. (1978) Single neuron analysis of human midbrain tegmentum, Applied Neurophysiol. in press.
7. Amano, K., Iseki, H., Kawabatake, H., Notani, M., Kawamura, H. and Kitamura, K. (1977) Applied Neurophsiol, 39, 202-211.

8. Nashold, B. S., Jr., Wilson, W. P. and Slaughter, D. G.
   (1969) J. Neurosurg. 30, 116-126.
9. Keller, H. H., Schaffner, R. and Haefely, W. (1976)
   Arch, Pharmacol, 294, 1-4.

© 1979 Elsevier/North-Holland Biomedical Press
Modern Concepts in Psychiatric Surgery
E.R. Hitchcock, H.T. Ballantine, Jr. and B.A. Meyerson, eds.

BRAIN MECHANISMS IN PSYCHIATRIC ILLNESS:
RATIONALE FOR AND RESULTS OF TREATMENT WITH CEREBELLAR STIMULATION

Robert G. Heath, Raeburn C. Llewellyn, and Alvin M. Rouchell

We have implanted electrodes for chronic cerebellar stimulation in
38 patients with a wide variety of behavioral pathology. The follow-up period
for the patients ranges from five months to two and one-half years. Criteria
for acceptance were: (1) a thorough trial with all other indicated forms of
treatment without beneficial results; (2) agreement of our staff with the
patient's referring physician that all possible therapeutic approaches had
been used and that the patient's illness was, indeed, intractable.

Our rationale for using the procedure to treat patients with behavioral
pathology was based on data from patients undergoing special therapeutic
procedures and animal experiments over the past 30 years.[1-3] In a large
series of intractably ill psychiatric and neurologic patients prepared with
deep and surface brain electrodes, recording and stimulation studies demonstrated sites where brain activity correlates with pleasure and other sites
where such activity correlates with adversive emotion (rage, fear, violence,
depression). Extensive animal experiments aimed at demarcating neural mechanisms for emotional expression had shown that the cerebellum is anatomically
connected to sites where neural activity has been correlated with pleasure
(principally the septal region and part of the amygdala), as well as to sites
where neural activity correlates with adversive emotion and onset of epileptic
seizures (principally the hippocampus and other sites in the amygdala).[4-9]
Physiologic studies in animals have shown that stimulation of certain cerebellar sites activates predominantly cells of the septal region, while generally inhibiting activity in the hippocampus and parts of the amygdala (Fig. 1).

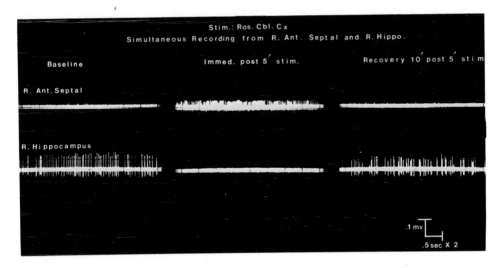

Fig. 1. Simultaneous oscilloscopic recordings of unit activity from the right
anterior septal region and right hippocampus of the cat with stimulation of the
rostral cerebellar vermis. Note the striking increase in firing of septal
units immediately following stimulation concomitant with almost complete inhibition of hippocampal activity. Ten minutes after the single five-minute
stimulation at 100 Hz, firing at each site returned to baseline.

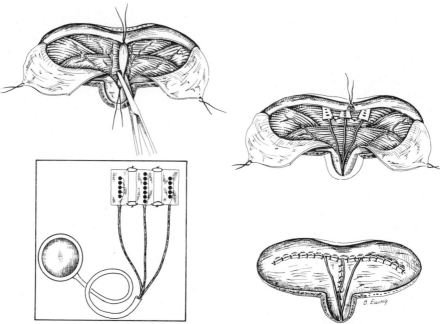

Fig. 2.   Drawing illustrating placement of the superior surface electrodes.
Upper left: exposure of the cerebellum.   Lower left: the electrodes – the
middle chain consists of seven platinum contacts, each 2 mm in diameter; the
lateral chains each consist of five platinum contacts, each 2 mm in diameter.
Upper right: electrodes in place.   Lower right: dural closure showing exiting
electrode wires.

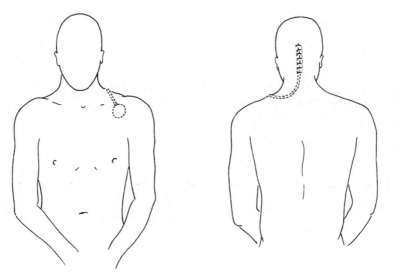

Fig. 3.   Drawing indicating path of electrodes from the posterior fossa to the
receiver implanted below the clavicle.

These effects were induced by stimulation of the rostral midline cerebellum, including the rostral vermis and fastigial nucleus, whereas lateral cerebellar stimulation was ineffectual.[10] Additional animal studies suggested a complex feedback loop among septal region-amygdala-hippocampus-cerebellum whereby activation of one site altered firing of neurons at other sites in the loop in a consistent way.[11]

In the first 29 patients in our cerebellar stimulator series, electrodes were placed over the vermal surface only (Figs. 2 and 3). In the last nine patients in the series, stimulation was through the cerebellum from the superior to the inferior surface so as to activate intervening folia and the fastigial nucleus (Fig. 4). The 2-mm contact points of the surface electrodes were alternating negative-positive. With superior-to-inferior electrodes, the superior surface was cathodal and the inferior surface anodal.

Many parameters of stimulation have been tried. The most effective is at 100 Hz with a pulse width of 150 to 250 microseconds at a voltage setting determined by sensory evoked potentials recorded from the scalp and by the patient's clinical response. The stimulator is set to apply the stimuli sequentially, five minutes on and five minutes off. Patients initially wear the stimulator during waking hours and some, depending on clinical disorder, wear it through the night as well. In our experience, epileptic patients with nocturnal seizures and profoundly disturbed psychotic patients require stimulation around the clock. Some of the less deteriorated patients, on the other hand, particularly the depressive ones, can determine with experience how much or how little they need to maintain the beneficial results.

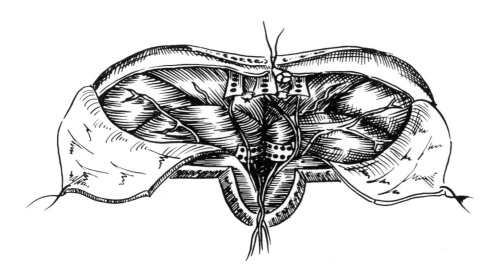

Fig. 4. Drawing of the superior-inferior electrode configuration with the inferior placements at the midline.

Results

Table 1 summarizes the results up until now in the 38 patients.

Table 1

Classification	Number of Patients Improved				Total
	Significant	Moderate	Minimal	None	
Schizophrenia	2	6	3	4[*]	15
Depression	5	0	0	1[**]	6
Epilepsy	5	2	1	0	8
Organic Brain Syndrome	1	4	0	0	5
Miscellaneous	2	0	2	0	4
Total	15	12	6	5	38

*   Three of the four patients are not wearing the stimulator.
**   Patient not wearing the stimulator.

Schizophrenic Patients

The 15 schizophrenics have had the poorest response among all the patients. Their responses are perplexing. Initially, even the most chronically ill patients, some of whom had been in state hospitals continuously for as long as 15 to 25 years, improved dramatically with diminution or disappearance of thought disorders and hallucinations. As a result, their neuroleptic medications were discontinued, but gradually signs and symptoms recurred to varying degrees. Those patients who have continued to use the stimulator have maintained some improvement over one to two years, but most have had to resume neuroleptic medications, although at reduced dosages.

Patients with Depression

All six patients with severe depression had had extensive trials on both antidepressant and neuroleptic drugs, as well as electro-convulsive therapy, without improvement. We classified these patients as chronic depressives because depression was the predominant symptom. Most of them, however, reported almost life-long histories of anhedonia. In four of the six, obsessive-compulsive symptoms were predominant. One was notably paranoid and had profound hyperchondriacal symptoms with his depression.

Five of the six patients in this group are largely free of depressive symptoms and require no medication. Stimulation promptly relieved symptoms in the sixth patient, the paranoid-hyperchondriacal man, but before long, however, the stimulator was incorporated into his hypochondriasis. He reported various discomforts and disconnected his unit, and we subsequently removed the device.

Epileptic Patients

All eight patients had gross behavioral abnormalities, both interictal and in association with their seizures. The most gratifying result in the epileptic group has been the elimination of behavioral symptoms with associated improvement in personality. The treatment has had only minimal effect, however, on grand mal or absence seizures, both of which, fortunately, are usually controlled with medications. We are treating grand mal seizures with phenytoin sodium (Dilantin) and absence seizures with valproic acid (Depakene).

Patients with Organic Brain Syndrome

Two of the five patients with organic brain syndrome had severe head trauma from automobile accidents and consequent psychotic behavior, which could not be controlled by neuroleptic drugs. Both patients had extensive brain atrophy, as demonstrated by computer axonal tomography (C.A.T. head scan), and severe spasticity. In both patients, the stimulation relieved the psychotic behavior, and neuroleptic medication was no longer required. Spasticity was only minimally reduced. After six months, one of the patients felt he no longer needed the stimulator and disconnected it. His signs and symptoms have partially recurred. In one of the five patients, spastic at birth, paranoid psychosis developed, with episodic violent behavior, a condition that remained uncontrolled with anticonvulsants and neuroleptic medications. With stimulation, he initially improved and required no medication, but after two months symptoms partially recurred.

Another patient, one of the earliest in the series, who had extensive brain damage from gunshot injury and consequent uncontrollable homicidal rage, remains well controlled 22 months after activation of her stimulator.

The fifth patient in this group had some mental retardation and poor coordination from birth, suggestive of mild organic brain syndrome. Decompensating obsessive-compulsive symptoms and antisocial behavior were unrelieved by medications and psychosurgical intervention. Since implantation of the pacemaker ten months ago, the patient's antisocial behavior has disappeared and his obsessive-compulsive symptoms have been reduced, but have not been completely eliminated.

Miscellaneous Group

Four patients are included in our miscellaneous group. One, a patient with hystero-epilepsy, continues to be essentially symptom-free. Two have shown only minimal improvement. One, with severe anorexia nervosa for 12 years and amenorrhea during most of the 12 years, had been continuously tube-fed and completely amenorrheic during the five years preceding operation. She displayed intense bizarre compulsive-ritualistic behavior and at times was catatonic. Since operation, compulsive rituals have been significantly reduced, and she states the stimulator makes her feel pleasant and relaxed. Her menstrual cycle returned to normal about four months after stimulation began. She steadfastly refuses, however, to eat, and tube-feeding therefore continues. The third patient in this group, with severe personality disorder, suffered depression, anxiety, and disturbances in visual and auditory perception subsequent to drug abuse. Stimulation has alleviated the anxiety and lessened the aberrations in sensory perception, but depression persists.

The fourth patient in this group, the first in whom we implanted a stimulator, is mildly mentally retarded and displayed extreme, uncontrollable violent-aggressive behavior. For two and a half years after operation, he remained free of violent-aggressive symptoms and attended rehabilitation school. Because this patient's subsequent course provides important data regarding control, he is discussed later.

Discussion

Cerebellar stimulation has consistently produced its best therapeutic results in patients whose principal symptoms are related to profound adversive
emotion, that is, in those with intractable depression and those with violent-
aggressive behavior consequent to epilepsy or an organic brain syndrome.
Results in schiozphrenic patients have been less gratifying. One obvious
cause of failure in three of the severely deteriorated, long-term chronically
ill schizophrenics was their refusal to wear the stimulator. On the other
hand, some patients who have conscientiously used the pacemaker have had only
limited beneficial effects.

We have considered two possible explanations for the poorer results obtained
in schizophrenics. It may be that the complex, underlying disease, that is,
the biochemical lesion of schizophrenia, impairs ability of certain cells
(particularly those in the pleasure-alerting system) to respond to the stimulation. Or, it may be that neuronal function has been damaged by prolonged and
heavy use of neuroleptic drugs. Every patient in the schizophrenic group had
been subjected to long-term maximal drug therapy.

Surgical complications encountered thus far have been bothersome rather than
serious: a third of the patients have temporarily had an accumulation of
spinal fluid in the electrode track between the receiver in the chest and the
electrodes in the posterior fossa.

Although the deliberate establishment of controls for this type of study is
difficult, a number of satisfactory controls have inadvertently developed.
With each patient, there is, for comparison, a long preoperative course involving many forms of treatments. Serving as control for suggestion consequent
to this new treatment have been numerous and varied technologic failures. The
most dramatic controls were two uncontrollably violent patients who had breakdown in function of the implanted device. The first patient in the series, an
explosively violent young man who had made numerous suicidal and homicidal
attempts, was symptom-free for two years and four months, at which time essentially the same behavioral pattern recurred. Over a few weeks, he was increasingly restless and oppositional, and he then became extremely agitated.
Without precipitating cause, he attempted to kill both parents, necessitating
intervention by the police. Large doses of medications failed to control his
behavior in the hospital, and he injured a number of the personnel. Roentgeno-
grams showed that the cable connecting the implanted receiver to the cerebellar
electrodes was broken (Fig. 5). A new device was implanted in an emergency
operation. For about ten days after activation of the new stimulator, his
restlessness, agitation, and violence decreased, and later they completely
disappeared. He is now living at home, is taking no medication, and has resumed his vocational studies.

One of the early chronic schizophrenics in the series had had a long history
of violence. He often viciously attacked family members and hospital personnel. After activation of the stimulator, his violent behavior subsided, and
he did fairly well at home for one and a half years. When the episodic violent
behavior returned, stimulus artifact-testing indicated that the internal apparatus was not functioning, and the defect was traced to the receiver. It was
replaced and since reactivation of the system, the patient has remained free
of violent-aggressive behavior.

Other controls resulting from inadvertent technical failures include:
(1) inaccurate placement of electrodes in two patients -- in one, too far
laterally, and in the other, too far posteriorly. In both patients, stimula-

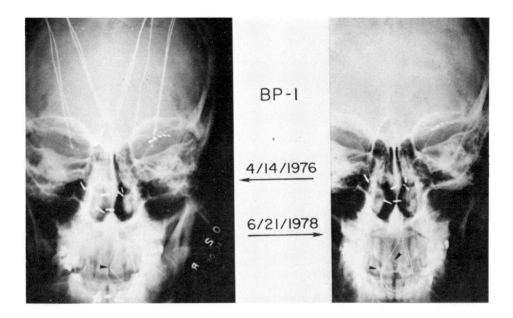

Fig. 5. Left: roentgenogram taken after the original operation, the arrow indicating a kink in the electrode. The deep electrodes implanted into selected subcortical sites for recording and stimulation were removed approximately one month later. Right: roentgenogram just before second operation, the arrows indicating the break in the cable.

tion was ineffectual. When the electrodes were repositioned (two months later in one patient and two weeks later in the other), stimulation produced beneficial results.

(2) antenna breakage, with recurring clinical symptoms.

In summary, results obtained with cerebellar stimulation continue to be encouraging. Most of the patients, all of whom were previously intractably ill, have benefited. We have gained more information about the types of patients who are most apt to respond. Those who are ill because of profound adverse emotion (depression, rage, violent behavior) benefit significantly. The stimulation also works well in patients with the clinical diagnostic entity of depression, including anhedonia. Psychotic manifestations of epilepsy have been largely eliminated by this technique. And the therapeutic procedure has removed many symptoms in patients with organic brain syndrome. Whereas the schizophrenics have been notably helped when stimulation has been possible, they have been less responsive as a group for reasons that are still obscure. Changes in techniques have been made, and more modifications are likely in the future as a result of technologic advances and further data from the animal studies.

Acknowlegment: The authors wish to acknowledge the technical assistance of Charles J. Fontana, Herbert J. Daigle, and Stanley B. John.

References

1. Heath, R.G., and the Tulane University Department of Psychiatry and Neurology (1954). Studies in Schizophrenia, Harvard University Press, Cambridge, Mass.

2. Heath, R.G. (1964). Developments toward new physiologic treatments in psychiatry. J. Neuropsychiat. 5:318-331.

3. Heath, R.G. (1975). Brain function and behavior: I. Emotion and sensory phenomena in psychotic patients and in experimental animals. J. Nerv. Ment. Dis. 160:159-175.

4. Heath, R.G. (1972). Physiologic basis of emotional expression: Evoked potential and mirror focus studies in rhesus monkeys. Biolog. Psychiat. 5:15-31.

5. Harper, J.W., and Heath, R.G. (1973). Anatomic connections of the fastigial nucleus to the rostral forebrain in the cat. Exper. Neurol. 39:285-292.

6. Heath, R.G., and Harper, J.W. (1974). Ascending projections of the cerebellar fastigial nucleus to the hippocampus, amygdala, and other temporal lobe sites: Evoked potential and histological studies in monkeys and cats. Exper. Neurol. 45:268-287.

7. Heath, R.G., and Harper, J.W. (1976). Descending projections of the rostral septal region: An electrophysiological-histological study in the cat. Exper. Neurol. 50:536-560.

8. Heath, R.G. (1976). Correlation of brain function with emotional behavior. Biolog. Psychiat. 11:463-480.

9. Heath, R.G. (1976). Brain function in epilepsy: Midbrain, medullary, and cerebellar interaction with the rostral forebrain. J. Neurol. Neurosurg. Psychiat. 39:1037-1051.

10. Heath, R.G., Dempesy, C.W., and Fontana, C.J. (1978). Cerebellar stimulation: Effects on septal region, hippocampus, and amygdala of cats and rats. Biolog. Psychiat. 13:501-529.

11. Heath, R.G., and Fontana, C.J. Feedback loop between cerebellum and septal-hippocampal-amygdala sites: Its role in emotion and epilepsy. Presented at the meeting of the Society of Biological Psychiatry, Atlanta, Georgia, May, 1978 and submitted for publication to Biolog. Psychiat.

© 1979 Elsevier/North-Holland Biomedical Press
Modern Concepts in Psychiatric Surgery
E.R. Hitchcock, H.T. Ballantine, Jr. and B.A. Meyerson, eds.

CHRONIC MEDIOTHALAMIC STIMULATION FOR CONTROL OF PHOBIAS

GERT DIECKMANN

Division of Stereotactic Neurosurgery, Department of Neurosurgery, Universität des Saarlandes, Homburg-Saar (West Germany)

ABSTRACT

This preliminary report deals with the clinical and electrophysiological data of a patient suffering from phobias successfully treated for 1 year by chronic stimulation within the sub-
dominant medial thalamus.

INTRODUCTION

In 1967 together with Hassler[1] we reported stereotactic
thalamotomy as a method for the surgical treatment of obsessive
and compulsive disorder. Circumscribed lesions in the rostral
intralaminar and dorsomedial thalamic nuclei were followed by an
improvement or relief from obsessive-compulsive and phobic
symptoms. Since that time we have used this treatment on
patients with intractable mental illness, most of whom suffered
from obsessive-compulsive neuroses, tics, erethisms and phobias[2].
Up till now patients with phobias always required a bilateral
thalamic intervention to obtain sufficient results but because
a bilateral procedure produces undesirable side-effects, a new
technique seemed necessary.

We reasoned that a new, non ablative technique might prevent
the complications that occurred after bilateral thalamic lesioning.
The therapeutic concept was that repeated stimulation of the non-
specific thalamic activating system could modify its disinhibited,
enhanced activity and thereby change the compulsive character of
the disease. In animals it is known that low frequency stimulation of different parts of the unspecific thalamic system induces
an inhibitory effect clinically and electrophysiologically. Since
the pathways of this system converge in the rostral intralaminar
nuclei as well as in the basal part of VA, this region was chosen
as the target point for stimulation.

MATERIALS AND METHODS

The technique of electrical selfstimulation by an implantable pacemaker was used in the treatment of a female patient suffering from necrophobia and phobic ideas of injuring children.

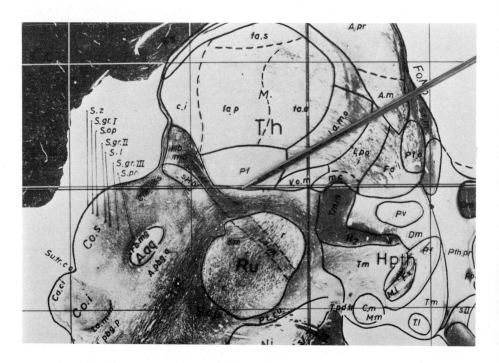

Figure 1. Sagittal section through human diencephalon, 5 mm lateral of the midline. The needle indicates site and approach of the stimulating permanently implanted electrode. The upper 2 poles of the electrode are estimated lying within the 2 intralaminar nuclei (La.m.o.). The length of one site of the grid is lo mm. (Using a picture of Schaltenbrand and Bailey[3], anatomical labelation by Hassler).

A deep brain stimulation electrode used in permanent self-stimulation in patients with chronic pain (Medtronic[R]), was implanted stereotactically in the medial thalamus of the sub-dominant hemisphere. A description of electrode position is given in Figure 1. The figure shows a sagittal section through

the human diencephalon in which site and approach of the
electrode is indicated by a needle. The tip of the electrode
reaches the parafascicular nucleus, 5mm lateral the midline.
The active surface of the electrode consists of 4 poles over a
total length of 12 mm. This arrangement permits bipolar stimulations of different sites involving both parafascicular nucleus
as well as rostral intralaminar nuclei.

Figure 2 represents an X-ray of the patient today. Besides
the permanent implanted electrode itself one sees the extra-
cranially, subcutaneously implanted chronic extension which leads
to a radio frequency receiver implanted in a subcutaneous subclavian pocket. Chronic stimulation is performed by the patient
herself with a radio frequency transmitter giving the current by
an antenna through the skin to the receiver by way of induction.

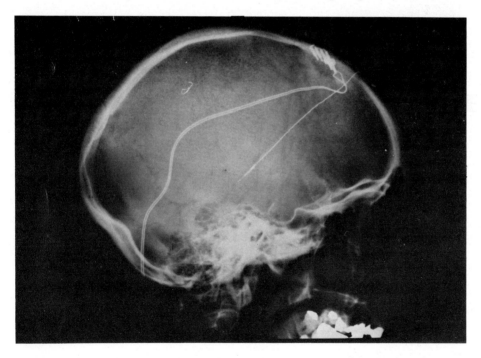

Figure 2   Sagittal X-ray of the patient. In the centre the
implanted deep brain stimulating electrode, at the
left the extracranial, subcutaneously implanted
chronic extension to a subclavian radio frequency receiver.

During the intraoperative as well as the postoperative trial
period low frequency stimulation of the upper 2 poles situated
within the intralaminar nuclei gave the most curative effect
for the patient. Therefore the internalization of the whole
system was performed over these 2 poles.

RESULTS
    First results in the EEG during stimulation were obtained
3 weeks after the test implantation. Evoked potentials were
found over both frontal poles, ipsilateral more pronounced than
contralateral (see Figure 3, 5th row) and the recruiting character
of the effect was evident. During this period, the patient
reported a sedative effect after 10 minutes of stimulation.
    2 months later, typical records resulting from repetitive
1/second, 3/second and 5/second stimulation were obtained. The

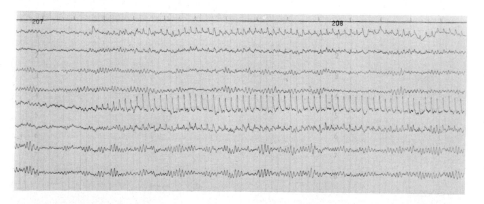

Figure 3   Monopolar EEG recording during trial period, 3 weeks
           after electrode implantation. The first 4 rows indicate
           the contralateral derivations, the other 4 ipsilateral
           to the stimulated hemisphere. A recruiting answer appears
           over the ipsilateral frontal region.

records in Figure 4 provide in all respects the standard surface
potentials of thalamic-induced recruiting responses. The 1/second
stimulation in the upper third of the figure produced slow negative
waves at a latency of about 50 milliseconds which are followed by
a large negative wave after 125 milliseconds. Particularly the

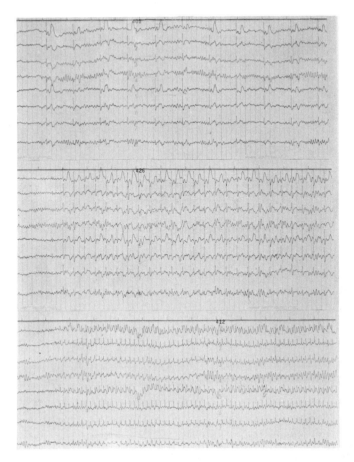

Figure 4   Monopolar EEG recording over both hemispheres during
unilateral (right) mediothalamic stimulation with
different frequencies. Upper third of the picture:
1/second stimulation; middle third: 3/second stimulation;
lower third: 5/second stimulation.

latter showed waxing and waning features, thus varying their
voltage between 80 and 120 microvolts. The recruiting phenomenon
is better obtainable with 5/second stimulation, the record of which
is shown in the lower third of the figure. The stimulation effects
were found over the frontal, precentral and parietal areas of
both hemispheres particularly ipsilaterally, while the occipital
region does not regularly show an influence. The 3/second stimulation shows the tendency to set up a general synchronization.
Such a general synchronization induced by 5/second stimulation

replacing the spontaneous bioelectrical activity occurred 3
months after implantation of the deep brain stimulation electrode
and is now the general effect of the 2 times per day stimulation
of the patient.

The upper third of Figure 5 shows the beginning of the stimulation, the middle part represents the recording after 5 minutes
stimulation while the lower part demonstrates the end of the
stimulation after 10 minutes. Immediately after stopping the
stimulation the usual bioelectrical activity recurred, with the
exception of a tendency to more desynchronized activity in both
frontal and precentral regions, as indicated by occasional faster
activity of lower voltage.

During the 5/second stimulation the patients phobias disappear.
She is then able to walk to a cemetery, to see hearses or to play
with children without fearing injuring them. All of this was,
and is not, possible without the stimulation. Furthermore, she
reported that she became quiet during the stimulation and 3 to
4 hours after it.

After this encouraging result during the trial period, the
final implantation of the device was performed 3 months after
the test implantation of the deep brain-stimulation electrode.
From that time the device failed. Clinical sedation was not
reported by the patient nor did electrophysiological features
of regular low-frequency stimulation occur. The EEG records
seemed not to be influenced. After several other trials, we
saw that a somewhat different kind of current reached the
patient's deep brain-stimulating electrode by way of the radio
frequency receiver belonging to the usual stimulating device
used in patients with chronic pain states. Since an interposition
of a condenser could not correct this failure sufficiently, we
continued to stimulate directly over transcutaneous wires which
are connected with the implanted device by-passing the radio
frequency receiver. In that way a good clinical result concerning
the phobias was again achieved, remaining so until the present
day.

A direct relation between correct current application and
the blood supply of the brain estimated by the measurement of
the peripheral blood pressure was observed, although the

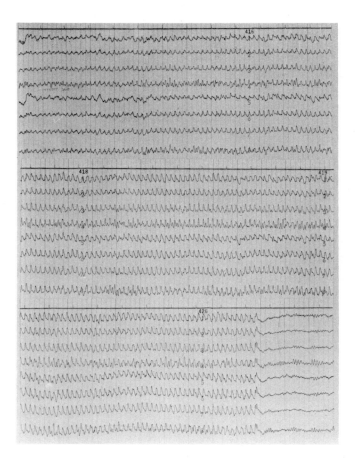

Figure 5   General synchronization of the EEG during permanent
           unilateral mediothalamic 5/second stimulation.   Upper
           part: at the beginning of the stimulation; middle
           part: after 5 minutes stimulation time; lower part: at
           the end of stimulation period, 10 minutes after the
           beginning.

influence of these variables is complicated by a lot of unknown
factors.   Several times when low frequence stimulation was used,
it was not possible to obtain a sufficient clinical effect as
well as a typical EEG-recording.

     As an example, Figure 6 shows 2 surface recordings from
different days, but in the arrangement as before.   In the days

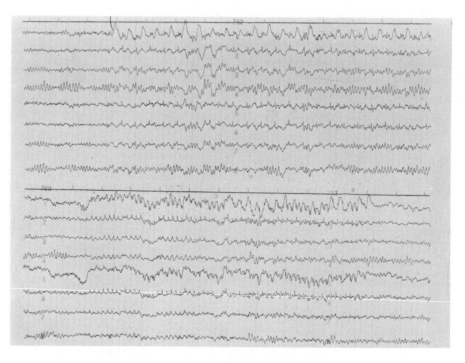

Figure 6   Monopolar EEG recording during 3/second stimulation
(upper part) and 5/second stimulation (lower part) of
the right medial thalamus during states of blood hypo-
tension.   The usual general synchronization does not
occur.

when the blood pressure of the patient was low, figures of 90 to
50 mm mercury were measured.   The electrophysiological effect
was remarkably restricted, practically only to the prefrontal
regions as shown in rows 1 and 5 of both parts.   In both examples,
showing a 3/second stimulation in the upper part and a 5/second
stimulation in the lower part of Figure 6, no clear general
synchronization occurred.   Only sometimes a tendcney to synchronization was recognised.   The same happened when a medical tran-
quilizer was given before the stimulation period.

     As far as the clinical result is concerned, the patient became
quiet during 5/second stimulation, she was free of phobic ideas
and had a satisfied expression on her face.   Recently she used
to stimulate herself 3 times per day and gained a state free of

phobic ideas by these stimulations. On the contrary, a 50/second
stimulation was experienced as being very disagreeable. In that
case one sees in the face of the patient that the stimulus obviously
induces unpleasant feelings. She herself reported anxiety and
some strange, inexplicable, unpleasant feelings depending on
stimulation with this frequency.

CONCLUSION

Using a commercial deep brain stimulating electrode device,
phobic symptoms of different kind and strength could be improved
or relieved by repetitive, low frequency self-stimulation within
the rostral intralaminar nuclei of the subdominant thalamus.
The patient reported here and followed over 1 year is able to
supress her phobic symptoms by self-stimulation on demand like
pain patients who can relieve their pain by such a deep brain
stimulation. Recordings of EEG surface potentials during stimulation periods showed typical effects known to be induced by
stimulation of non-specific thalamic structures in animal experiments. The aim of the intervention, to relieve the patient of
her phobic ideas, was obtained, although several technical problems
still exist.

REFERENCES

1. Hassler, R. and Dieckmann, G. (1967) Confin. Neurol. 29,
153-158.

2. Hassler, R. and Dieckmann, G. (1973) in Surgical Approaches
in Psychiatry, Laitinen, L.V. and Livingston, K.E. eds., Medical
and Technical Publishing Co. Ltd., Lancaster, pp. 206-212.

3. Schaltenbrand, G. and Bailey, P. (1959) Introduction to
Stereotaxis with an Atlas of the Human Brain, Thieme, Stuttgart,
pp. 230-290.

© 1979 Elsevier/North-Holland Biomedical Press
Modern Concepts in Psychiatric Surgery
E.R. Hitchcock, H.T. Ballantine, Jr. and B.A. Meyerson, eds.

ANALYSIS OF CERTAIN RESPONSES TO THERAPEUTICAL ELECTRICAL
STIMULATION OF THE BRAIN.

S. OBRADOR and J.G. MARTIN-RODRIGUEZ.
Department "Sixto Obrador" of Neurosurgery. Centro Especial
"Ramón y Cajal" of the Spanish Social Security. Madrid. Spain.

During the course of therapeutical stimulation of the brain
(TESB) in patients with chronic intractable pain a period of
test stimulation is performed before a decision will be taken
regarding which cases could benefit from a permanent implantation of a subdermal stimulator. Days or even weeks of trans-
dermal test stimulation may be needed before this decision is
drawn and meanwhile, a series of responses to different parameters of stimulation are being recorded to which probably
much attention is not paid at the time. We have looked "at
posteriori" into these recordings and the analysis of some
responses will be the subject of this short presentation.

MATERIAL and METHODS.- The records of the 5 patients that
form our second series of cases with intractable pain treated
by TESB have been jointly analysed from the point of view of
their responses to stimulation. Details of the cases as well
as their routine studies in our "pain clinic" were given in
our presentation this morning and could be found in the previous presentation (pag.47).

Once the decision regarding surgery was taken in each individual case, a 4 contacts schriver type Medtronic electrode
was implanted stereotaxically using the recent model of the
Leksell frame, allowing easy intraoperative x-ray control of
electrode insertion and position in both the lateral and AP
projection. Two patients were operated under local anaesthesia and 3 under general. The selected target was demonstrated by positive contrast ventriculography with emulsified
Conray injected through an Ommaya reservoir with its catheter

placed in the III Ventricle. The width of the posterior part of the III Ventricle was evaluated with 1cc of Myodil and the target calculated as usual with the Leksell tecnnique.[1,2] Electrode insertion was achieved from a coronal burr-hole contra-lateral to the side of the pain and directed towards the target formed by the "Posterior Commisure-periventricular-Parafasci-cular-Centre Median" area (Fig. 1). Check lateral and AP

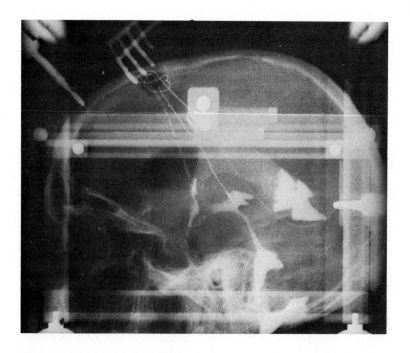

Fig. 1. Intraoperative lateral x-ray demonstrating the tip of the electrode just in front of the posterior commisure and run-ning upwards towards the coronal burr-hole where the electrode is twisted as a coil before fixation to avoid electrode dis-placement by brain pulsation.

x-rays were taken at this point. The electrode was fixed to the edge of the burr-hole and twisted as a coil between its fixation point and the surface of the brain in a attempt to

minimize electrode dislodgement by brain pulsation. Intraoperative stimulation was not performed. The electrode was
then externalized through a puncture incision placed in a different scalp site. New control x-rays were taken and the
stereotaxic frame removed.

Post-operative test stimulation was initiated once the patients regained their original pain, as all 5 patients expe-
rimented immediate post-operative pain relief lasting between
1-5 days. This may be interpreted as a result of the insertion injury produced at the time of surgery.

Stimulation was applied either using a Grass S 88 coupled
to a Grass Stimulus Isolation Unit PISU 5 or by means of a
Medtronic Neuromod stimulator with a 50% current reduction
device. A bridge circuit linked to an oscilloscope was introduced to measure electrode impedance. Pulse and respiration
rate were continuously monitored but skin impedance was not
measured.

Cathodic bipolar derived monophasic square pulses were used
either in a single or train mode. Pulse width (PW) varied
between 0.2-1 ms and frequencies ranged from 10-100 Hz. When
train was used the patterns of 5 sec "on"- 5 sec "off" was
followed, although continuous stimulation was used as well.
Current intensities varied between 0.1-0.8 mA.

Each session of stimulation never lasted more than one hour
and was tried only once per day, although the time of the day
when it was applied changed at random as well as the surrounding conditions in what stimulation was to be performed.

Response to stimulation was carefully recorded both by direct and indirect observation as well as tape-recordered.
Placebo stimulations were performed without knowledge of both
the patient and the observer.

A variable course of test stimulation was carried out for
days or weeks until enough data were collected to make an
analysis in base of which the contacts and parameters most likely to control pain could be selected. Test stimulation was
then followed again during a few days to prove their benefit.

RESULTS.- A full study of all responses recorded in the 5
patients was recently iniciated and this is just a preliminary
report. Responses from 1000 combined stimulation parameters
averaging some 200 responses per patient were analysed. Only
those responses found to be reproducible in more than 2 stimulation sessions in the same contacts with the same parameters
were selected for analysis.

All sensations reported were subjective ones with the only
exception of those referring either to muscle tightness or
relaxation, that was graphically verified in one of the cases
by means of muscle tone and active plus passive contraction
studies.

Autonomic responses were not analysed but in a quick survey
they were found to be extremely infrequent.

Diziness could be elicited in all patients in the most posterior periventricular areas at frequency ranges 30-50 Hz with
high current intensities. When frequency increased above 50
Hz it will change to a sensation of nausea and pressure in the
stomach. This sensations were accompanied some times by a
feeling of either "floating" or "falling in the emptyness"
that the patient described as a very unpleasant sensation.
In the same area at PW between 0.6-1 ms, frequencies of 80-
100 Hz and currents of 0.3-0.6 mA, four of the five patients
described blurring of vision with a feeling of "empty head-
iness". The remaining patient, that was the only one in whom
the tip of the electrode was not aimed to the posterior commisure but to 2 mm forward of it in the AC-PC line, described
jumping of vision, similar to that referred in nistagmus, although neither type of ocular movements could be observed.
Nistagmography was not performed. However, the referred jumping rate would increase or decrease by changing the frequency
rate up or down.

There were critical sites where stimulation produced a feeling of "anguish or anxiety" accompanied in one patient by a
sensation of precordial pressure without particular changes
in the ECG. In this patient the effect could be reproduced
time and time again between electrode points 2-1 at any pa-

rameters with point 2 as a cathode. Curiously enough the response will disappear when the polarity was reversed and it could not be elicited if the stimulation was performed between electrodes 0-3 and 0-1. A similar sensation was elicited between points 2-3, 2 again as cathode, if high frequency-high current intensity was used. Definite implantation was however performed at points 1-2, 1 as cathode, as these two points gave the maximum control on pain relief. She is the same patient in which the plotings of the contacts in the Van Buren and Borke atlas were presented this morning (pag.). Up to date, 8 month following internalization, she has kept a good pain control without any untowards effects on mood.

In 2 patients a sensation of "falling asleep without feeling sleepy" was reproduced at frequencies of 30-50 Hz in a point thought to be in Centre Median (CM). We had previously reported a sensation of "sleepiness" in one of our patients with cancer pain belonging to the first series of cases and in whom a post mortem study showed the stimulation point to be in CM.[3] This sensation was reported as pleasant in all three patients.

Sensation of hot or cold was reported by two patients and in both referred to a contralateral lower limb affected by pain. Objective temperature changes were not confirmed. The effect was obtained from a point presumably in CM and at a frequency of 50 Hz with low current intensity. One of these patients is the one with cancer pain from a Ca. of the uterus controlled until death by TESB. Her brain is being processed at present.

To end this report we would like to comment in a common pattern that emerged from data collected in all the 5 patients. "Vibratory" and "tingling" paraesthesia some time referred as a feeling of "electric current", was reported by all the patients in those areas affected by the pain but it did never extend to any other area of the same hemibody. In the four cases that benefited from stimulation this paraesthesia was followed by a sensation of muscle tone relaxation that the patients described with different expressions such as "soft, relieving,

relaxed, unhardenned, smoothed", but always referring to a previously present feeling of "tightness or pressure". When ever
this relaxion appeared pain relief did followed TESB. In one
case, however, PW and frequency parameters, together with length
of TESB, were so critical that stimulation could produce a completely opposite sensation worsenning his pain: this was the
case with a thalamic syndrome.

DISCUSSION.- I have no doubts that Prof. Obrador, who worked
deeply in this paper during his final illness would have produced today a profound and critical discussion regarding central
mechanisms of brain stimulation. However we cannot count today
with his usual dynamic discussion and will just comment on some
of the points that have been presented.

It could be said that stimulation in this periventricular
area would interfere with mechanisms of consciousness, a fact
already pointed some years back by several authors at least with
regards to CM. Dizziness, floating, falling, sleepiness, etc.
could be interpreted somewhat as disturbance of consciousness,
but the fact is that in many cases we have destroyed the CM-Pf
complex bilaterally at a single surgical session for the treatment of chronic pain, without consciousness being affected at
all: a contradiction of the results obtained by stimulation,
that could suggest a mechanism involving transmission to distant
areas of the brain.

A note should be made of the difference between pleasant and
unpleasant sensations (reward versus punishment) caused by stimulation and how critical is the point where stimulation is being applied within the same nucleus. This fact is in accordance
to the reports made by Delgado[4] in the primate brain where moving the electrode fractions appart will change from a reward-
ing area to an unrewarding one.

Perhaps the most interesting fact is the relationship presented between the production of paraesthesia and the appeerence of
analgesia. The changes in motor activity could be related to
spreading into the anterior part of Pulvinar, and we have pre-

viously shown by microelectrode recordings the role played by
this area in motor mechanisms [5]. However, what cannot be explained is why the paraesthesia is circunscribed to the area
of pain and does not follow a topographic distribution. We
think that the feeling of muscle tone relaxation preceeding
pain relief is again directly related to a possible feed-for-
ward mechanism triggered by spread stimulation into the ante-
rior-medial part of Pulvinar, inducing changes in the effective perception of pain and somewhat in body image representation.

What seems to be made again clear is the fact that mechanisms
of analgesia induced by cerebral stimulation cannot be accounted only in chemical changes and that direct electrical stimulation plays a role as important as the chemical one.

REFERENCES

1. Leksell, L. (1949) Acta Chir. Scand., 89, 229-233.

2. Leksell, L. (1971) Stereotaxis and Radiosurgery: An operative
   System, Charles C. Thomas, Springfield, Ill.

3. Obrador, S., Delgado, J.M.R. and Martín-Rodriguez, J.G.
   (1975) in Cerebral Localization, Zulch, K.J., Creutzfeldt,O.
   and Galbraith, G.C. eds., Springer-Verlag, Berlin, Heidelberg, New York, pp. 171-183.

4. Delgado, J.M.R. and Bracchita, H. (1972) Int. J. Psychobiol.,
   2, 233-248.

5. Buño, W., Martín-Rodriguez, J.G., García-Austt, E. and
   Obrador, S. (1975) Acta Neurochir., Suppl., 24, 109-119.

© 1979 Elsevier/North-Holland Biomedical Press
Modern Concepts in Psychiatric Surgery
E.R. Hitchcock, H.T. Ballantine, Jr. and B.A. Meyerson, eds.

ALTERING MEMORY WITH HUMAN VENTROLATERAL THALAMIC STIMULATION

GEORGE A. OJEMANN, M.D.
Department of Neurological Surgery RI-20, University of Washington,
Seattle, Washington 98195 (U.S.A.)

A mechanism in human ventrolateral thalamus (VL) that facilitates
later retrieval of material entering short- or long-term memory, and acts
as a gate determining access to memory at any point in time is discussed
in this paper. This mechanism in left VL is concerned principally with
information that can be verbally coded, that in right with visuospatial
information. The relative intensity of this mechanism in right or left
VL may determine, at a point in time, the degree to which verbal or
visuospatial features of the environment will be remembered, and the degree to which previous verbal or visuospatial memories are available.
This mechanism is available for surgical manipulation, as it is activated
by electrical stimulation of right or left VL, and an initial observation
of potential therapeutic usefulness is discussed.

The evidence for this mechanism comes from studies of language and
memory changes during and after VL thalamotomy for dyskinesias. Initial
studies[1,2,3] measured the effects of VL stimulation on short-term verbal
memory using a single item paradigm adapted from Peterson and Peterson[4].
This test consisted of 60 consecutive trials, each trial having four
achromatic slides. The first, the _input_ to memory, is a picture of an
object with a common name. The patient names the object pictured on this
slide aloud. After four seconds, a second slide appears. It pictures a
two-digit number greater than 30 that the patient reads aloud and then
counts backwards by threes from it aloud. Counting is paced by an audi-
ble pulse each second. The counting acts as a distraction, preventing
rehearsal during the six seconds this slide is shown. This is the time
that the object name must be stored in short-term memory. The third and
fourth slides are two different modes of _output_ from short-term memory,
each shown for four seconds. The third slide measures output by cued recall. It has the word "recall" on it. In response to this the patient
is trained to say aloud the name of the object pictured on this trial.
The fourth slide measures output by recognition. Four words are on this
slide: the correct name, the name of the immediately preceding object,

and two names from elsewhere on the list. The patient says aloud the correct name.

The patient is trained in this test the night prior to operation. During operation electrical stimulation was delivered in a monopolar mode through a 1 x 5 mm electrode after its initial insertion into the VL target, using 60 Hz 2.5 msec total duration biphasic square wave pulses in four second trains at currents less than the threshold for any disturbance of naming, motor or sensory responses. Average maximum stimulating current was 6.1 milliamps (range 4 to 14 ma) measured between pulse peaks. Stimulation is applied during the input slide only on some trial (I), the storage slide (S) or output slide (O) only on others, or the input and output slides (I + O) on the same trial. These were arranged pseudorandomly along with interspersed trials without stimulation that measure control performance.

Data on the effects of stimulation during the various parts of the test on recall are available from 37 consecutive operations in 35 right handed patients, 17 in left brain, 20 in right. Only trials where objects were correctly named were analyzed. Right VL stimulation had no consistent effect on verbal recall. Left VL stimulation applied during input decreased recall errors to about half control levels. This effect is statistically significant at the .025 level (Wilcoxsin Matched Pairs Sign Rank Test, two tailed) and was seen in 14 of the 17 patients. Applying the same current at the same sites but at the time of output had a different effect, increasing errors markedly (to nearly double control levels). This effect is also statistically significant at the 0.01 level and was present in 15 of 17 patients. Combining stimulation during input and output on the same trial had the algebraic sum of these effects and is indistinguishable from control performance[1,2]. Storage stimulation also had no significant effect. These same effects of left but not right VL stimulation are also present in a series matched for control performance and there, both input and output stimulation have statistically significant differential effects between right or left VL[2]. In addition, the latency of correct recall responses is shortened during output stimulation[5]. Electrodes showing this effect were localized by radiologic landmarks, referred to VanBuren and Borke's[6] atlas, that shows the mean location and range of variability of thalamic structures about the same landmarks, and indicates that these electrodes were in VL.

We called this effect a "specific alerting response" and noted that
when it was activated by left VL stimulation, verbal information in the
external environment entered short-term memory in such a way that its
later retrieval was more accurate. But simultaneously, verbal material
already internalized into short-term memory could not be readily retrieved, a gating effect determining what enters or leaves short-term
memory at any point in time.

The effects of VL stimulation on short-term memory for non-verbal material, nonsense shapes, was next determined in another consecutive
series of right handed patients. A continuous recognition rather than
recall task was used; the effects of stimulation on recognition of a
second presentation of shapes with few verbal associations, adapted from
Vanderplas and Garvin[7], was compared to the effects on recognition of
object names, in both cases after a six to eight second interval occupied
by an appropriate distractor, in a series of 14 thalamotomies in 11 patients, six in left brain, and eight right. The details of the non-
verbal recognition test have been published elsewhere[3]. In summary, it
has input, storage, and output phases like the verbal memory test, and
also includes a check on perception of the shapes with each recognition.
Only when a shape had been correctly perceived and correctly recognized
as not being seen before at the time of input was the trial included in
the analysis of non-verbal memory. Stimulation occurred during input,
output or input and output on the same trial for both the verbal and non-
verbal tests. Performance on control trials without stimulation did not
differ significantly between right and left sides (verbal recognition:
left, 25%, right, 19%; non-verbal recognition: left, 50%, right, 50%),
nor is there any significant difference in maximum stimulating currents
(mean left, 6.3 ma; right, 5.3 ma). Figure 1 shows the changes in recognition evoked by stimulation during the various parts of the verbal (object name) and non-verbal (shapes) tests in this series of patients with
right or left VL electrodes. Note that both the decrease in errors with
stimulation during input and increase with stimulation during output, the
major features of the specific alerting response are present for the non-
verbal test with right brain stimulation as well as on the verbal test
with left.

In addition, an unexpected finding was an effect of left VL stimulation on the non-verbal test. Right VL stimulation evokes no changes in

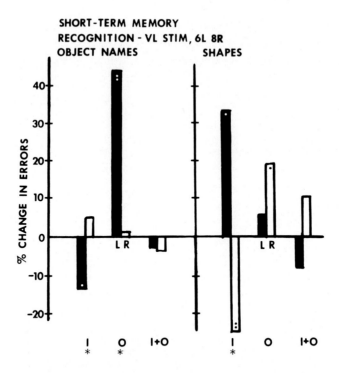

Fig.1 Effects of ventrolateral thalamic stimulation on short-term recognition memory for object names and shapes with few verbal associations.
Bars show % change in recognition errors from control levels (given in
text), associated with stimulation during input (I), output (O) or input
and output (I + O) on the same trial, for six patients with left (solid
bars) and eight with right (open bars) VL electrodes. Dots on bars indicate statistical significance of change: double, p < .05 single .05 < p
< .10. No dot, p > .10. Stars indicate right-left difference is statis-
tically significant at 1.05 level or less. Note decrease in errors (improved performance) with input stimulation, and differential effects of
right or left VL stimulation on verbal and non-verbal tasks.

the verbal test, but left VL stimulation during input to the non-verbal

test substantially increased later recognition errors. This is the re-

verse of the effect of right VL stimulation during input on this test,

and also the reverse of left VL stimulation during input on the verbal

test. The "specific alerting response" evoked from left VL seems to be

highly specific to verbal material; when evoked in the presence of an in-

put of only non-verbal information, that information is ignored. Right

VL stimulation effects may be less modality specific (or the verbal test has more non-verbal features) or this may be true dominance where verbal processes preclude functioning of similar non-verbal processes.

Evidence that at least some features of the "specific alerting response" also modulate long-term memory is also available. A transient anomia is sometimes seen several days after left VL thalamic lesions. When this appeared, naming of those objects that had stimulation during naming at operation (input stimulation to long-term memory for that object) was compared to naming of those objects without such stimulation at operation. At testing two to four days after operation, naming of objects with stimulation at operation showed only 57% of the errors that would have been expected from performance on trials without stimulation at operation. This effect was present in six of the seven patients with postoperative anomia, and is statistically significant (p < 0.05)[2]. The effects of input stimulation of VL in enhancing later retrieval extend into long-term verbal memory.

The name of a pictured object must be retrieved from long-term verbal memory. We would expect left VL stimulation also to interfere with such correct retrieval if the "specific alerting response" can be detected in long-term memory. And it does, though such errors in object naming are evoked only from more discrete areas of left VL and at higher currents than is disruption of short-term memory[2,3,8].

Some evidence for "specific alerting response" phenomena in non-verbal long-term memory are now also available (Mateer and Ojemann, unpublished observations). Two patients have been shown a series of standard colored shapes during right VL operations. During the presentation of some, right VL stimulation occurred. Twenty-four hours later, the patient is tested for recognition of which shapes have been previously seen. The shapes presented at operation with or without stimulation are mixed with shapes not previously seen. In one case, at 24 hours, 83% of the shapes with stimulation at operation were correctly recognized as previously seen, only 33% of the shapes without stimulation at operation. In the other, all shapes presented with stimulation at operation were recognized, but only 67% of those without stimulation. This suggests that the enhancement of non-verbal memory effects of right VL input stimulation also extend to long-term memory.

The relative activation of this VL system in right or left brain then would determine the ease with which verbal or non-verbal features of an input will be later recalled and the difficulty of retrieval of previous verbal or non-verbal memories. The electrodes producing this effect are clearly within the ventrolateral thalamus. Within VL there seems to be some localization of the major features of the specific alerting response. The enhancement of later recall is more readily evoked anteriorly, the disturbance of retrieval of previous memory posteriorly, extending into anterior superior pulvinar[3,9]. These effects may reflect local VL neuronal activation, or more distant effects on a portion of the thalamocortical activating system, such as intralaminar nucleus or its efferent fibers that pass across VL. Why the specific alerting response can be evoked from a nucleus whose major anatomic connections and other known functions are related to the motor system is not entirely clear. Perhaps VL coordinates alerting and motor processes in a mechanism phylogenetically important for animal motor learning, that in man has also been adapted to lateralized verbal or visuospacial learning[3].

Manipulation of this system by stimulation through an electrode implanted in one or the other VL may be of therapeutic value. A patient undergoing thalamotomy for a dyskinesia secondary to a left hemispheric stroke also had a mild anomia, making 20% errors on our simple object naming task prior to operation. At operation, left VL and pulvinar were stimulated during naming. At testing, four days after operation, naming of objects with no stimulation at operation or with pulvinar stimulation was unchanged, with an error rate similar to the preoperative one. But objects with VL stimulation were all named correctly. This suggests that such stimulation of VL during input can be used to increase the accuracy of language function in some patients with at least mild aphasias, and may be of assistance in rapid retraining of some of those patients.

ACKNOWLEDGEMENTS

Supported by NIH research grant NS 04053, National Institute of Neurological and Communicative Disorders and Stroke, USPHS/DHEW. The author is an affiliate of the Center for Child Development and Mental Retardation, University of Washington.

REFERENCES

1. Ojemann, G., Blick, K. and Ward, A. (1971) Improvement and Disturbance of Short-Term Verbal Memory with Human Ventrolateral Thalamic

Stimulation. Brain 94: 225-240.

2. Ojemann, G. (1975) Language and the Thalamus: Object Naming and Re-
    call During and After Thalamic Stimulation. Brain and Language 2:
    101-120.

3. Ojemann, G. (1977) Asymmetric Function of the Thalamus in Man. Ann.
    N. Y. Acad. Sci. 299: 380-396.

4. Peterson, L. and Peterson, M. (1959) Short-Term Retention of Individ-
    ual Verbal Items. J. Exp. Psychol. 58: 193-198.

5. Ojemann, G. (1974) Mental Arithmetic During Human Thalamic Stimula-
    tion. Neuropsychologia 12: 1-10.

6. VanBuren, J. and Borke, R. (1972) Variations and Connections of the
    Human Thalamus, Vol. 2. Variations of the Human Diencephalon.
    Springer-Verlag, Berlin.

7. Vanderplas, J. and Garvin, E. (1959) The Association Value of Random
    Shapes. J. Exp. Psychol. 57: 147-154.

8. Ojemann, G. and Ward, A. (1971) Speech Representation in Ventrolater-
    al Thalamus. Brain 94: 669-680.

9. Ojemann, G. and Fedio, P. (1968) Effect of Stimulation of the Human
    Thalamus and Parietal and Temporal White Matter on Short-Term
    Memory. J. Neurosurg. 29: 51-59.

© 1979 Elsevier/North-Holland Biomedical Press
Modern Concepts in Psychiatric Surgery
E.R. Hitchcock, H.T. Ballantine, Jr. and B.A. Meyerson, eds.

RECOVERY OF HOMEOSTASIS BY CINGULUMOTOMY IN MONKEY

Eldon L. Foltz, M.D. and Joan Lockard, Ph.D.

INTRODUCTION

Laboratory research concerning behavioral effects of manipulation or alteration of the limbic system as applied to clinical needs in psychosurgery is difficult[1]. Only recently have clinicians widely recognized the need for this type of research[2,4]. This type of research, however, required special facilities, special interests and is therefore rare. However cingulumotomy as a valuable technique in psychiatric surgery has become recognized without in-depth animal laboratory research[2,3].

During the past twelve years, considerable data has been accumulated in the chronic animal behavioral or psychophysiological laboratories (Department of Neurological Surgery, University of Washington) from which certain groups of data have been extracted for purposes of supporting the broad concept that the limbic system is the second or even third level control system on the autonomic effector systems which produce autonomic effects inherent in emotional expression. Thus, "emotionality" in the laboratory animal has been studied by the use of psychophysiological methods including behavior observations with measurements of motor (somatic) and gut (autonomic) activity in certain induced "emotional" or "psychosomatic" disease states in monkey[4,5,6,7,8]. These studies also included morphine withdrawal attenuation[1,9].

PSYCHOPHYSIOLOGIC CONCEPTS OF THE LIMBIC SYSTEM BASIC TO PRIMATE RESEARCH ON CLINICAL PROBLEMS

The limbic system is an ancient part of the brain represented well in all mammals, and anatomically indentifiable in rabbit, cat and monkey with relatively direct correlation to human brain[10]. Such acceptable correlation has long been recognized (Fig. 1).

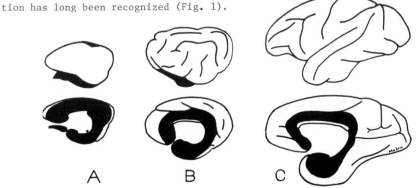

Fig. 1. Lateral and medial surfaces of brains in rabbit (A), cat (B), and monkey (C), showing that limbic lobe (black) forms a common base in brains of all mammals (10).

112

This system has classically been identified as a midline "lobe" consisting of cortex areas and nuclear masses connected and underlain with fiber pathways which conduct ascending influences from brainstem structures to neuronal groups where presumably such input is modulated in a complex manner and, after being affected by this multiple positive feedback system, is then projected back to the limbic midbrain area of Nauta to effect or modify autonomic effector systems involved in emotion[10,11,12]. Classically, this system affects emotionality and is a system wherein balancing subsystems may function to facilitate or inhibit overt emotional expressions [11]. The widespread nature of self-augmenting activity within the limbic system has been well studied by electrophysiologic[4,13] techniques and by anatomical methods[10,12] (Fig. 2). White modified these limbic system concepts to identify the "inner limbic ring" and "outer limbic ring"[14,15,16] (Fig. 3).

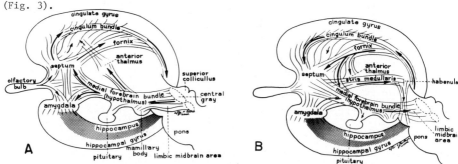

Fig. 2. Diagrammatic limbic system: A, ascending pathways; B, descending pathways (after Mac Lean (10)).

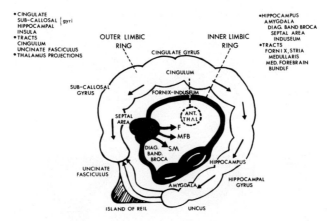

Fig. 3. Diagram of morphological concept of inner limbic ring and outer limbic ring which functionally interact and can be considered the limbic lobe (after White (14) and Foltz (16)).

These rings are anatomically closely adjacent and interconnected but have different outflow pathways signifying separate but interacting functions. Both "rings" consist of structures which have been targets of surgical ablations to modify behavior. These are brain areas of the psychosurgeons' domain.

The inner limbic ring (made up of the circular arrangement of amygdala, septal area, hippocampus, and the tracts of the fornix, median forebrain bundle and stria medullaris) is conceived as the emotion-activated system directly influencing autonomic effectors and expression through immediate brainstem activation. This implies a phylogenetic basis for the inner ring of "protective activation," a concept postulated by Yakovlev[12] early in the recognition of this system.

On the other hand, the "outer limbic ring" (made up of cingulate gyrus, hippocampal gyrus, uncus and Island of Reil cortex areas with cingulum and uncinate faciculus as connecting fiber pathways as well as pathways to the anterior thalamus and pituitary) may function as a control system to the inner ring[14]. Anatomically it is situated to do so; electrophysiologic studies clearly show the close relationship required for such a relationship. In the evolution of the primate brain, this entity developed later than the inner limbic ring. The outer limbic ring may, therefore, act primarily as an evaluator and modifier of basic emotional forces of the "inner limbic ring."

For some years we have considered that this system must function "in balance" with emotional reactions produced appropriate to whatever stimuli are presented to the individual, either from internal environment or from external environment[12,17,18]. Homeostasis is thereby maintained, the individual functions effectively and reacts in a normal degree of life insults and challenges. Mood and emotion swings do occur based largely on neurophysiology within the system, and at times such swings are vigorous--but overall balance is maintained and the individual remains effective and productive. Such homeostasis in this broad sense is essential to a productive and effective existence[16,17,18,19].

Loss of homeostasis does occur when this system becomes overloaded or decompensates, in our view. The system, very sensitive to its own activity because of the extensive positive feedback loops involved in its structure and function, may self-augment to the extent of complete loss of control and cycling of emotional output may occur, or complete breakdown of control or varying degrees of control loss appear. All of these crude

clinical behavior concepts do have electrophysiologic correlates. When
such breakdown of the system occurs due to severe protracted emotional insults to the patient, such as pain, fear of death, loss of family, economic
ruin, protracted stress of any kind, then overactivity of the self-augmenting outer limbic ring may cause severe loss of homeostasis[19]. The result
is inappropriate or over-reaction, often of a cycling nature, in the emotional sphere and producing functional incapacity of the individual. This
loss of homeostasis is due to over-activity of the control system and
should be correctable by reducing that system activity through volume reduction anatomically of structures involved, i.e., by destruction of the
cingulum, cingulate cortex, or any other structure of the outer limbic
ring. Likewise, destruction of structures within the inner limbic ring
would control the effectiveness of this direct autonomic effector system,
probably with more profound results than by destruction of outer ring
structures.

Such a thesis should be susceptible to laboratory research in monkeys
in addition to continued clinical research in patients suffering from
chronic pain or severe mood disturbances associated with emotion correlates[20].

EXPERIMENTAL CINGULUMOTOMY IN MONKEY

Laboratory self-contained projects extracted from a large amount of data in a large series of monkey experiments undertaken in "experimental psy-
somatic disease states in monkey" project, all designed to study the function of the cingulum, include:

I.   Effects on social dominance in the monkey[4,19];

II. Morphine withdrawal effects in monkey[1,4];

III. Effects of cingulumotomy in "conditioned stress," as measured by
     lever pulling behavior in avoidance (somatic), and gut motility in
     avoidance (autonomic);

IV. Cingulumotomy effect on learning (active avoidance and passive
     avoidance).

The major goal of these projects was to investigate the physiologic-
behavioral function of the cingulum fasciculus. The function of this
structure, however, appeared more accesible to observation if the limbic
system was overloaded and a disease state similar to clinical problems produced, such as morphine withdrawal and the "conditioned stress" syndrome
in monkey[15]. It should be emphasized that these laboratory projects were
conducted in time simultaneously with continued neurosurgical clinical
projects on the cingulum (Fig. 4)[4,19].

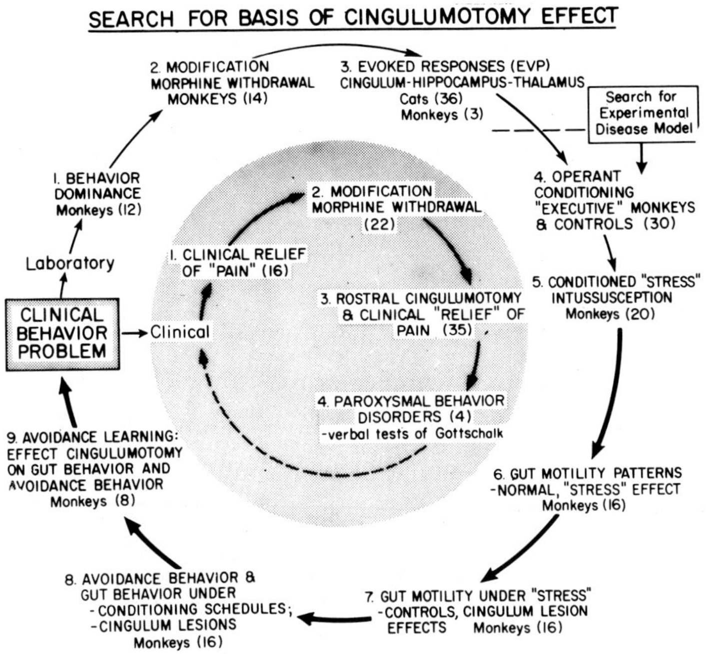

SEARCH FOR BASIS OF CINGULUMOTOMY EFFECT

2. MODIFICATION MORPHINE WITHDRAWAL MONKEYS (14)

3. EVOKED RESPONSES (EVP) CINGULUM-HIPPOCAMPUS-THALAMUS
Cats (36)
Monkeys (3)

Search for Experimental Disease Model

I. BEHAVIOR DOMINANCE Monkeys (12)

Laboratory

2. MODIFICATION MORPHINE WITHDRAWAL (22)

I. CLINICAL RELIEF OF "PAIN" (16)

4. OPERANT CONDITIONING "EXECUTIVE" MONKEYS & CONTROLS (30)

CLINICAL BEHAVIOR PROBLEM → Clinical

3. ROSTRAL CINGULUMOTOMY & CLINICAL "RELIEF" OF PAIN (35)

5. CONDITIONED "STRESS" INTUSSUSCEPTION Monkeys (20)

4. PAROXYSMAL BEHAVIOR DISORDERS (4)
-verbal tests of Gottschalk

9. AVOIDANCE LEARNING: EFFECT CINGULUMOTOMY ON GUT BEHAVIOR AND AVOIDANCE BEHAVIOR Monkeys (8)

6. GUT MOTILITY PATTERNS -NORMAL, "STRESS" EFFECT Monkeys (16)

8. AVOIDANCE BEHAVIOR & GUT BEHAVIOR UNDER - CONDITIONING SCHEDULES; - CINGULUM LESIONS Monkeys (16)

7. GUT MOTILITY UNDER "STRESS" -CONTROLS, CINGULUM LESION EFFECTS Monkeys (16)

Fig. 4. Summary of simultaneous and/or sequential cingulum clinical and laboratory studies.

I. EFFECT ON SOCIAL DOMINANCE IN NORMAL ANIMAL

Twelve animals in a standard quality care facility were paired in cages.

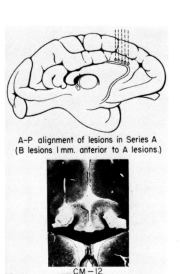

A-P alignment of lesions in Series A
(B lesions I mm. anterior to A lesions.)

CM-12

These animals were carefully observed and their behavior patterns were recorded with respect to dominance; parameters included self-cleaning, companion preening, food dominance, threat reactions (external), etc. Pairs were of males or of females--not mixed. Cingulumotomy lesions were made by standard stereotaxic methods (Fig 5). The animals were studied thereafter for 8 weeks to observe the effect on

Fig. 5. Cingulum lesions in monkeys, social-behavioral dominance study; CM-5 lesions not adequate; anteroposterior axial lesions (diagram) at five points in each animal assured adequate cingulumotomy lesions (19).

social dominance. The lesions were satisfactory at postmortem study but no consistent effect on dominance was observed. Those animals which had been dominant remained so; those which had been undominant had variable responses.

Conclusion: This study on normal animals probably had little clinical relevance. Rostral cingulum lesions are considered for patients who are disabled by their complaints and who therefore have disease of at least a functional nature. Cingulum lesions should be evaluated in the experimental animal ONLY on animals with presumed disease states thought to be similar to the clinical problems encountered.

II. EFFECTS ON MORPHINE WITHDRAWAL ATTENUATION

In a series of 14 monkeys, morphine addiction was produced and then acute withdrawal symptoms were studied, using both simple withdrawal of the drug and Nalline-induced withdrawal. The symptoms of withdrawal in the monkey have been well recorded and include progression of autonomic hyperactivity (Fig. 6). This may progress to right-sided cardiac failure

SIGNS OF MORPHINE WITHDRAWAL IN THE MONKEY:
PROGRESSION OF AUTONOMIC HYPERACTIVITY

1.Pilorection	5.Anorexia	8.Yawning	11.Cyanosis
2.Salivation	6.Diarrhea	9.Abdominal	12.Possible death
3.Rhinorrhea	7.Conjunctival	cramps	(autonomic
4.Lacrimation	Inflammation	10.Agitation	collapse)
		Fig. 6.	

and death. This is an experimentally produced disease state in the monkey with considerable "emotional" overtones, and is a severe reaction.

The syndrome in monkeys is markedly attenuated by rostral cingulumotomy. The "emotionality" (psychic factors) associated with morphine withdrawal is not obvious after operation. The autonomic signs (somatic factors) present in withdrawal after cingulumotomy are often difficult to identify. The animals show only a modified effect of the withdrawal if any at all.

Conclusion: The autonomic hyperactivity associated with emotionality in morphine withdrawal in the monkey is markedly attenuated by cingulumotomy. This is probably secondary to reestablishment of homeostatic capabilities and reduction of feedback loop activity in the limbic lobe functions which produce the unattenuated withdrawal in the normal monkey. Thus, action of the limbic lobe to augment such autonomic effects of withdrawal is prevented because the limbic lobe volume of activity is markedly reduced by the cingulumotomy lesions. Homeostatic capacity is thus reattained by balancing the system involved. The system had been thrown out of balance by the withdrawal of morphine in the addicted monkey. Although we still do not understand the physiology of withdrawal or its modification by cingulumotomy in complete detail, homeostasis capacity seems to be reattained after the cingulum lesions as demonstrated by clinical observations. Such modification has been studied in other brain lesions as well, but cingulumotomy lesions are the most discrete and smallest lesions effective in this regard. It may be that the electrophysiologic effect is the primary cause of this phenomenon, but it may also be that such lesions produce B-endorphin within the brain itself. Recent studies may ultimately support the concept that endogenous morphine-like substances are produced as a result of cingulumotomy, and therefore are responsible for the striking attenuation of withdrawal.

III. THE "CONDITIONED" STRESS RESPONSE IN MONKEY AS EMOTION-RELATED (PSYCHOSOMATIC DISEASE):

Background: In a behavioral laboratory designed for such purposes, monkeys were conditioned or taught to respond to certain signals (colored light) in order to avoid uncomfortable body shocks, given in unpredictable sequence. Monkeys responded to such studies by developing peptic ulcers and became known as "executive monkeys"[21]. Further studies with evoked controls indicated that the gut activity became very abnormal even producing intussusception and death[5]. Because gut activity has long been recognized as associated with certain emotional responses and psychosomatic disease states including morphine withdrawal[1], it seemed important that this system be instrumented in an attempt to record data which might be significant relative to emotional state in the monkey which had been conditioned to "stress." Such an "autonomic" factor (gut motility) could then be correlated with the relative efficiency of the monkey in lever pulling in avoidance activity, considering this activity as a somatic factor in emotion. A lengthy sequence of involved experiments, well balanced on a statistical basis, included a number of interesting studies some of which are as yet not clearly interpretable. Several of these studies, however, have clinical pertinence, and two are presented here.

A. Avoidance lever-pulling under "stress"--modification by cingulumotomy[6,7,8,19]:

Thirty-two monkeys, instrumented for conditioning responses and gut motility recording over weeks, were studied extensively (Fig. 7). These

118

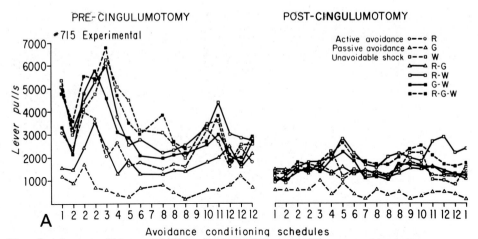

PRE-CINGULUMOTOMY   POST-CINGULUMOTOMY

A   Avoidance conditioning schedules

Fig. 7. Lever-pulling activity: Number of lever pulls on avoidance conditioning schedules, pre- and post-cingulumotomy. In postcingulumotomy state, much less divergent rates for different schedules and improved efficiency (all conditions showed lever pulling closer to the optimum for active avoidance along, which is the ideal response)--does this show much less "emotionality"? (6,7,8,19)

animals were trained to active avoidance response (pulling a lever to avoid a body shock when the red light was on), passive avoidance response (avoiding the lever because of a mild hand shock when touching it when the green light was on), and unavoidable punishment (inevitable body shock 15 seconds after a white light appeared). These animals were in a yoked control design and were subjected to aperiodic schedules of these epochs after adequate training to criteria. Lever pulls under all conditions were automatically recorded and gut activity was recorded continuously by three small gut strain gauges placed at operation.

The ideal lever-pulling response was found to be just enough pulls to avoid the body shock. Thus, an efficient response in the active avoidance epoch was equated to a lever pull every 10 to 15 seconds to avoid the body shock which otherwise would occur every 15 seconds. On this basis, efficiency of lever pulling could be calculated and overpulling could therefore be recognized (Fig. 7).

In this study, the divergence of pulling rates in the several epochs (red light, green light, white light combinations) was marked (Fig. 7), but after cingulumotomy, the statistical study indicated considerably more efficiency in lever pulling. This clearly was not a learning effect caused by the experimental design.

B. Gut motility under "stress"-modification by cingulumotomy[6,7,8,19]:

Gut response of normal animals under these conditions, such as response to daily food patterns, etc., has been well established. Gut motility responses under these experimental conditions were correlated with each epoch of the complex schedule, comparing the normal data with the gut activity under conditioned stress and then as affected by cingulumotomy. The results in this study before cingulumotomy showed that each animal had his own particular pattern of response to the "conditioned stress"--both in the lever pulling and gut motility. Some animals showed immense overpulling response; others were less so.

In the gut activity, some animals showed a hypermotile response to the stress conditioning and others showed a hypomotile response (Fig. 8A,8B). After adequate control schedules, cingulum lesions were made in certain animals and control lesions in others. The statistics clearly showed a change in response in the animals who had the cingulum lesions. The hyperresponders (both gut and lever-pulling) became hyporesponders, and the hyporesponders became hyperresponders. The lever pulling and gut activity effects were parallel.

Conclusions: The effect of cingulumotomy in these animals appeared based on their original reactivity both in lever pulling and gut activity. They might be correlated with augmentors and reducers, a classification of personality in man by Petrie[21]. The retrospective assumption that emotionality in some of these animals had been lessened whereas in others emotionality had been increased seemed at least logical. It seems that homeostasis loss in some had been modified or at least improved, whereas in others such homeostatic loss had been worsened. The change induced by cingulumotomy appeared to be based on the preoperative reaction of the animal to the behavioral situation.

IV. CINGULUMOTOMY EFFECT ON LEARNING

Background: Emotional drive and ability to learn have long been associated. If emotional drive is reduced, possibly the ability to learn is likewise reduced. Emotionality may be equated to ineffective leverpulling as demonstrated in previous responses to "conditioned stress," of this emotionality already demonstrated might be associated with reduced capacity to learn. Likewise, if gut motility is associated with emotionality, gut motility change by cingulumotomy might also indicate a reduced learning capacity if the basic thesis is valid[7,8,19].

Therefore, a series of animals instrumented to study gut motility and lever pulling was studied under learning conditions of active avoidance response. (Fig. 9.10).

120

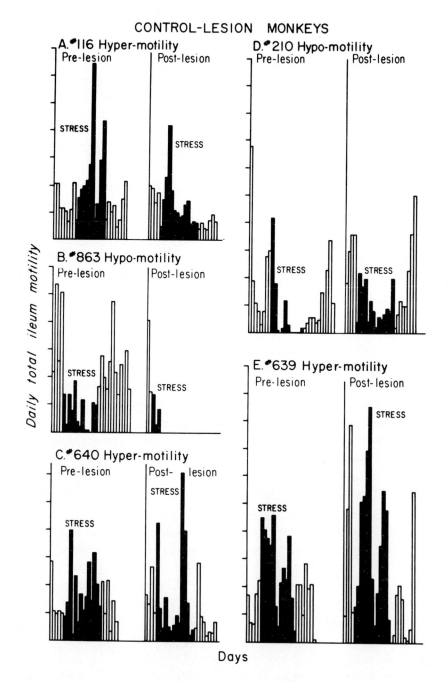

Fig. 8A
Gut motility histograms to show effect of stress on gut motility and then
modification of this stress effect by cingulum lesions in the same animal:
A, control lesion animals—no effect.

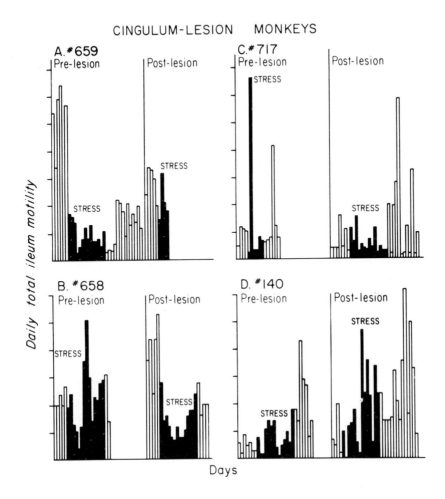

Fig. 8B

B: cingulum animals-reversal of motility effect (i.e., hypomotile became hypermotile response-nos. 659, 140; hypermotile became hypomotile response-nos. 658, 717) (6,7,8,19).

122

Acquisition of AAR				Acquisition of PAR				Extinction of AAR			
Monkey #	Control	Cingulum	Monkey #	Monkey #	Control	Cingulum	Monkey #	Monkey #	Control	Cingulum	Monkey #
296	3	10	295	296	20*	20*	295	296	18	15	295
83	4	5	84	83	6	20*	84	83	27	17	84
155	7	4	158	155	3	20*	158	155	20	20	158
49	18	12	102	49	20*	20*	102	49	26	26	102
	M=8	M=8			M=12←p < .001→M=20				M=23	M=20	
					*failed to reach criterion						

Fig. 9. Table of comparison of control versus cingulum monkey in learning (acquisition and extinction of avoidance): AAR, active avoidance response (lever pull avoids heavy body shock); PAR, passive avoidance response (mild shock of lever touched). Note: None of 4 cingulum monkeys
acquired PAR (no emotional drive to learn?). AAR learning unimpaired,
presumably because of more significant and larger stimulus relationship;
more "emotional" drive? (6,8,19).

A. Lever pulling under avoidance conditions:

Eight naive male monkeys in two lesion groups were adapted to
chair confinement after which either cingulum or control brain
lesions were made. Ten days later, conditioned avoidance training was started. This training included active avoidance response (red light, to avoid body shock), passive avoidance response (lever shock avoidance, associated with green light) and
a combination of these two. Training was continued up to 20 days
on each animal. Extinction of the active avoidance response was
then recorded as an additional learning parameter. Lever pulls
in each of these situations was recorded constantly to interpret
the nature of the monkey response.

The results were clear:

1. Control and cingulum monkeys showed no difference in learning
or extincting the active avoidance response (body shock)(Fig. 9).
2. Cingulum lesion monkeys did not acquire passive avoidance response even after 20 days, a statistically significant finding(Fig. 9).
3. Cingulum lesion monkeys demonstrated a rate of lever pull
more efficient than the high inefficient rate of the control
monkeys (Fig. 10).

Conclusion: To clinicians, these results indicate that significant

LEVER PULLS DURING AAR(a) (red), CONTROL GROUP

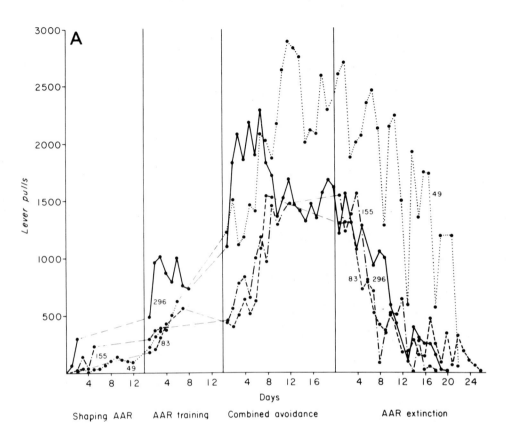

Fig. 10A
Lever pulls of monkeys under training: A: control group-excessive activity;

124

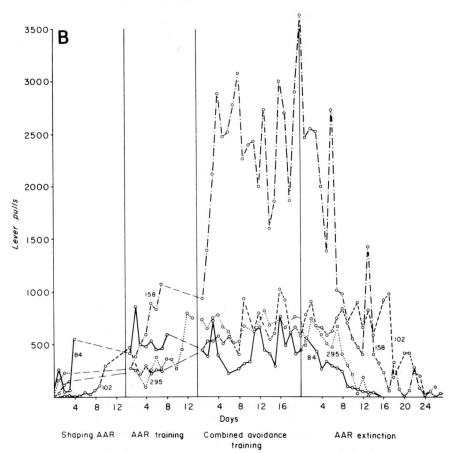

Fig. 10B
Lever pulls of monkeys under training: B; cingulum monkeys—except for one inadequate lesion, markedly improved efficiency for all schedules or epochs.
(6,8,19).

factors in learning are not impaired by cingulum lesions because the animals rapidly learned active avoidance responses, including extinction. However, more subtle learning did <u>not</u> occur in the passive avoidance response which involved avoiding a small hand shock every time the lever was touched. This effect appeared unrelated to any change in threshold of sensation response since all animals quickly took their hand off of the lever whenever they touched it. However, the cingulum lesioned animals may have had a small emotional response to this minor inconvenience to an extent that it did not promote learning--at least that is one interpretation.

During this learning sequence, the cingulum lesion monkeys showed a more efficient rate of lever pull. This may indicate less emotional titer in their response to the active avoidance response.

B. <u>Gut motility studies</u>

At the same time as lever pulling was being studied in this learning project, gut motility was recorded. Thus, gut motility was recorded continuously and data collated on each time epoch to the percentage of daily motility[6,7,8,19]. Gut motility was decreased in the cingulum animals during learning and was less variable than in the control animals. This extensive statistical analysis has a high level of validity in view of the enormous amount of normative data on gut motility already recorded.

<u>Conclusions</u>: Certain conclusions from this learning study are presented. Animals with adequate cingulum lesions were <u>less reactive</u> autonomically (gut motility) and <u>less reactive</u> behaviorally (lever pulling) under these conditions of active avoidance acquisition, passive avoidance learning and, extinction. This can be interpreted as less emotionality and reactivity in the animals with cingulum lesions than in the control animals. <u>Learning was not impaired</u> if a significant stimulus was present, but a small stimulus, as in passive avoidance response, apparently was not as meaningful-- and again this may be important when viewed from a bias of emotion relationships.

DISCUSSION

These experimental techniques were intended to produce psychological states of high emotional tone, and they seem to have been effective. Projects III and IV indicate the cingulum ablation did have an effect on monkey by reducing an overactive, inefficient response to a more optimum level as measured by lever pulling. The gut motility studies probably mean the same thing since gut motility is recorded as a percent of normal activity.

We can possibly say that this is recovery of homeostasis capability and that it is not associated with reduced learning or less retentive capability. Emotionality may have been reduced to a lower level, thus allowing homeostasis to be reestablished and resulting in more appropriate behavior.

Our experimental efforts with experimental psychic disease states were, of course, basic to our concepts that the limbic lobe function is altered under such conditions and that cingulumotomy may produce an effect quite different from the effects of the same lesion in a normal animal. Emphasis must be placed on the many variables in the problem studies, but the relatively large number of animals used did appear to give statistical control of such variables.

These experimental studies may give support to the clinical neurosurgeon, psychologist and psychiatrist who seek support for the use of behavior-modifying methods for patients whose incapacity from intractable pain or intractable behavior disability is believed to result from inadequate homeostatic capacity and a resultant compensatory factor breakdown.

SUMMARY AND CONCLUSIONS

1. A concept of limbic lobe function is presented, modified from previous longstanding neurophysiologic and behavioral data, to indicate that homeostasis in this highly sensitive, emotionally related system, is lost in certain disease states with high emotional components, such as intractable pain and intractable mood disturbances.

2. Normal monkeys showed no change in "social dominance" after cingulumotomy.

3. Morphine addiction in monkeys is markedly attenuated by cingulumotomy.

4. Experimentally produced emotion related disease states, "conditioned stress," has been developed in monkeys in which cingulum lesions appear to have reestablished a level of homeostasis, or recovery of lost homeostasis in this concept. Such lesions are associated with recovery of efficient lever pulling and near normal gut activity.

5. Cingulumotomy is associated with no impairment of learning for an adequate stimulus but some impairment of inadequate stimulus learning (passive avoidance) in monkey.

REFERENCES

1. Foltz, E.L. and White, L.E., Jr. (1957) Experimental cingulumotomy and modification of morphine withdrawal, J. Neurosurg. 14: 655-673.
2. Psychosurgery, report and recommendations: The National Commission for Protection of Human Subjects of Biomedical and Behavioral Research; DHEW Publication No. (OS77-0001).
3. Psychosurgery, Appendix: The National Commission for Protection of Human Subjects of Biomedical and Behavioral Research; DHEW Publication No.

(OS77-0002).
4. Foltz, E.L. (1972) Clinical problems and primate research in the limbic lobe--a 12 year project report. In treatment of Pain Symposium, Hahnemann Medical College, Philadelphia; unpublished.
5. Foltz, E.L., Millett, F.E., Jr., et al. (1964) Experimental psychosomatic disease states in monkeys. II. Gut hypermotility. J. Surg. Res. 4: 455-453.
6. Lockard, J.S., Ehle, A.L., et al (1972) Diurnal variation of ileum motility in monkey during different feeding and avoidance-conditioning schedules. Physiol. Behav. 8: 195-200
7. Haller, R.G., Lockard, J.S. and Foltz, E.L. (1976) "Avoidance behavior and ileum motility post-cingulumotomy in monkey. Biol. Psych.,11: #2.
8. Lockard, J.S., Foltz, E.L., et al (1977) Ileum motility of monkey during chronic avoidance-conditioning pre- and post-cingulumotomy. Physiol. Behav. 18: 111-117
9. Foltz, E.L. (1968)Current status in use of rostral cingulumotomy. Southern Med. J. 61: 899-908
10. MacLean, P.D. (1958) Contrasting functions of limbic and neocortical systems of brain and the development of gastrointestinal ulcer. J. Exp. Anal. Behav. 1: 69-72
11. Papez, J.W. (1937) A proposed mechanism of emotion. Arch. Neurol. Psychiatr. 38: 740-743.
12. Yakovlev, P.I. and Locke, J.S. (1961) Limbic nuclei of thalamus and connections of limbic cortex. III. Corticocortical connections of the anterior cingulate gyrus, the cingulum, and the subcallosal bundle in monkey. Arch. Neurol. 5: 364-400.
13. White, L.E., Jr., Nelson, W. and Foltz, E.L. (1960) Cingulum fasciculus study by evoked potentials. Exp. Neurol. 2: 401-421.
14. White, E.L., Jr. (1965) A morphologic concept of the limbic lobe. Int. Rev. Neurobiol. 8: 1-34.
15. Chronister, R.D., and White, L.E., Jr. Limbic lobe morphology; an approach to a new system. In Advances in Neurology, edited by J.K, Penry and D.D. Daly, Vol. 11, pp. 15-25. Raven Press, New York, 1975.
16. Foltz, E.L., and White, L.E., Jr. (1968) The role of rostral cingulumotomy in pain "relief." Int. J. Neurol. 6: 353-374.
17. Foltz, F.L., and White, L.E., Jr. (1966) Pain "relief" by frontal cingulumotomy. In pain, edited by R.S. Knighton and P.R. Dumke. Little, Brown and Co., Boston.
18. Foltz, E.L. and White, L.E., Jr. (1973) Affective disorders involving pain. In Neurological Surgery, edited by J. Youmans, Vol. III., Chapter 101. W.B. Saunders, Phila.
19. Foltz, E.L. (1977) Psychosurgical approach to chronic pain (Cingulumotomy). In Management of Pain, edited by Charles C. Thomas, Springfield, Ill., Chapter 7.
20. Ballantine, H.T., Jr., Cassidy, W.L., et al. (1967) Stereotaxic anterior cingulumotomy for neuropsychiatric illness and intractable pain. J. Neurosurg. 26: 488-495
21. Brady, J.R., Porter, R.W., et al. (1958) Avoidance behavior and the development of gastroduodenal ulcer. J. Exp. Anal. Behav. 1: 69-72.
22. Kohler, W., and Walloch, N. (1944) Figural after effects. Proc. Am. Phil. Soc. 88: 269.
23. Gottschalk, L.A. (1972) An objective method of measuring psychological states associated with changes in neural function: content analysis of verbal behavior. Biol. Psychiatr. 4: 33-49

EPILEPSY, PERSONALITY AND LIMBIC SYSTEM

© 1979 Elsevier/North-Holland Biomedical Press
Modern Concepts in Psychiatric Surgery
E.R. Hitchcock, H.T. Ballantine, Jr. and B.A. Meyerson, eds.

PERSONALITY STUDIES IN SURGERY FOR EPILEPSY

Claudio Rossi, Raul Marino Jr., Latife Yazigi +
FUNCTIONAL NEUROSURGERY RESEARCH CENTER, UNIVERSITY OF SÃO PAULO MEDICAL SCHOOL-
INSTITUTO DE PSIQUIATRIA - CAIXA POSTAL 8091 -CEP 65403 SÃO PAULO - BRASIL

ABSTRACT

The authors studied in a structural and dynamic approach the personality changes observed in patients submitted to temporal lobectomies for treatment of epilepsy.

Ten cases, of a series of forty, were psychiatrically and psychologically examined before and after surgery. Their study was completed with data collected by neurologists, neuropsychologists, and social workers.

The personality changes observed were classified in 1- primary: a) relief of seizures and improvement of reflex and voluntary attention, attributed by the authors to the removal of the "focus"; b) useful changes in emotional response and in mood that through the phenomenological study of aggressiveness and the results of Rorscharch test, were considered as constitutional changes (in the biologic basis of personality) and attributed to the disconnection of temporo-limbic circuits which occurred during surgery; 2- secondary: better adaptation to work and to personal relationships, that were interpreted as a consequence of psychodynamic interaction between primary changes, previous personality structure and environmental opportunities in the post-operative period.

A block diagram was prepared to show graphically the interrelationship of the personality changes observed.

INTRODUCTION

Several authors have reported on psychiatric studies of temporal lobe epileptics, operated upon for the treatment of epilepsy.

Jensen[1], Slater and Glithero[2], Serafetinides and Falconer[3], showed that the number of psychotics decreases post-operatively. They also showed that the schizophrenia-like patients had less florid psychiatric pictures post-operatively.

Hill et al[4], and Hill[5] also verified that paranoid traits of epileptics are not relieved by surgery.

Not only psychotics have benefited from surgery, but also neurotic and epileptoid psichopaths, as Taylor[6] has shown:

+ Respectively psychiatrist, neurosurgeon and psychologist.

The normal group was increased mainly by the psychopaths, in which aggression was their main characteristic.

Other effects of epilepsy surgery were also studied in other aspects of mental functioning, independently from the psychiatric diagnosis of the patients. Thus, Taylor[6] is in agreement with other authors, that aggression is one of the aspects more often altered by surgery. Walker and Blumer[7] reported that aggressive traits (impulsive, irritable behavior and violence) improved, even in cases with persistent seizures post-operatively; marked sexuality changes were noticed: patients that were hyposexuals become normal or hypersexuals, and these are early post-operative changes, where duration depends on the presence or absence of seizures. When seizures recur, hyposexuality also returns. Sexually normal subjects have not shown any changes post-operatively. The same authors have shown that religiosity and viscosity were not altered after surgery. Taylor[6] reported that in neurotics there was a significant improvement of anxiety, phobias, and depression, while the hysterical traits were not modified.

Horowitz et al[8] have shown that "remission or improvement in seizures cannot immediately allow the individual to function normally. If the patient had not learned adaptation skills, identity and facility in interpersonal processes to cope with "normal" life, he must be helped in these areas before any social change can be detected".

Ferguson and Rayport[9] have reported on an "identity crisis" post-operatively. These authors have interpreted certain depressive states found post-operatively as "symptom substitution" (depression instead of seizures).

Objective. Our objective was to describe the personality changes of the patients, and to try to understand their interrelationships, from a structural and dynamic point of view. Our purpose was also relating them to well known facts about the functions of the brain circuits involved in the surgery and to the physiopathology of epilepsy.

MATERIALS AND METHODS

Our subjects are epileptic patients submitted to temporal lobectomies for relief of intractable seizures.

The present study is based on the first 10 cases of a series of 40, that had pre-operative psychiatric examination and at least one year of post-operative evolution.

Table 1 shows age and sex of our patients, side of operation, and date of surgery.

TABLE 1

DATA OF PATIENTS

Case nr	Age	Date of surgery	Later.	Sex.
1	38	03.19.75	R	F
2	20	06.18.75	L	F
3	28	03.31.76	R	M
4	33	04.07.76	R	F
5	28	05.05.76	L	M
6	39	08.25.76	L	F
7	31	12.15.76	L	F
8	30	12.22.76	R	F
9	21	02.02.76	R	M
10	27	06.23.76	R	M

The psychiatrist based his observations on the direct examination of patients and their families and also on the data collected by the social worker and by the nurses who have observed the patient in the hospital environment.

Subjective experiences and feelings of the patients were studied with special care, and special attention was given to the way the patients elaborated and described such facts.

The psychologist used the Rorscharch test as a method of personality study of patients, interpreting the data according to the criteria adopted by Silveira[10], similar to those used by Piotrowski.[11]

All these proceedings were performed before surgery and in the follow-ups, these latter occurring after 6 months, one year, and two years after surgery. Special attention was given to the first year of post-operative evolution, since we were interested in observing changes that might be dissimulated by reorganization of functions that occur in a more extended evolution time.

RESULTS

The changes in psychiatric diagnosis, personality traits, and symptoms are in agreement with those mentioned in the literature (Table 2).

TABLE 2

CHANGES IN DIAGNOSTIC, TRAITS AND SYMPTOMS

	Number of patients	
	PRE	POST
Psychotics	2	2
Hyposexuals	6	5
Normosexuals	3	3
Hypersexuals	1	0
Paranoid traits	3	3
Hysteric traits	1	1
Viscosity	3	3
Religiosity	3	3
Anxiety	10	5
Depression	5	2

This table indicates that the psychotics remain psychotic, although the psychiatric pictures are less florid mainly due to a reduction of aggressiveness. The number of patients with normal sexual response has increased in the follow-up period. The patients presenting paranoid and hysterical traits, viscosity and religiosity, did not present changes as to these characteristics, and the number of patients presenting anxiety and depression was reduced.

As to the seizures, 7 patients are controlled, 2 presented reduction in the seizure frequency and 1 remained unchanged.

The study of aggressiveness was more detailed and this trait was more frequently and more intensively changed by surgery. During the pre-operative period the majority of patients described themselves as being nervous, explosive, impulsive, irritable. Their emotional experiences were of hate, irritation, drive to attack, frequently judged by themselves as abnormal and unpleasantly intensive. We classified as: a) "aggressive mood" the occurrence of these subjective experiences in the absence of qualitative adequate environment stimuli to produce them. Some patients already woke up in this mood or turned so before or after a seizure. In this mood the patient sometimes provoked the others creating opportunities to quarrel. We classified as: b) excessive emotional response to frustration when, after a stimulus adequate to induce rage (e.g.- humiliations, professional and affective frustrations, frequently caused by social consequences of the desease, provocative behavior of another person, rivalry, jealousy etc.), the patient response is excessive. We classified as: c) excessive duration of the emotional response to frustration, when after a frustrating situation the patient remains during hours or days with strong anxiety, with aggressive or guilty ruminations, various aggressive fantasies, psychomotor excitation, resentment and insomnia. Often the patient obtained relief only after discharging the rage over the person who had provoked him or over a target that had nothing to do with the initial stimulus. We have also found: d) verbal and e) physical aggressive behavior where violence was frequent. Finally we considered as having f) ability to restrain aggression when there was a subjective tendency to attack without overt aggression. Table 3 shows the occurrence of these manifestations during pre-operative period and during the early and late follow-ups. The characteristic was considered to be present when it occurred during the given period of time, even if it presented lower intensity than before the surgery, what in fact occurred with all patients, except 2 (cases nr. 1 and 2).

TABLE 3

AGGRESSIVENESS PRE- AND POST-OPERATIVELY

		Number of cases	
	PRE	POST OPERATIVE PERIOD	
		3 to 9 mo	after 12 mo
a) aggressive mood (subjective)	9	3	6
b) excessive emotional response to frustration	9	4	8
c) excessive duration of the emotional response to frustration	8	2	5
d) verbal aggressiveness	8	4	7
e) physical aggressiveness	5	0	4
f) ability to restrain aggression	4	2	6

The table shows that all these aspects of aggressiveness were strongly present before surgery. In the early post-operative period we notice a dramatic decrease of them. In the late post-operative period there is a tendency to a new increase of these characteristics without attaining the pre-operative levels. The only exception was the control ability which surpassed the pre-operative level after 12 mo of follow-up.

The following reports of patients illustrate how they felt some of these changes.

Report of case nr 6 (20 months after surgery): "-The feeling is that the surgery removed an evil I had. Before surgery I felt like aggression coming from the inside, I can't even remember the reason for the last quarrel which put an end to my engagement. I was always looking for pretexts for quarreling.

^{O}nce I was so angry that I bit the engagement ring! Several times I had hurt my fiancé, slaping him and hitting him with my purse on his face. All this disappeared and I can't explain why... I'm not impulsive nor aggressive any longer and that's all I can say." Soon after she added that now she is able to count until 10 before exploding and can control herself. "-Before I couldn't count up to 1." Eventually she still "explodes" and then she stated: "-After a quarrel I used to be irritated during hours and the irritation kept growing. Now it is different. Soon after exploding I'm calm again and free of resentments." (As this patient still gets irritated and occasionally presents verbal aggression, in table 3 she is classified as having this behavior.)

Report of the patient nr. 10 (3 months after surgery): "-Now I feel more calm. Anything made me explode before the surgery. I can talk better with people. I'd never take an insult home. Anything that happened used to make me quarrel. Now this is not any longer. If someone insults me I'd rather forget. This was something impossible to do before. Now it is better." We have also observed an improvement of the intellectual functions in 3 patients (cases nr. 3, 5 and 10) due to the improvement of attention and concentration. The report of our patient nr. 5 (24 months after surgery) exemplifies this fact: "-Before, when I was going to do something, and I needed to concentrate, any little thing was able to make me loose my point and I had to start all over again. If someone gave me a suggestion to do something in another way, I'd get irritated and I had to continue doing the way I had planned. Now this is not so. If I'm doing something for you and you suggest I do it in a different way, I follow your suggestion and wait to see what happens. I've learned many new things this way."

The involuntary passive attention has also improved; fact which is exemplified through the report of patient nr. 3 (25 months after surgery): "-Now I am more lucid. I can think faster and it is easier to remember things. I used to be somewhat drowsy. If I was doing something I could pay attention only on that thing. Now this is not so. If I am working on my weaver's loom, I can even observe what is happening around me.

This other report of patient nr. 3 (6 months after surgery) exemplifies the greater interest in adequating to social situations and a better insight of his limitations. "-Before, I used to say everything that came to my mind. I didn't care about the opinion of others. Now I prefer to speak less and to think more about what I say. I don't want to talk many foolish things."

As to their social adaptation, the patients were classified from A to F.

Under A we classified patients having frequent admittance in mental hospital
for their inability to live in society due to severe behavior inadequacies.
Under F we classified the patients who have an active participation in society
through work, good affective contacts and community activities according to
their social-cultural possibilities. Under B, C, D, and E we classified those
whose social adaptation is between these two extremes. Table 4 indicates what
happened with these aspects before and after surgery.

TABLE 4

SOCIAL ADAPTATION OF PATIENTS

Pattern	Period			
	Pre	3 to 6 mo	7 to 12 mo	after 12 mo
A	–	–	1	1
B	4	1	1	1
C	3	6	–	–
D	2	2	7	4
E	1	1	1	2
F	–	–	–	2

It may be observed that as time passes, greater number of patients were classified under D, E and F, which is the opposite of what happened before surgery.
We have also observed that the patients having families better structured and
those having better social opportunities after the surgery, were the ones that
had a better development from the ADAPTIVE point of view.

Rorschach's results

With the purpose of deepening our study of patient's affective alterations
and their changes on the social adaptation, some Rorschach's indexes were
selected and compared pre- and post-operatively. Thus, for the affective alterations we used the Silveira's[15] affective (Af) and impulsiveness (Imp)
indexes. We also made a study of the other Rorschach's indexes and components
(R.m.i., Con., λ) and of their relationship on the color and monotone plates
separately; and inside the color series confronting plates II and III as a group
with VIII to X as another. Among the results obtained through that comparison,
we examined the phenomenon of the psychological shock that on Silveira's[10] conception means an assemblage of deviations in the indexes that can appear in the
color plates (affective shock) or in the monotone ones (emotional shock).

TABLE 5

RORSCHARCH RESULTS

	INDEX	PARAMETER	PRE	EARLY P.O.	LATE P.O.
Form Responses	% F	64.0 ±8.0	77.09	81.83	72.33
Good Form Responses[a]	% F+	75 to 90	67.86	69.00	77.54
Popular Responses[a]	% P	27.0 ±4.0	14.89	20.55	28.04
Animal Responses[b]	% A	37.0 ±4.0	34.58	39.55	46.28
% F+ + % P + % A /3[b]	R.m.i.	50.0 ±5.0	40.97	42.26	50.57
% F+ - % (R-F)[c]	Con.	50.0 ±3.0	44.96	51.29	49.87
R - F / F[d]	λ	0.50±0.10	0.35	0.24	0.45
R color /R mono[e]	Af.	1.20±0.10	1.36	1.27	1.62
R II+III /R VIII to X[f]	Imp.	0.34±0.05	0.86	0.82	0.65

a- according to Small[12]; b- Silveira's[14] index for the intellectual rapport with the outer world; c- Silveira's[13] conative index for measuring the explicit action; d- Beck's Lambda index for measuring the personal resources; e- Silveira's[15] affective index; f- Silveira's[15] impulsiveness index.

Comparing the results of the affective sphere of the personality of the pre--operative with the 6 months of follow-up we observed:

1) a decrease of the affective sensitiveness that still remains above the average, and that corresponds with a certain reduction of the affective excitement, that allows an inter-personal relationship where the intensity of the affective response became more adequate to the stimulus (this interpretation is a consequence of the relationship between the fall of the Af and Imp indexes with the disappearance of the affective shock and with the increase of the % F+ in the color plates).

2) a small decrease of the intensity of the instinctive impulsions (primary, archaic affectiveness linked to biological constitution). This decrease is very helpfull, since the excessive intensity of them disturbs the rationality and the possibility for responsible and reasonable behaviors. We also noted that the patients started to act in a more adapted way to the environment with more conscious control in their action, suffering less interference of the abnormal mechanisms of thinking. So, they start managing their instinctive reactions and their sociability in a better way, since they become socially more appropriate and controlled (reduction of the Imp. index; increase of the R.m.i. index; and % F+, followed by the fall of Confabulation, Condensation Contamination on the plates II and III; increase of the % F+ and % P on the plates VIII, IX and X).

3) disappearing of a deep and unconscious anxiety which causes inharmonies and troubles on the affective relationship with others (disappearing of the psychological affective shock caracterized by a structural disarticulation

of the perception while facing the color plates).

Comparing these affective alterations between the pre- and the late follow-
-up (more than one year of evolution) we observed that:
1) the patients react moreand with more interest and spontaneity to the
situations with affective involvement with other people and to those situations
having a more social significance (increase of Af index due to the increase of
R and RC in the plates VIII to X);
2) there is still a greater reduction in the intensity of the instinctive impulsions at the same time that they start having towards them a more self-
-assertive, self-controlled and independent behavior, not being so commanded
by such subjective pressure, which before surgery used to impell them to
immediate reactions (in short circuit) and to motor outlets face the milieu
(diminishing of the Imp. index; raise of RM and of % F+ in the plates II and
III):
3) it reappears a deep and unconscious anxiety that occurs in situations of
affective involvement with other people and in those situations having a more
social significance, originated from the difficulty to handle those situations
that previously had little interest to the patients, since they reacted to
them in a more primitive way (psychological affective shock reappers due to
the deviations of the indexes in the plates VIII to X).

We have also studied the intellectual rapport with the outer world by
Silveira's[14] R.m.i. index. This index depends on: the individual's capacity
to make an objective and impartial examination of the facts, as a consequence
of the conative effort to stabilize the attention (% F+); the motivation and
interest in a rapport with the reality (% A); the way of accepting the values
on which everyone agrees, thus standing for the use of logical and conventional
thinking in the process of assimilation of the patterns of conduct adopted by
the social group (% P).   The capacity to perceive and to accept the limitations and impositions of the outer reality -social and physical- depends on
these three factors in association. During the pre-operative period this index
was much below the normal average, because despite the interest in the rapport
with the reality was adequate, the patients failed in the apprehension of the
social patterns and in maintaining an objective examination of the outer world.
On the precocious follow-up (6 months) this index got better, getting closer
to the normal average levels, due to an improvement in the adoption of the
social rules, but still remaining the lack in having a good judgement of the
reality. On the late follow-up this index reaches the normal area, but revealed a higher emotional tension (% A surpassed the normal area), revealing that

the patients started to accept the limitations imposed by the external world, with more and better conative control of the impulses, but with emotional tension, because they were now extremely worried about their social adequation.

DISCUSSION

Our results are in agreement with those of the literature mentioned in the introduction. The psychosis, the paranoid and hysteric traits, the viscosity and religiosity were practically not affected by the surgery. On the other hand, the anxiety, the depression, sexuality, and aggressiveness presented significant changes. We concluded therefore, that it is in the affective side of the personality that these changes take place. We observed also improvement in the control of seizures, that disappeared in the majority of the patients, and better cognitive performance resulting from improvement of attention and concentration. This latter result is in agreement with those obtained by Camargo et al[16] through the neuropsychologic study of a sample similar to ours. Finally we observed better social adaptation of the patients in the follow-up.

The phenomenologic study of the early affective changes and mainly of the aggressiveness indicated that these occur in the emotional pattern of response to stimuli. They occurred as if the patient had changed his temperament. His way of seeing the world remained the same. However, despite interpreting the situation the same way as before, they started to react with less intensive emotions, even though somewhat above the normal levels. They felt more serene and were able to control themselves easily when facing stimuli that would previously leave them overwhelmed with rage. With reference to these alterations, the Rorscharch test also indicated that they were due to a decrease of the affective sensibility and of the instictive impulsions which previously blocked the adequate functioning of the patients personality. All these facts lead us to interpret that the changes would be due to constitutional alterations (and on biologic basis) of the personality.

If we consider that:

"The relationship between aggression and limbic disfunction is now supported by a substantial literature. In particular the amygdala has been considered responsible for governing this emotion." (Papez 1937, McLean 1949, 1954) quoted by Taylor[6].

"There is now extensive evidence that destructive lesions within the temporal lobe of primates may act to disconnect emotion mediating, limbic structures (such as the amygdaloid complex and hippocampus) from sensory association cortices of the visual or auditory system, resulting in a loss of learned emotional associations"(Geschwind).[17]

"Surgical disconnection appears both to disrupt "old" emotional bonds, and to inhibit formation of new stimulus-reinforcement (or sensory-limbic) linkages" (Jones B, and Mishkin M.)[18]:

Bear[19] speculated that changes in emotional association, in temporal epileptics, may be a consequence of the stimulation of the limbic structures and adjacent association cortex, by an active epileptic focus, perhaps resulting in new adventitious emotional bonds.

The surgical remotion of the temporal lobe in the lobectomized patients, interrupt these circuits, the normal as well the possible pathologic ones, leading to a desorganization of the aggressive response as well as to the loss of old and distorted emotional bonds, which could be on the basis of an abnormal aggressive response. As the lobectomy is unilateral, it does not occur a real "taming" with loss of motivation, since the other side compensates such functions.

If our hypothesis is correct, the described effect can be considered as "psychosurgical," and would occur as an immediate consequence of the surgery.

On the other hand the remotion of the focus, that either disturbed the functioning of the brain as a whole, or parts of it, causing "intermittent functional disconnections" of variable intensities, reflects not only in the reduction or disappearing of seizure, but also in the intellectual functioning that becomes more flexible, with better attention and concentration and better functioning of memory, as it occurred with some of our patients.

These three phenomena that are observed soon after surgery: change of aggressiveness, improvement of cognitive functions and the reduction of seizures, are, therefore, from our point of view, the primary consequences of lobectomy and can be related neurophysiologically with the brain functions.

The primary consequences entering in a psychodynamic interaction with the remaining personality, will permit a reorganization which will depend however on its previous structure and on the experiences and social opportunities that the patient had after surgery.

The following report, 4 months after surgery of the patient nr 1, who had a chronic paranoid psicosis, shows how a personality with rigid structure can react badly to a change that the majority of the patients considered useful and pleasant:

"-I feel more like talking and it seems that I please more. The people don't recognize me - I am affraid of becoming too nice and they make a fool of me -

142

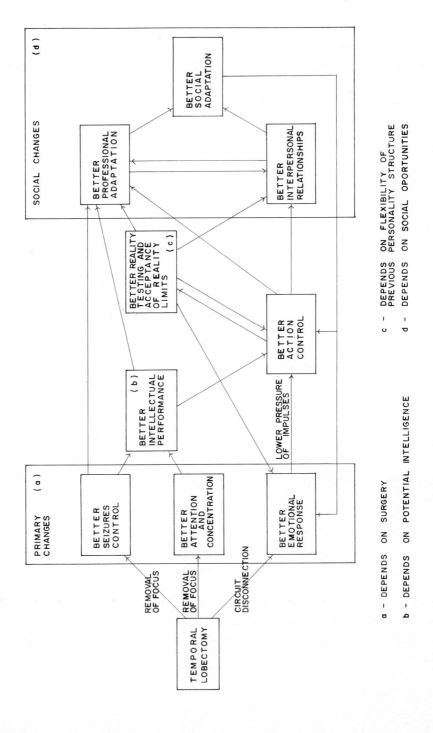

a - DEPENDS ON SURGERY

b - DEPENDS ON POTENTIAL INTELLIGENCE

c - DEPENDS ON FLEXIBILITY OF
    PREVIOUS PERSONALITY STRUCTURE

d - DEPENDS ON SOCIAL OPORTUNITIES

FIGURE 1   PERSONALITY   CHANGES   BLOCK   DIAGRAM

I don't want to be nervous as before, but I'm not so sure I can defend myself. If I want, I can attack, but I prefer to let things go. I'm affraid I'll let things go too much. I don't have anyone to defend me. I'm affraid the others will step on me. They envy too much that I got well."

We observe therefore that there is an addition of effects which influence each other resulting after some time a great variety of results.

We would like, however, to mention some other relationships that our study allowed us to notice. It was observed that the reduction and normalization of aggressiveness also contribute to the improvement of the intellectual function-ing. Therefore, during the early follow-ups the Rorschach test showed that the reduction of the instinctive pressure levels allowed a more adequate function-ing of the perception, that often became better structured and less distorted by emotions. This in a long term result, facilitated a better intellectual insight and reality testing, observed through the R.m.i. index.

As the patient adapts himself better and is able to do things with less anxiety and more efficiency, he gets less frustrated and therefore has less stimuli for his aggressiveness.

On the other hand, if through a better social adaptation the patient obtains gratification he has more to loose if he gets uncontrolled. This fact associat-ed with the previous ones explains, from our point of view, why there was a greater tendecy to control the physical and verbal aggressiveness after the surgery compared to the pre-operative levels.

(Among 9 patients with subjective aggressivenes, 4 could control themselves before surgery, while after surgery, among 7 patients with subjective aggres-siveness 6 were able to restrain it.)

The report of our patient nr. 7 (15 months after surgery) exemplifies what we just said: "-When a person feels himself inferior, full of drugs in his head, with the life without any purpose, it does not make any difference to control oneself or not. When Dr. Raul proposed surgery, what I really wanted was to die during operation. When someone starts enjoying to live, it is worth doing the best to control oneself, since there is more to lose."

The block diagram in figure 1 shows graphically the interrelationships proposed by the authors, of the personality changes observed.

BIBLIOGRAPHY

1. Jensen, Inge (1975) Temporal lobe surgery around the world.   Acta Neurol. Scandinav. 52, 354-373.
2. Glithero, Eric and Slater, Eliot (1963) The schizophrenia-like psychoses of epilepsy; IV Follow-up record and outcome. Brit. J. Psychiat. 109, 134-142.
3. Serafetinides, E.A. and Falconer, M.A. (1962). The effects of temporal lobectomy in epileptic patients with psychosis. J. Mental Sci., 108, 584-593.
4. Hill, J.D., Pond, D.A., Mitchell, W. and Falconer, M.A. (1957). Personality changes following temporal lobectomy for epilepsy. J.Mental Sci., 103, 18-27.
5. Hill, J.D. (1958). Proc.R. Soc. Med., 51, 610.
6. Taylor, D.C. (1972). Mental State and Temporal Lobe Epilepsy. Epilepsia, 13, 727-765.
7. Walker, A.E. and Blumer, D. (1977). Long term behavioral effects of temporal lobectomy for temporal lobe epilepsy. McLean Hosp. J., 85-103.
8. Horowitz, M.J., Cohen, F.M., Skolnikoff, A.A., Saunders., F.A. (1970). Psychomotor epilepsy: Rehabilitation after surgical treatment. J. Nerv. Ment. Dis. 150, 273-190.
9. Ferguson, S.M. and Rayport, M. (1965). The adjustment to living without epilepsy. J. Nerv. Ment. Dis., 140, 26-37.
10. Silveira, A. (1964) Prova de Rorschach: elaboração do psicograma. Edanee: São Paulo.
11. Piotrowski, Z.A.(1965): Perceptanalysis. Ex-libris: Philadelphia.
12. Small, L. (1956): Rorschach Location and Scoring Manual. Grune & Stratton: New York.
13. Silveira, A. (1958): Conative Index: an empirical evaluation of affective-emotional level of overt behavior. Comptes rendus, 4. Rorschach Internat. Congress. Brussels.
14. Silveira, A. (1965): Un indicateur pour le rapport intellectuel avec le monde exterieur. Comptes rendus, 6. Congrès Internat. Rorschach, Paris.
15. Silveira, A.(1970): Impulsiveness and ways of mastering it. Rorschach data with 100 adults. Rorschach Proceedings. VIIth Internat. Rorschach Congress, London, 1968. Hans Huber Publishers, Bern.
16. Camargo, C., Riva, D., Marino Jr, R. (1978): "Epileptic cognitive dysfunction" (E.C.D.) and psychiatric effects of epilepsy surgery. In this volume p. 145-150.

17. Geshwind, N. (1965): Disconnexion syndromes in animals and man. Part 1. Brain 88:237-294.
18. Jones, B., Mishkin, M. (1972) Limbic lesions and the problems of stimulus-reinforcement association. Experimental Neurology 36:362-377.
19. Bear, D. (1977) The Significance of Behavioral Change in Temporal Lobe Epilepsy. McLean Hosp. J. 9-21, June 1977.

© 1979 Elsevier/North-Holland Biomedical Press
Modern Concepts in Psychiatric Surgery
E.R. Hitchcock, H.T. Ballantine, Jr. and B.A. Meyerson, eds.

EPILEPTIC COGNITIVE DYSFUNCTION
AND THE PSYCHIATRIC EFFECTS OF EPILEPSY SURGERY.

Camargo C.P.,   Riva D.,   Radvany J.   and   Marino R.

Ten patients were submitted to temporal lobectomy for epilepsy. All were refractory to medical treatment. Selection
for surgery was based on very close follow-up, multiple drug
trials and determinations of serum anticonvulsant levels.

Besides the demonstration of the epileptic focus in the
left or right temporal lobes, all patients had extensive neuropsychological evaluation which revealed a cognitive dysfunction, suggesting involvement of frontal, parietal and temporal
lobes. The question was raised whether this dysfunction resulted from an interictal reticulo-cortical disturbance, determined by clinically undetectable epileptic discharges, or by
a diffuse cortical lesion. Neuropsychological re-evaluation
twelve to twenty-four months after surgery showed improvement
in all tests in most patients, suggesting that the dysfunction
was reticulo-cortical and not due to diffuse cortical lesions,
and that this reticulo-cortical disturbance was responsible
for the abnormalities found in testing higher cortical functions (1,2).

Three neuropsychological tests and a quantitative test of
attention were selected to illustrate this abnormality:

The first test was a test of word repetition. Series of
two to five simple unrelated words were presented verbally
and the patient was requested to repeat them after a pause of
15 seconds. This pause was either silent or filled with unrelated conversation.

Normal individuals repeated five to six words with no difficulty in any of these two conditions.

Abnormal responses consisted of less than five repeated
words, disordered sequence, perseveration, contamination of

From the Department of Functional Neurosurgery of the University of Sao Paulo Medical School and the Department of
Neurology, Boston University School of Medicine.

one word by an unrelated syllable and substitution of a word by another one presented to the patient in a previous series.

The second test ("word learning") consisted of showing the patient a card with a series of ten unrelated simple words. The patient was supposed to say how many words he expected to remember and then proceed to write them down in any order. This procedure was repeated ten times with the same card. At each time the patient's expectation as well as the number of words actually recalled were registered.

Normal individuals expected to recall seven to eight words at the first presentation of the card and this was the number they did recall indeed (congruent expectation = C). At each subsequent presentation of the same card the expectation and the number of words recalled increased in a parallel manner. With two or three presentations all ten words were learned and could consistently be recalled until the end of all the ten presentations of the card.

Abnormal responses consisted of a low number of words recalled at the first presentation, slow increase in the number of words recalled at each subsequent presentation, or a fluctuation in the number of words in subsequent presentations of the card. The expectation of the patients very often did not correspond to the number of words actually recalled (incongruent expectation = I).

These two tests involved the use of language. The abnormalities found, however, were the same in our patients no matter whether their epileptic focus was in the left or the right temporal lobe. Therefore, one could not attribute the poor performance in the tests to lesions of the left temporal lobe. So, we can conclude that word span, that is, immediate recall of words in these patients, was mostly a test of attention.

In the third test the patients had to perform two tasks: Block Design (Kohs' Cubes) and copy a cube in perspective (a Necker's cube). The purpose of these tasks was to detect constructional apraxia.

Kohs' Cubes evaluated the ability to transfer a bi-dimensional model into three-dimensional space. The intention was to check the patient's capacity to elaborate a strategy of approach and how he transferred the strategy from one model to the next. Necker's cube consisted of copying the drawing of the cube in perspective and of reproducing it from memory.

Normals had no difficulty in either task. Abnormal findings in Kohs' Cubes consisted of:

1. Apparently purposeless manipulation of the cubes (●).

2. Trial and error in all models without transference of strategy from one model to the next (■).

3. Errors of spacial inversion (▼).

4. No resemblance between model and construct (☉).

Abnormal findings in copying the drawing of the cube or in reproducing it from memory, consisted of :

1. Repeated trials and errors erasing the lines and arriving nowhere in spite of repeatedly consulting the model (□).

2. Loss of the perspective or the angles (▽).

3. No resemblance between model and drawing (○).

These tasks require adequate function of the temporo-parieto-occipital junctions and the frontal lobes. We thought we would find qualitative differences in the strategy of approach and the type of error, made by left as opposed to right temporal lobe epileptics. There was no difference found and there was marked improvement in constructional praxis after removal of the affected temporal lobe, without interference by surgery in the anatomy of the aforementioned temporo-parieto-occipital junctions and frontal lobes. We had to conclude that constructional apraxia before lobectomy was determined by a dysfunction in the maintenance of the level of the reticulo-cortical activation of these areas, and not due to focal lesions.

The fourth test used was Toulouse-Pieron's Test of Attention. This test allowed us to measure the speed and quality of a task in which attention is very much required. In this test the patient was presented a page filled with little individual squares. A small line touched either any one side or any one angle of each square. Of the eight possible combinations of square and its small line, the patient was supposed to cross-out four kinds which were represented in the upper left corner of the page. In five minutes the number of correctly crossed-out squares (speed) and the number of mistakes and omissions (quality) were counted.

NAME	AGE	SEX	DURATION	SIDE	WORD REPETITION — BEFORE: REPEATED WORDS	DISORDERED SEQUENCE	SUBSTITUTION	WORD REPETITION — AFTER: REPEATED WORDS	DISORDERED SEQUENCE	SUBSTITUTION	WORD LEARNING — BEFORE: EXPECTATION *	INSTABILITY IN LEARNING	PERSEVE-RATIONS	IRRELEVANT ASSOCIATIONS	WORD LEARNING — AFTER: EXPECTATION *	INSTABILITY IN LEARNING	PERSEVE-RATIONS	IRRELEVANT ASSOCIATIONS	ATTENTION B — CONSTRUCTIONAL	APRAXIA	ATTENTION A — CONSTRUCTIONAL	APRAXIA	ATTENTION B — SPEED	QUALITY	ATTENTION A — SPEED	QUALITY
JOP	28	♂	22	R	4			5			C			+	C				■◀	□ ○	■		110	110	16 18 84 2 1	21
GS	33	♀	21	R	5	+	++	5	+		C				C								130	101	60 8	8
JRA	27	♂	13	R	4	+	+	3	+		I	+			C				●■▶	▷		▷	94	101	07 6	6
MHZ	30	♀	29	R	4			5	+		I	+		+	C				●■▶	▷	■		unable	unable	80	6
JCM	21	♂	19	R	5	+	+	3		+	I	+			C				⊙	○	■		unable	unable	61	4
CS	27	♂	25	R	5	+	++	4		+	I	+			C	+			■▶●		●□	○	80	13	51	4
RC	28	♂	21	L	2		++	4		+	I	+	+		C				⊙●■▶	□□			67	8	68	0
HM	31	♀	26	L	4	++	++	4		+	I	+			C								115	19	126	2
MBC	29	♀	10	L	5	++	+	3			C				C								160	3	210	5
MRP	29	♀	17	L	4		++	4		+	I	+			I	+			■		▷		61	4	61	2

Normals reached at least half of the page and scored above 116 with four mistakes or omissions.

Abnormal responses consisted of low number of correct cross-outs along with omissions and errors. Although some patients had normal speed, the quality (omissions and errors) was abnormal.

After lobectomy, there was marked improvement in the ratio speed/quality, demonstrating an improvement in attention.

All patients were tested before and after surgery while still taking the same anticonvulsants, kept within therapeutic serum levels.

The results for each individual patient are shown in the table. The numbers indicate the best performance of examinations within the same or on subsequent days. This was necessary because this performance varied from one testing to the next, even within the same sitting. This fluctuation was marked before the operation and became negligible in the follow-up evaluations.

Two patients constituted exceptions:
MRP showed great stability in her equally poor performance before and after surgery. We believe that this stable poor performance was due to multiple cortical lesions caused by well documented repeated anoxic episodes during status epilepticus. Her pneumoencephalogram did indeed show diffuse cortical atrophy and generalized ventricular enlargement.

The post-operative performance of CS was poorer and showed more marked fluctuations than before the right temporal lobectomy. This became explained to us when follow-up electroencephalograms revealed a left temporal epileptic focus which was not detected on scalp recordings in his pre-operative tracings. It is important to note that CS had no clinical seizures after right temporal lobectomy, was kept on the same anticonvulsants with approximately the same serum levels within therapeutic range. Thus this patient illustrates that epileptic cognitive dysfunction has little to do with the frequency of overt clinical seizures.

The results above point to a disturbance in the function of structures that maintain an adequate level of attention for the performance of tasks even as simple as these. It was shown that this disturbance was independent from the side of the discharging focus, therefore, being related to a functional interference at the level of the reticular system. This involvment is of the most elementary function, indispensable for the performance of more complex tasks by the nervous system.

It was seen that this defective performance improved after surgery.

This disturbance has received very little attention in the study of temporal lobe epilepsy, the emphasis in most studies being on the frequency of seizures and on the personality disorder of these patients. However, subjecting the performance of these patients, and for that matter of any epileptic, to a qualitative analysis, it is possible to notice under close scrutiny the presence of subtle pervasive subclinical interictal abnormalities in attention. This interferes with mental activities such as orientation in complex situations, concentration, listening, memorizing, understanding and sequential planning. This results in an ongoing cognitive dysfunction that impairs performance and learning in school, in work, or in the patient's environment contributing to a feeling of failure and low self-esteem. The majority of these patients avoid significant interpersonal relationships or participation in social activites because they feel professionally and culturally disadvantaged.

The improvement of these patients after temporal lobectomy, associated with a reduction in this cognitive dysfunction, allowed many of them to return to school or to a profession, ultimately leading to better interpersonal relationships and social reintegration.

This raises the question whether we should extend the indications of epilepsy surgery to patients who exhibit this pattern of non-focal cognitive dysfunction in neuropsychological testing and an associated personality disorder by psychiatric evaluation, but who are otherwise well controlled as far as their seizures are concerned.

References:

1. Luria, A.R. (1966) Higher Cortical Functions in Man - Basic Books, Inc. Publishers.

2. Luria, A.R. (1966) The Working Brain - Penguin Books.

© 1979 Elsevier/North-Holland Biomedical Press
Modern Concepts in Psychiatric Surgery
E.R. Hitchcock, H.T. Ballantine, Jr. and B.A. Meyerson, eds.

AMYGDALA CHOLINERGIC HYPERSENSITIVITY:

IMPLICATIONS FOR PSYCHOMOTOR (LIMBIC) SEIZURES AND EPISODIC

BEHAVIOR DISORDERS

MAKRAM GIRGIS & LEOPOLD HOFSTATTER

University of Sydney, Australia, and University of Missouri-
Columbia, School of Medicine, Department of Psychiatry at
Missouri Institute of Psychiatry, U.S.A.; & University of
Missouri-Columbia, same as above.

This investigation is an attempt to create an experimental
model of temporal lobe epilepsy; as such it should not only
replicate some of the clinical and electrophysiological manifestations of temporal lobe epilepsy but allow conclusions as
to the underlying physiopathology, to its relationship to known
anatomical changes in the temporal lobes in that condition and
to possible therapeutic application.

The basal amygdaloid nucleus was made the target organ of
our experimental approach first because of its clinically and
experimentally well-established part in temporal lobe epilepsy
(DeFlorida & Delgado, 1958[1]; Grossman, 1963[2]; Belluzzi & Grossman, 1969[3]), of the successful surgical treatment of children
with temporal lobe epilepsy and related behavior disorders by
Narabayashi, et al (1963)[4] by means of stereotoxic amygdalectomy,
of the classical description of its relationship to violent
behavior by Mark and Ervin (1970)[5] in the framework of the
fight or flight response system for survival. of its hierar-
chical organization along an amygdala-hypothalamus-central gray
axis (Fernandez de Molina and Hunsperger, 1959[6]; 1962[7]; Girgis,
1971a[8]); of the production of a well co-ordinated attack behavior indistinguishable from ordinary one, with amygdaloid
stimulation (Kaada, et al, 1954 [9]; Zbrozjna, 1960[10]; Egger &
Flynn, 1963[11]), of the critical role of the muscarinic-cholinergic
mechanism in the modulation of rage and aggression (Karczmar,
1976[12]; Allikmets, 1974[13]) and of generalized convulsions
induced by cholinergic drugs.

The amygdala has furthermore the lowest threshold for EEG
seizures following electrical stimulation, also the lowest
threshold of excitability for overt convulsions, i.e. lower
than other brain structures (Goddard, et al, 1969[14]; Belluzzi,

152

1973[15]). The kindling effect of daily repeated electrical
stimulation, namely the gradual lowering of the convulsion
threshold, was found to be specific for limbic structures and
occurred far more readily in the amygdala (Goddard, et al,
1969[14]; and Delgado, et al, 1971[16]).

Histochemically, the amygdala is characterized and easily
identified by high acetyl-cholinesterase (AChE) enzymatic content and activity.

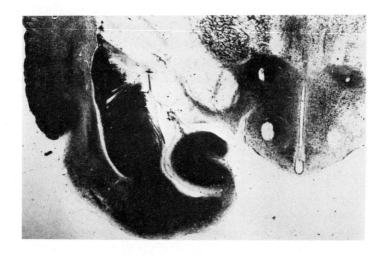

Fig. 1.   AChE in basal amygdala of monkey brain.

The stabilizing and protective role of AChE on the Acetycho-
line system by safeguarding the physiological threshold of
sensitivity to endogenous ACh and by preventing the development
of pathological cholinergic hyperactivity, hyper-reactivity, or
hypersensitivity was pointed out (Hofstatter, et al, 1973)[17].
The implication of ACh in head injuries, its release on the
surface of the cortex on cortical stimulation, into extracellular
spaces, the ventricles and cerebro-spinal fluid in convulsive
seizures and electroconvulsive treatment and the synergistic
aminergic-cholinergic neurotransmitter balance was presented
before. Increased sensitivity to topically applied ACh and
spontaneous epileptic discharges by chronically isolated cortex

because of local enzymatic AChE deficiency was demonstrated by
Echlin, et al, 1963[17a].

We were motivated in our investigations by the possibility of
obtaining EEG and possibly behavioral pattern in the monkey
comparable to those of psychomotor epilepsy in man by an experimentally produced local imbalance of neurotransmitters that
could be expected to bring about dysfunction of the underlying
structure, the amygdala, with associated behavioral and electrophysiological manifestations.

METHOD

In order to explore the relationship of histochemical, biochemical, neurophysiological and clinical findings, the behavioral and EEG effects of a single microinjection of neostigmine
into the basal amgdaloid nucleus were studied. Neostigmine
inhibits AChE and causes accumulation of ACh and facilitation
of ACh activity. Three months were allowed for observation of
the animals' normal behavior in individual cages.

Chemitrodes (Girgis, 1975)[18] that allowed not only injection
of isotonic saline solution or neostigmine through a cannula
guide but also to obtain EEG recordings from the amygdala and
the brain above, were implanted stereotaxically into the skulls
of 10 adult cebus monkeys (Cebus apalla) of 2½ kg weight under
aseptic conditions and intraperitoneal pentobarbital sodium
(45 mg/kg) anesthesia.

The bipolar teflon insulated stainless steel wire electrodes,
each 0.08 in. in diameter, were fixed in a miniature electric
connector (9-pin Winchester socket). The recording cable was
fabricated from individually shielded wires fixed to a Win=
chester 9-pin plug, which mated with the chronic electrode
connector on the skull. The cannula guide was constructed from
a 25 gauge lumbar puncture needle which extended about 8 mm
deep to the cerebral cortex.

For 2 or 3 weeks after stereotaxic brain surgery EEG tracings
were obtained and compared with those following injection of a
normal (isotonic) saline solution into the target and after
the same experimental amount of neostigmine was deposited 2
to 3 mm above the predetermined target area in two other monkeys.

154

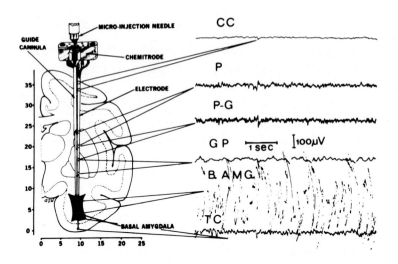

Fig. 2. Chemitrode in basal amygdala and paroxysmal EEG
discharge in response to intracerebral (amygdala) neostigmine
injection.

Then 5-8 ul of neostigmine bromide (1 μg/1 ul) was slowly,
over a period of 4 minutes, injected into the basal amygdaloid
nucleus by means of a Hamilton microsyringe and a very fine
microneedle. EEG activity from the basal amygdala at a depth
of 18 mm and of 4 layers above 2 mm apart was recorded with
the aid of an 8 channel electroencephalograph (Beckman Polygraph)
immediately prior to, during the injection of neostigmine, after
the injection, and subsequently every 15 minutes for a total
of three hours and at weekly intervals over a period of 3 months;
in three animals EEG studies were extended over 6 months. At
the end of our correlative observations of the dramatic, though
temporary and gradually subsiding, electroencelphalographic and
the continuing and persistent behavioral changes consequent to
the neostigmine dose injected, the effect of i.m. atropine
injections (0.5 mg to 1.0 mg/kg, occasionally 2.5 mg/kg) on
these monkeys were studied.

Histological examination of frozen sections through the area
of the chemitrode, stained with luxol-fast blue, confirmed the
intended placement of the electrode loci in all animals. A

small area of necrotic tissue was found within 1/2 mm of the tip of the implanted cannula guide, about 20 mm above the intact amygdala, 8 mm below the cerebral cortex.

RESULTS

The surgical stereotaxic procedure of implanting the chemitrodes as such had no immediate and subsequent effect on electrical and behavior activities. The effects of intracerebral neostigmine microinjection on the animals' behavior and on the EEG, however, was impressive. After a latency of about two hours a series of complex behavioral phenomena made their appearance. The animal became restless, protrusion of the tongue, rhythmic smacking,licking, and chewing, i.e. an automatism of masticatory movements became manifest; this was associated with considerable salivation and occasional turning of the head in one direction, myoclonus in the opposite muscles of facial expression, particularly in the orbicularis-oculi and orbicularis oris. Occasional evidence of angry expression occurred during this initial period.

An episode of true rage reaction became more apparent after a few hours whenever the monkey was approached. These episodes lasted about 2-3 minutes and were followed by (post-ictal) loss of tone and a period of confusion during which the animal was unresponsive and looked around aimlessly. After regaining its usual alertness the animal became aggressive and remained so throughout the period of experimentation.

During the first few weeks after the neostigmine injection, the aggressive reaction required no special provocation. The aggressive animal would attack another Cebus monkey in the same cage and inflict severe wounds. The animal would also try to attack any person approaching the cage and was too dangerous to be handled except after an intramuscular injection of the anesthetic ketamine. Therefore, the animals were housed in squeeze back cages. After repeated injections of atropine a real rage reaction of these aggressive animals occurred only upon direct provocation. No overt epileptic convulsions were ever observed in these animals; their attack behavior, that persisted and outlasted electrical changes, resembles, to a great extent, the clinical behavior of patients with temporal epilepsy, particularly those with episodic behavior disorders.

EEG changes also started to occur after a latency of 2 hours and continued for several days, up to seven weeks, as the result of one single intracerebral injection of neostigmine. They consisted in bursts of paroxysmal discharges (high voltage spike, sharpwave, polyspike and wave). Three weeks later, spikes occurred and still showed high amplitude slow wave patterns; one pattern was characterized by high voltage waves at a frequency of 8-10 Hz, a second pattern was characterized by polyspikes of 10-12 cps frequency. The paroxysmal activity remained always restricted to the area of the neostigmine application. Neither saline injection nor neostigmine above the predetermined amygdaloid site had brought about any electrophysiological nor behavioral responses.

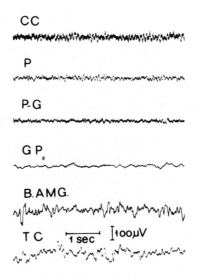

Fig. 3. Dampening effect of i.m. Atropine upon the EEG seizure pattern elicited by neostigmine micro-injection into the amygdala.

Intramuscular administration of the anticholinergic atropine
(0.5 mg/kg) slightly reduced the amplitude and frequency of
spiked discharges in the amygdala and induced slow waves in the
remaining areas of the brain. A consistent shift to low
voltage slow activity of the EEG (after a delay of about 25
minutes) resembled drowsiness, although the animals were
awake, a dissociation of electrical pattern and behavior
(Wikler, 1952)[19]. Larger amounts of atropine (1 mg/kg) obscured
the high amplitude spike discharges, temporarily, with slow
waves; 2 mg/kg of atropine produced even more prominent slow
waves, further obscuring the spike discharges, that would
reappear the next day. In the interval between atropine injections that were given for about two months at weekly intervals
with the identical results (Fig. 3), the EEG activity at the
amygdaloid site showed always high amplitude activity. Toward
the end of the second month the EEG records gradually diminished and returned to normal. The electrophysiological changes
produced by neostigmine injected into the amygdala nucleus of
the monkey bear close resemblance to those observed and
described in temporal lobe epilepsy in humans.

DISCUSSION

The method of liquid neostigmine intracerebral microinjection
has the advantage over cristaline carbachol injection (Grossman, 1963)[2] of exact dosage without the hazards of its hygro-
scopic properties, of being reproducible, of restriction of
spike activity to the amygdala, of avoidance of electrophysiological spread to other areas of the brain, resemblance of the
EEG response to the pattern of human psychomotor seizures and
absence of overt generalized epileptic seizures. Bandler, Jr.
(1970)[20] and Igic, et al (1970)[21] also described persistent
behavioral changes, hyperactivity and aggression, not associated with overt convulsions following cholinergic stimulation
of certain limbic structures such as the hypothalamus and some
amygdaloid nuclei.

The latency of electrophysiological and behavior manifestations appears to reflect the slow and gradual inhibition of
AChE enzyme activity by the injected neostigmine and the
resulting slowly increasing amygdaloid ACh levels.

Behavior effects and EEG changes in animals comparable to

those of temporal lobe epilepsy in humans could be produced by
interfering with the neurotransmitter balance i.e. increasing
the local concentration, availability and activity of ACh by
injecting a minimal amount of neostigmine, an AChE inhibitor,
into the amygdala and could be antagonized by cholinergic
blocking agents, like intramuscular atropine or scopolamine.
They both apparently are mediated by the acetyl-choline system,
the significance of which for the physiopathology of psychomotor seizures and episodic behavior disorders in man becomes
apparent.

The biochemical mechanism responsible for the precipitation
of temporal lobe epilepsy may rest in either uninhibited abnormal cholinergic hyperactivity, possibly due to a primary defect
or decrease of the protective AChE that no longer counteracts
the development of bizarre sensitivity in susceptible cells
(Hofstatter, et al, 1973)[17] and parallels the increased sensitivity to endogenous ACh.(Hebb, et al, 1963[22]; Rosenberg, et
al, 1968[23]).

Supersensitivity may moreover play an important part in
those instances, where associated or underlying structural
pathology in the temporal lobe (Glaser, et al, 1963[24]; Falconer, et al, 1958[25]; Falconer, et al, 1963[26]), may have led to
disconnection of nerve pathways and isolation with decreased
cholinesterase activity (Echlin, et al, 1962)[17a] and increased
reactivity to ACh i.e. to denervation or disuse supersensitivity (Cannon, et al, 1949)[27] to endogenous ACh. This raises
the practical possibility of appropriate use of anticholinergic
drugs in temporal lobe epilepsy as a rational therapeutic
measure.

CONCLUSION

We have attempted to experimentally lay the foundation of
an animal model of temporal lobe epilepsy, including psychomotor (limbic) seizures and episodic behavior disorders that
not only replicates the behavioral and electrophysiological
manifestations but also allows a better understanding of the
underlying biochemical mechanism, namely of the ACh system
through either ACh hyperactivity possibly due to a primary AChE
deficiency or, where structural pathology is concerned, through
denervation or disuse supersensitivity to endogenous acetyl-

choline.

REFERENCES

1. DeFlorida, F.A. & Delgado, J.M.R. (1958) Amer. J. Physiol. 193, 223-229.
2. Grossman, S.P. (1963) Science 142, 409-411.
3. Belluzzi, J.D. & Grossman, S.P. (1969) Science 166, 1435-1437.
4. Narabayashi, H., Nagao, T., Saito, Y., Yoshida, M., & Nagahata, M. (1963) Neurol. (Chic) 9, 1-16.
5. Mark, V.H. & Ervin, F.R. (1970) in: Violence and the Brain, Harper & Row, New York, pp 170.
6. Fernandez de Molina, A., & Hunsperger, R.W. (1959) J. Physiol. 145, 251-265.
7. Fernandez de Molina, A. & Hunsperger, R.W. (1962) J. Physiol., 160, 200-213.
8. Girgis, M. (1971a). Int. J. Neurol. 8, 327-351.
9. Kaada, B.R., Andersen, P., & Jansen, J. (1954) Neurology (Minneap) 4, 48-64.
10. Zbrozyna, A.W. (1960) J. Physiol. 153, 27-28.
11. Egger, M.D. & Flynn, J.P. (1963) J. Neurophysiol. 26, 705-720.
12. Karczmar, A.G. (1976) in: Biology of Cholinergic Function A.M. Goldberg & I. Hanin, eds., Raven Press, New York, pp 395-449.
13. Allikmets, L.H. (1974) Med. Biol. 52, 19-30.
14. Goddard, G.V., McIntyre, D.C., & Leech, C.K. (1969) Exp. Neurol. 25, 295-330.
15. Belluzzi, J.D. (1972) J. Comp. and Physiol. Psych. 80, 269-282.
16. Delgado, J.M.R., Rivera, M.L., & Mir, D. (1971). Brain Res. 27, 111-131.
17. Hofstatter, L. & Girgis, M. (1973) in: Surgical Approaches in Psychiatry. L.V. Laitinen & K.E. Livingston, eds., Univ. Park Press, Baltimore, Chap. 31.
17a. Echlin, F.A. & Battista, A. (1963) Arch. Neurol. (Chic) 9, 154-170.
18. Girgis, M. (1975) J. Electrophysiol Tech. 5, 42-46.

19. Wikler, A. (1952) Proc. Soc. Exp. Biol. 79, 261-265.

20. Bandler, Jr.,R.J. (1970) Brain Res. 20, 409-424.

21. Igic, R., Stern, P., & Basagic, E. (1970) Neuropharmaco. 9, 73-75.

22. Hebb, C.O., Krnjevic, K., & Silver, A., (1963). Nature (London) 198, 692.

23. Rosenberg, P. & Echlin, F.A. (1968) J. Nerv. Ment. Dis. 147, 56-63.

24. Glaser, G.H., Newman, R.J., & Schafer, R. (1963) in: EEG and Behavior. G.H. Glaser, ed.. Basic Books, New York, pp 345-365.

25. Falconer, M.A., Hill, D., Meyer, A., and Wilson, J.L. (1958) in: Temporal Lobe Epilepsy. M. Baldwin & P. Bailey, eds., Thomas, Springfield, pp 396-410.

26. Falconer, M.A. & Serafetinides, E.A. (1963) J. Neurol. Neurosurg. Psychiat. 26, 154-165.

27. Cannon, W.B.A. & Rosenblueth, A. (1949) in: The Supersensitivity of Denervated Structures; a Law of Denervation. McMillan, New York, pp 245.

© 1979 Elsevier/North-Holland Biomedical Press
Modern Concepts in Psychiatric Surgery
E.R. Hitchcock, H.T. Ballantine, Jr. and B.A. Meyerson, eds.

TEMPORAL LOBE DYSFUNCTION TREATED BY MINUTE
SURGICAL LESIONS *

Dr. MANUEL VELASCO-SUAREZ, F.A.C.S.
INSTITUTO NACIONAL DE NEUROLOGIA Y NEUROCIRUGIA
Mexico - 1978

Past interest in temporal lobe dysfunction has centered
largely on epileptic phenomena. However careful clinical
observation of interictal behavior may aid in selection of
drug resistant patients for surgery and in determining lateralization of the lesion. Of assistance also are deep electrode
placements for recording, stimulation and, on occasion, the
production of minute radiothermic or electrolytic lesions.

It is generally believed that the left temporal lobe is
related to intellectual activity and the right to emotional
content and altered behavior.

The pioneer work of Klüver and Bucy[15] on temporal lobe
function demonstrated emotional changes including aggression
and sociopathic behavior. Extrapolations from their studies
suggested limbic dysfunction and the possibility of treatment through deafferentation of the amygdala.

Our studies as well as those of others have suggested
lateralization of certain symptoms[1,2,10,9,24, 21, 17,19,20]
and that the left lobe specializes chiefly in intellectual
activities: linguistics, memory, analytic processing, self-
deception and personal dependence.[12] In contrast, the right
lobe specializes in the less intellectual functions though
capable of synthesizing affective tone. Should there be
some doubt about the lateralization of abnormal discharge
and related symptoms Wada's test, using unilateral intra-
carotid injection of barbiturates, may be of assistance
in further interpretation of the depth recordings.

The limbic differentiated subcortical apparatus is known
to be involved in the regulation of endocrine-visceral effector mechanisms and their functional patterns are expressed

---

* Controlled recently by CT SCAN - and assisted by Dr. A.
F'dez-Guardiola of our Brain Research Unit INNN.
FIFTH CONGRESS OF PSYCHIATRIC SURGERY - BOSTON,
August 21-25, 1978

POSTOPERATIVE RESULTS*

Problem	Patients No.	Operations	Results	Side Effects	Evolution
Psychomot Epilepsy -Periodic aggressiveness	5	Open unilateral amygdalectomy	50% acceptable, good 50% paradoxical behavior improved, seizured recurred	Hyperactivity & iteration; floating sensation in 2	19 years 1 15 years 2 10 years 2
Psychomot Epilepsy -Permanent abnormal	4	Stereotaxic medial Amygdala lesion, dorsomedial Thalamus (Unilat) in one	2 markedly good 1 improved 1 not improved	(Transient) 1 insomnia 1 hyperphagia 4 increased libido	8 years 7 years 50% 1 1/2 years
Schizoids -aggressiveness -destructiveness - violence -hallucinosis	3	Amygdala & dorsomedial Thalamus or GI.Pallidus	2 moderately improved 1 markedly improved (working)	overdependence	8 years to 3 months

* From two groups of 36 patients, the remainder have been treated also with chemicals (intracerebral carbachol, atropine, L Dopa and opiates).

through behavioral motivation and correlated attitudes.[32]
The endocrine system serves as a modulating agent of
amygdaloid-hippocampal activities, potentiated by a great
chain of hormones acting on enkefalin or endorfin receptors.

The structures implicated in long circuits linking the
temporal complex to a fairly well defined subcortical neural
continuum from the septal region to the mid-brain[13]
receive discharges from the hippocampus and amygdala via
the fornix, thence by way of the thalamus and the medial
forebrain bundle to the cingulum and orbital cortex.[4,5]

The frontal lobe and the limbic-subcortical axis[14]
encompass brain activities that allow man to be human.
Its dysfunction compromises the SELF and may make social
life impossible. Surgical lesions in the system, as
emphasized by Nauta[18], even though minimal and productive
of therapeutical benefit may be accompanied by some other
"minimal" loss.

Subjects:

Selection of patients for operation depended primarily
on the nature of the seizures and the EEG patterns.[8,11,23,25]
However operation was carried out in some patients with
characteristic behavioral patterns in whom it was possible,
through stimulation of implanted electrodes, to produce
anger, to stop rage or to alter a disturbed mood. From
two groups of patients, totalling 36 individuals[29] we
we have selected 12 cases, some with long term follow-up.

Five of these underwent open amygdalectomy (one left
for right) between 1959 and 1966. Of this initial group
of five all are working and are earning a living. Prior
to operation all had had intractable seizures associated
with unilateral positive temporal EEG foci.

In the other seven deep electrodes were placed for
stimulation recording and the subsequent creation of
minute lesions.[27-31] Bilateral recordings and stimulation were carried out in the amygdala, hippocampus,
the thamalic nuclei and the globus pallidus before
choosing the side for creating a minute lesion.

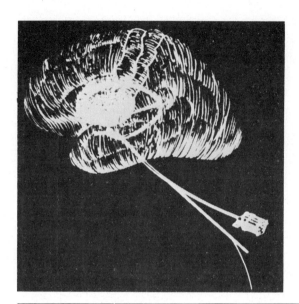

Fig. 1. Left amygdaloid phantom with deep electrode.

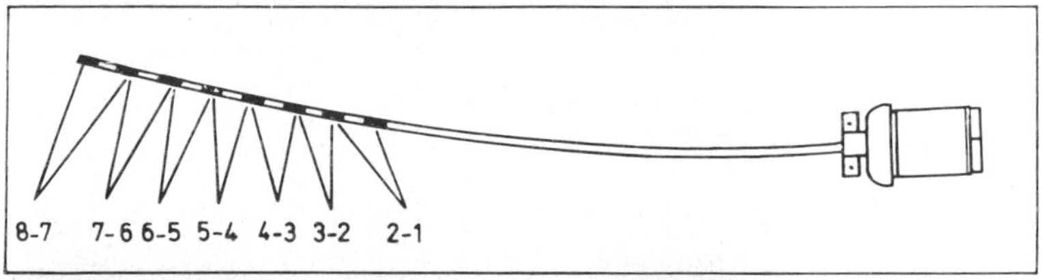

8-7   7-6 6-5 5-4 4-3 3-2 2-1

Fig. 2.

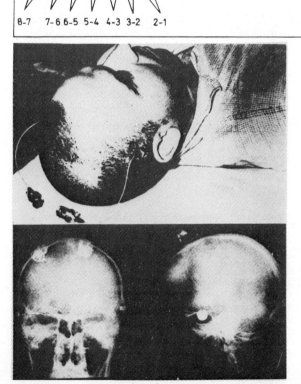

Fig. 3. Cannulated screws and electrodes in place for recording and stimulation.

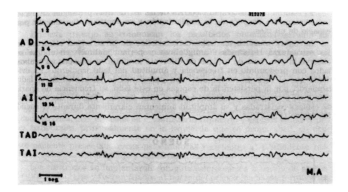

Fig. 4. Preoperative tracing.

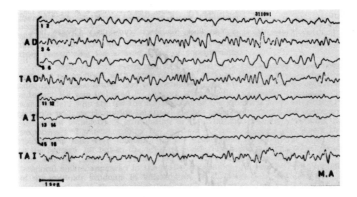

Fig. 5. Postoperative tracing.

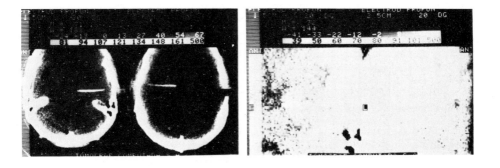

Fig. 6. Tc scan with deep electrodes.

Operative Technique:

The electrodes were implanted under local anesthesia
utilizing the "INN" stereo-apparatus. Using the tube-
guides, burr holes were placed in the temporal region bilaterally, 1.5 cm above the zygoma and 2.5 cm behind the
external orbital arch. The target area lay 15 to 20 mm
anterior to the center of the pineal gland in the frontal
plane and 15 mm lateral to the sagital plane. The
electrodes were directed toward the posterior clinoid
and positioned with the aid of x-ray visualization, in
the last case by CT scanning. Bipolar square wave
stimulation (1 ms., 50Hz) was used, the current being
gradually increased. Stimulation was stopped when
electrical or clinical seizures were produced or when
post discharge activity was recorded.

Observations:

In almost all cases of left amygdalo-hippocampal
stimulation there were observed confusion and vague
auditory hallucinations accompanied occasionally by
reminiscent phenomena (motion picture). Simultaneously
there were noted tachycardia, increased blood pressure,
polypnea, opening and closing of the eyes, elevation of
the arms, and sometimes spitting and perseveration of
movements.

The affective content of verbal responses was constant
when the same point was stimulated, Thus, as has been
recorded in the motion picture of one of our patients,
she experienced a pleasant moment at kindergarten.

There were manifestations of pleasures and joy. The next
stimulus, however, 5mm laterally, produced the panic of
being raped, assulted and injured with a knife.

Discussion:

Depth electrodes making possible both focal stimulation
and EEG observations are helpful in deciding whether to
create a lesion, not where the stimulus elicits memory
responses, but where it produces rage, compulsive tics,
aggressiveness and/or epileptic seizures. We believe that
minute central amygdala lesions of the dominant hemisphere
are apt to cause confusion and memory disturbance.

It should be emphasized that whenever we work with the amygdala or the thalamus we are affecting the limbic system as a whole and in regulating behavior we may influence other physiologic responses within the limbic system.

Conclusion:

One can justify only minimal surgically produced lesions of the limbic system in the efforts to control anxiety, negative mood changes, aggressive behavior or intractable psychomotor epilepsy. Limbic dysfunction manifests itself as disorders of electrical and chemical changes reflected as mood, personality and behavioral disturbances.

REFERENCES

1.   Bear DM, Fedio P: Quantitative analysis of interictal behavior in temporal lobe epilepsy. Arch Neurol 34:454-467, 1977.

2.   Blumer D: Temporal lobe epilepsy and its psychiatric significance, in Benson DF, Blumer D (eds): Psychiatric Aspects of Neurologic Disease. New York, Grune & Stratton Inc., 1975.

3.   Donnelly EF, Dent JK, Murphy DL, et al: Comparison of temporal epileptics and affective disorders on the Halstead-Reitan test battery. J Clin Psychol 28:61-62, 1972.

4.   Escobedo F, Fernandez-Guardiola A, Solis G: Chronic stimulation of the cingulum in humans with behaviour disorders, in Laitinen L: Surgical Approaches in Psychiatry. Baltimore, University Park Press, 1973.

5.   Personal Communication: A. Fernandez-Guardiola.

6.   Feindel W, Penfield W: Localization of discharge in temporal lobe automatism. AMA Arch Neurol & Psychiat 72:605-630, 1954.

7.   Flor-Henry P: Psychosis and temporal lobe epilepsy: a controlled investigation. Epilepsia 10:363-395, 1969.

8.   Williams JM, Freeman W: Amygdaloidectomy for suppression of auditory hallucinations; preliminary report of theory and its application in one case. M Ann District of Columbia 20:192-196, 1951.

9.   Gazzaniga MS: The Bisected Brain. New York, Appleton-Century-Crofts, Inc., 1970.

10. Geschwind N: Disconnexion syndromes in animals and man:II Brain 88:585-644, 1965.

11. Gloor P: The pattern of conduction of amygdaloid seizure discharge: an experimental study in the cat. AMA Arch Neurol & Psychiat 77:247-258, 1957.

12. Harris RJ: A Primer of Multivariate Statistics. New York, Academic Press, 1974.

13. Hassler R, Deickmann G: Relief of obsessive-convulsive disorders, phobias and tics by stereotactic coagulation of the rostral intra-luminal and medial-thalamic neuclei, in Laitinen L:Surgical Approaches in Psychiatry. Baltimore, University Park Press, 1973.

14. Kim YK, Umbach W: Combined stereotactic lesions for treatment of behavior disorders and severe pain, in Laitinen L: Surgical Approaches in Psychiatry. Baltimore, University Park Press, 1973.

15. Klüver H, Bucy PC: Preliminary analysis of functions of temporal lobes in monkeys. Arch Neurol & Psychiat 42:979-1000, 1939.

16. MacLean PD, Rodriguez Delegato JM: Electrical and chemical stimulation of the frontotemporal portion of limbic system in waking animal. Electroencephalog & Clin Neurophysiol 5:91-100, 1953.

17. Mark VH, Ervin FR: Violence and the Brain. New York, Harper & Row, 1970.

18. Nauta WJH: Connections of the frontal lobe with the limbic system, in Laitinen L: Surgical Approaches in Psychiatry. Baltimore, University Park Press, 1973.

19. Penfield W, Jasper H: Epilepsy and the Functional Anatomy of the Human Brain. Boston, Little, Brown and Company, 1954.

20. Penfield W: Functional localization in temporal and deep sylvian areas. Res Pub Ass Res Nerv Ment Dis 36: 210-226, 1958.

21. Rossi GF, Rosadini G: Experimental analysis of cerebral dominance in man, in Darley FL, et al (eds): Brain Mechanisms Underlying Speech and Language. New York, Grune & Stratton Inc., 1967.

22. Schwab RS, Sweet WH, Mark VH, et al: Treatment of intractable temporal lobe epilepsy by stereotactic amygdala lesions. Trans Amer Neurol Ass 90:12-19, 1965.

23. Spiegel EA, Wycis HT (eds): Advances in stereoencephalotomy, Vol. 2. Pain, convulsive disorders, behavioral and other effects on stereoencephalotomy. White Plains, New York, Albert J Phiebig, 1966.

24. Sperry RW: Lateral specialization in the surgically separated hemispheres, in Schmitt FO, Worden FG (eds): The Neurosciences: Third Study Program. Cambridge, Mass. MIT Press, 1973.

25. Talairach J, Szikla G, Tournoux P, et al: Atlas of stereotaxic anatomy of the telencephalon. Paris, Masson, 1967.

26. Velasco-Suarez M: Amygdaloidectomia en el tratamiento de desordenes mentales de predominio alucinatorio. Cir Cir 20:225-249, 1952.

27. Velasco-Suarez M: Epilepsia Psicomotora Temporal Amigdalina Asambleas. Mexico 2: 37-43, 1962.

28. Velasco-Suarez M, Guzman-Flores, et al: Epilepsia Temporal, Estimulacion, Registro y Cirujia de Profundidad. Simpsio Internacional "Lobulo Temporal" actividades cientificas inaugurales del Instituto Nacional de Neurologia y Neurocirugia (Velasco-Suarez y Escobedo). Memoria Nov 1964, Edit. Progreso, Mexico, D.F.

29. Velasco-Suarez M: Electrical and chemical stimulation of limbic structures within the temporal lobe. Confin Neurol. Wycis Supplement, Stereoencephalotomy. Basel, Karger, 1964.

30. Velasco-Suarez M: Stereotaxic neurosurgery in Latin America. Confin Neurol 23:516-519, 1963.

31. Velasco-Suarez M: Temporal epilepsy: deep electrodes and amygdaloidectomy. Med Ann DC 33:251-253, 1964.

32. Walker AE, Thomson AF, McQueen JD: Behavior and the temporal rhinencephalon in monkey. Bull Johns Hopkins Hosp 93:65-93, 1953.

© 1979 Elsevier/North-Holland Biomedical Press
Modern Concepts in Psychiatric Surgery
E.R. Hitchcock, H.T. Ballantine, Jr. and B.A. Meyerson, eds.

TEMPORAL LOBE SEIZURES AND HYPERSEXUALITY

(TESTOSTERONE EFFECTS)

O. J. Andy, T. Kurimoto, and S. Velamati

Department of Neurosurgery

University of Mississippi Medical Center

INTRODUCTION

The present investigation is a further attempt to elucidate underlying
mechanisms of seizure induced hypersexuality. It was previously demonstrated that repeatedly induced limbic seizures elicited postical hypersexual behavior in the adult male cat.[1] It was also noted that
dopaminergic mechanisms facilitated the development of the postictal
hypersexual state.[2] Since circulating androgens are not elevated during
hightened sexual activity[3] and since the cortex appears essential for
initiating mating behavior in most male mammals[4,5] the question
arises as to whether a neural circuit, once established, can be activated
in the absence of circulating androgens. It was previously observed that
the postictal hypersexual behavior induced by repeated limbic stimulations was abolished following castration.[6] The present study attempts to
more critically determine whether the hypersexual response to androgens
is an "all-or-none" phenomenon or a graded response related to the available hormone.

PROCEDURE

Animals. Eleven adult male alley cats were used for this study.

Electrode Insertion. Bipolar electrodes 1.5 mm apart, 1 mm bare tip
were placed under general anesthesia. Electrode placements were histo-
logically verified as indicated (table 1) in limbic, basal ganglia and
diencephlic structures.

Electrical Stimulation and Recordings. Electrical stimulation was
performed with a glass square-wave stimulator. The stimulation consisted
of a constant current, 60 cps, 1 msp applied for a period of 15 sec.
Each brain site was stimulated with three different levels of progressively increasing increments of current, during one session. The threshold for inducing seizures was established for each subject. Parameters
used for seizure induction consisted of current values at threshold in
addition to two additional levels of stimulation, each of which was at a
0.2 MA higher interval than the lower one. The brain structures were
stimulated in rotation. The interval between each applied stimulus was
three minutes. A daily stimulation session consisted of stimulating 2 to
4 structures in a fixed sequence. Each structure was stimulated one to

TABLE 1

INTRACEREBRAL TESTOSTERONE INJECTION (▲) AND STIMULATION (X,O) SITES

SUBJECTS	HYPERSEXUAL						NON-HYPERSEXUAL				
	30	31	32	35	40	43	36	37	41	42	44
L. SEPTUM											X
R. SEPTUM	X			X		±▲			X▲		
L. AM	X		X	o▲	X▲	X▲	X		X▲	X▲	
R. AM	X		X	X		o	▲		X▲		X▲
L. AAA		▲									
L. HIPP		±									
R. HIPP			X								
L. A HY					±	o		X			
L. L HY				o							
R. A HY		X					±▲				±
R. L HY		X		o▲			±▲				
R. M HY	±						o▲				
L. THAL											o▲
R. THAL							X▲				
R. L GEN		X									
L. PUT							X▲	o▲			
L. GP							X▲	o▲			
R. CN		X		o			±▲				
R. MES TEG		o					X▲				
L. PED		o								o	
SEIZURES (N)	162	35	67	99	55	22	78	15	56	6	15
STIMULATIONS	567	864	444	1,224	171	225	588	324	288	36	81
TOTAL SEIZURE DURATION	9,174	3,166	5,899	7,491	4,819	724	5,685	1,000	3,156	148	354
STIM. DAYS	63	96	37	102	57	25	49	27	32	4	9

X = SEIZURES O = NO SEIZURES ▲ = INTRACEREBRAL TESTOSTERONE

three times daily. Stimulation days were grouped in sets of 3 to 5 days. A rest period of at least two days occurred on the weekend. The total number of stimulations were 4,812. The total number of seizures induced were a total of 610. Bipolar recordings were made with a glass electro-encephalograph.

Behavior. The subjects were allowed to move freely in a chamber (3.5'x 1.5'x 1.5') with a transparent window. The behavior of the animal was evaluated before and after the applied drugs and stimulations. Sexuality was evaluated by exposing the male to another male cat. The hypersexual drive was rated from one to 5 plus as follows: 1 plus vocalization and approach, 2 plus biting, 3 plus mounting, 4 plus pelvic thrust and 5 plus intromission. In the present experiment 5 plus was not accomplished since the animals were not exposed to female partners.

Drugs. The following drugs were given individually or in sequential combinations at a given session before the onset of the applied stimulation. D-amphetamine 1 mg/lb., 1 mg/lb. (1 to 4 doses) systemically and testosterone (intracerebral) 0.1 mg/lb. Following the drug injections the subjects were observed for 15 to 30 minutes before stimulations were induced. Intracerebral injections were performed through chronic inplanted "chemode" made from 20 gage needles. Testosterone propionate in oil and saline were used. In some instances, a 22 gage properly insulated "chemode" also served for recording and stimulation.

Histology. The animals were sacrified with a general anesthetic and brains prefused with a 10% Formalin, serially sectioned and stained for cells.

RESULTS

Onset Day of Hypersexuality. Postictal hypersexuality developed within 3 to 27 stimulation days (fig. 1). Subject A-32 displayed the best example of progressively increasing seizure duration over time, termed "seizure-maturation period", leading to postictal hypersexual behavior (A-32, fig. 1). The "seizure-maturation period" tends to be longer if after-discharges are infrequently elicited, as in subject A-31, (fig. 1). The discharge durations coinciding with the hypersexuality "onset-day" are usually longer than previously elicited discharges. In subject A-35 an abrupt change occurred on the 5th to 7th day suggesting a change from one discharge system to another, which under the influence of amphetamine, progressively peaked in duration from the 5th to the 9th day.

Testosterone, Catecholamine and Stimulation Treatment Modalities. Testosterone administered as a single treatment when injected intra-cerebrally in 5 subjects and systematically in 6 did not induce hyper-sexuality (table 2). Administration of catecholamines alone did not

TABLE 2

HYPERSEXUALITY RELATED TO SINGLE AND COMBINED TREATMENTS

SUBJECT	Single treatments				Combined treatments							
	CT	ST	C	S	S+ST	S+C	S+ST+C	S+CT	S+CT+C	CT+ST	CT+C	ST+C
30	NT	o	o	o	o	o	●	NT	NT	NT	NT	o
31	o	o	o	o	o	o	o	●	●	o	o	o
32	NT	o	NT	o	●	NT	●	NT	NT	NT	NT	o
35	o	NT	NT	●	NT	●	●	●	●	NT	NT	●*
36	o	NT	o	o	NT	o	o	o	o	o	o	o
37	o	o	o	o	o	o	o	o	o	o	o	o
40	NT	o	NT	●	NT	o	●	NT	●	o	●*	o
41	o	o	NT	o	o	o	o	o	o	o	NT	o
42	NT	NT	NT	o	NT	NT	NT	o	NT	NT	NT	NT
43	NT	NT	NT	o	NT	o	o	NT	o	o	o	●*
44	NT	NT	NT	o	o	o	o	o	o	o	o	o

ST = Systemic Testosterone CT = Intracerebral Testosterone NT = Not Tested
C = Catecholamine - (amphetamine and/or apomorphine) ● = Hypersexuality
o = No Hypersexuality S = Stimulation-seizures * = Hypersexuality attenuated

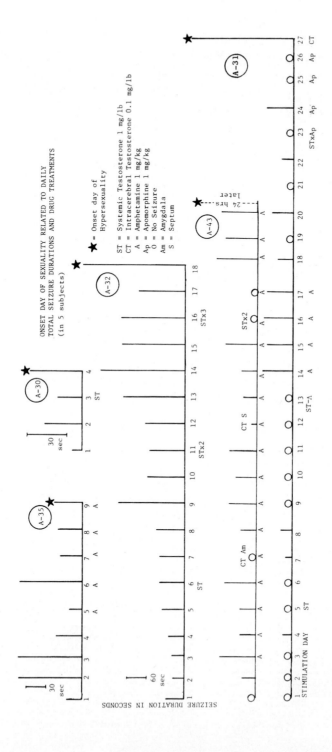

Fig. 1. Total daily seizure duration in sec. is graphed for 5 subjects identified by encircled numbers. The 60 sec. calibration also applies to subjects A-43 and A-31.

induce hypersexuality. Stimulation with associated after-discharge was
the only single treatment which induced hypersexuality, 2 of 11 subjects (18%).

Among the combined treatment modalities electrical stimulation plus
systemic testosterone and catecholamine elicited hypersexuality in (40%)
of the subjects. Electrical stimulation plus intracerebral testosterone
plus catecholamine elicited hypersexuality in (38%) of subjects. The
percent frequency among subjects obtained from other combined treatments
were as follows: electrical stimulation plus intracerebral testosterone
(29%), electrical stimulation plus systemic testosterone (17%), electrical stimulation plus catecholamine (11%), intracerebral testosterone plus
catecholamine (16%), systemic testosterone plus catecholamine (20%), and
systemic testosterone plus intracerebral testosterone (0%).

Although the numbers are too few for statistical analysis they suggest
that administration of either systemic or intracerebral testosterone at
the dose levels used, does not induce hypersexuality unless one or more
additional treatment also is applied. The most effective treatment for
inducing hypersexual behavior is testosterone, either intracerebral or
systemic, plus electrical stimulation and a catecholamine agonist.

Testosterone Potentiated Effects. An increased amount of available
testosterone was accompanied by an increased magnitude of hypersexuality.
For example, a 3 plus postictal sexual response became 4 plus when the
dose of testosterone was doubled in subject A-40, (compare sessions 43-47
and 48-52, fig. 2).

Catecholaminergic drugs also tended to enhance the testosterone
effects. A lower dose of testosterone when combined with apomorphine
elicited the same response which previously necessitated a greater
amount of testosterone as a single treatment (fig. 3, A-32 sessions
16-20 and 29-33).

Testosterone Inhibited Effects. In 3 subjects spontaneous hypersexuality was present in 23 of the test trials before the treatments were
applied. ELectrical stimulation and after-discharges abolished the
hypersexual state in 13 of the 23 trials. These observations suggest
that the "sexual system" which is already "overactive," tends to be
dampened by superimposed subsequent treatments such as electrical stimu.
lations and discharges (fig. 2, sessions 1-5, 20-23, 28-30, 31-34).

Catecholamine antagonists also tended to attenuate the electrically
induced discharge and to prevent the development of postictal hypersexual
behavior. In subject A-31, hypersexual behavior did not develop in
response to intracerebral testosterone when combined with haloperidol

176

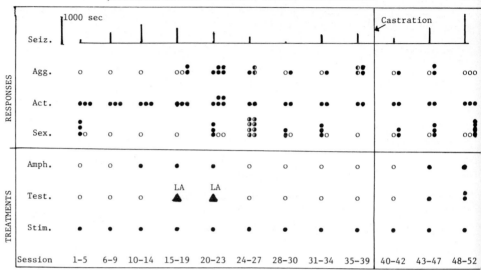

Fig. 2.   Treatment modalities and responses are related to weekly
cumulated test sessions for a period of 52 sessions in subject A-40.
Seizures (Seiz.), Aggression (Agg.), Activity (Act.), Hypersexual (Sex.),
Amphetamine (Amph.), Testosterone (Test.), Stimulation (Stim.).   The
vertical bars represent seizure durations for each group of test
sessions.   Three consecutive dots and/or circles in horizontal sequence
under responses refers to a specific behavior observation made (1) before
a drug is injected (first symbol); (2) after the drug is injected (second
symbol); and (3) after the electrical stimulation and seizure (third
symbol).   The number of vertically oriented black dots refers to the
magnitude of the behavior response (1 to 4 black dots equal 1 to 4 plus
response) and for testosterone it refers to magnitude of the dose, (1 to
3 dots equal single to triple dose).   Session (24-27), a 4 plus hypersexuality before stimulation (4 solid dots) was unchanged in session 24
and abolished in session 27 (both) identified by 4 half filled dots.

and phenoxybenzamine (fig. 4 insert 4).   However, postictal hypersexuality

developed in response to intracerebral testosterone when combined with

amphetamine (fig. 5 insert 5).

Endogenous Androgen Reduction Effects.   Castration was used in 5

subjects to abruptly reduce the major source of endogenous testosterone in

addition to other androgens.   A 24 to 48 hr. period of increased sexual

response to limbic stimulation and seizures usually occurred after

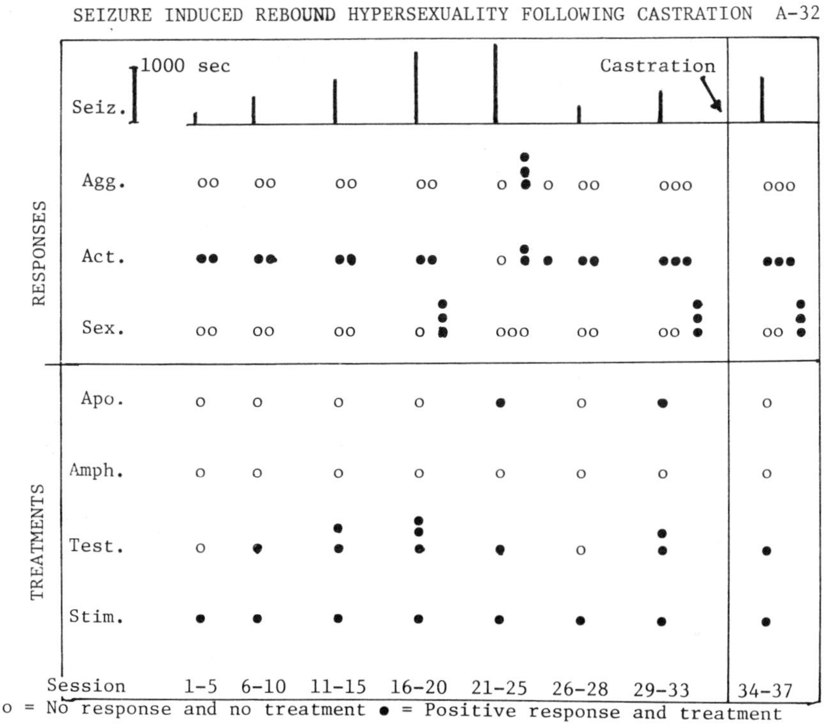

SEIZURE INDUCED REBOUND HYPERSEXUALITY FOLLOWING CASTRATION   A-32

							Castration	
Seiz.								

RESPONSES

Agg.	oo	oo	oo	oo	o ●● o	oo	ooo	ooo
Act.	●●	●●	●●	●●	o ●● ●	●●	●●●	●●●
Sex.	oo	oo	oo	o ●●	ooo	oo	oo ●●	oo ●●

TREATMENTS

Apo.	o	o	o	o	●	o	●	o
Amph.	o	o	o	o	o	o	o	o
Test.	o	●	●	●	●	o	●	●
Stim.	●	●	●	●	●	●	●	●

| Session | 1-5 | 6-10 | 11-15 | 16-20 | 21-25 | 26-28 | 29-33 | 34-37 |

o = No response and no treatment ● = Positive response and treatment

Fig. 3.   Subject A-32 Apomorphine (Apo.).   For further details refer to fig. 2.

castration. Hypersexuality became pronounced and could be elicited with decreased treatment magnitudes. Following castration, subject (A-35) developed spontaneous hypersexuality (fig. 5 compare inserts 1 and 2). Subject (A-40) went from zero to 2 plus hypersexuality (fig. 2). Subject (A-30) went from 2 plus to 3 plus, and subject (A-32) displayed 3 plus postictal sexuality with one dose of testosterone whereas before castration 2 doses of testosterone were needed, in addition to apomorphine, to elicit the same response (fig. 3). In subject (A-40) stimulation and seizures alone, immediately after castration resulted in hypersexuality whereas similar treatments before castration were ineffective (fig. 2, compare sessions 35-39 and 40-42).

The percent number after-discharges elicited from a given limbic structure within 24 hrs. after castration, were either (1) increased; (2) unchanged or (3) decreased. In 4 of 8 stimulated structures the

178

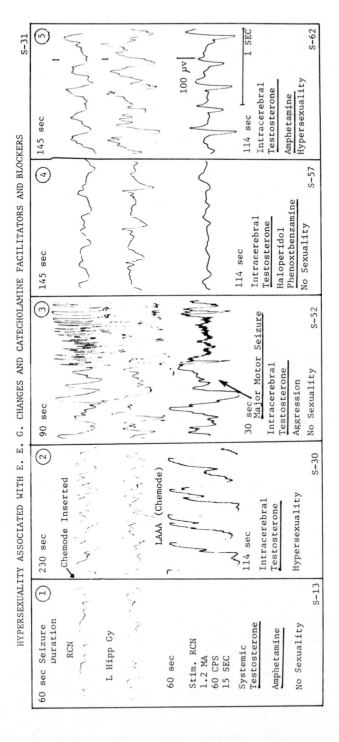

Fig. 4. Subject A-31. Inserts 1 through 5 represent 1.5 sec. strips of 5 independent limbic system after-discharges. Note that testosterone injected in the left anterior amygdaloid area (LAAA) potentiated the after-discharge and was conducive to postictal hypersexual behavior (insert 2), whereas systemic testosterone did not have similar effects (insert 1). Amphetamine (insert 5) reversed the effects of haloperidol and phenoxybenzamine. Following a major motor seizure there was no postictal hypersexuality, it was replaced by aggression (insert 3). Left hippocampal gyrus (L Hipp Gy), right caudate nucleus (R CN).

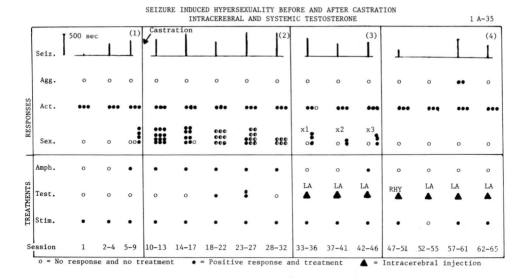

SEIZURE INDUCED HYPERSEXUALITY BEFORE AND AFTER CASTRATION
INTRACEREBRAL AND SYSTEMIC TESTOSTERONE   1 A-35

o = No response and no treatment   ● = Positive response and treatment   ▲ = Intracerebral injection

Fig. 5. Subject A-35. Treatment modalities and responses are related to weekly cumulated test sessions for a period of 102 sessions. Left amygdala, (LA), right posterior hypothalamus, just lateral to the mammillary body (RHY), number of stimulation trials which displayed hypersexuality (X1 to X5). Refer to fig. 2 for further interpretation of symbols.

percent number of seizures elicited after castration more than doubled. In 3 of 8 structures the percent number of seizures after castration was unchanged. In 1 of 8 it was decreased. The after-discharge duration before and after castration averaged 108.7 and 91.0 sec. respectively for structures displaying increased number of seizures. Structures displaying no change in the number of seizures reflected increased seizure durations after castration, going from an average of 50.2 sec. before, to 77.4 sec. after castration

Seven to 14 days after castration, postictal hypersexual behavior could not be elicited, unless testosterone replacement therapy was also administered. The effect of testosterone replacement therapy peaked at 2 to 4 days after injection. The postictal hypersexual responses gradually decreased in magnitude and frequency of occurrence over a period of 7 days, following which they were no longer elicitable. In order to repeatedly elicit postictal hypersexuality after castration, it was necessary to administer weekly injections of testosterone, starting one to two weeks after the castration.

180

Brain Structures Associated with Postictal Hypersexuality. The
amygdaloid nucleus was implicated by electrical stimulation and/or testosterone injection in the 6 of 11 subjects which developed hypersexual
behavior (table 1). The amygdala also was represented in 3 of 4 subjects
which did not develop hypersexuality. Several factors were thought to
account for the lack of hypersexuality in those 3 subjects. In two
subjects (A-42 and A-44, table 1), the number of stimulations and
seizures were relatively very few. In addition, testosterone injected
in the thalamus of subject A-44 could have counteracted the anticipated
amygdaloid hypersexual response. This possible mechanism, in part, was
supported by the observation that one subject, (A-36), with testosterone
in the thalamus, hypothalamus, putamen, globus pullidus mesencephalon
and amygdala also did not develop hypersexuality. In A-37 hypersexuality
did not occur following injection of the hypothalamus and basal ganglia.
That the amydgala is involved with development of the behavior and that
extra amygdaloid structures may be inhibitory is also suggested by the
following observation. Testosterone injection in the right
posterolateral hypothalamus of subject A-35 abolished hypersexuality
which was previously induced by testosterone injected in the amygdala
(fig. 5, compare inserts 3 and 4). Following the subsequent return of
hypersexuality in response to systemic testosterone in the same subject,
a repeat injection in the right posterolateral hypothalamus reproduced
the inhibitory effects on sexuality (fig. 6, compare inserts 5 and 6).
The remaining subject which lacked hypersexuality, A-41, developed
intractable recurring seizures immediately after the testosterone
injection in the amygdala. The spontaneously recurring motor seizures
continued for 10 days. Electrical stimulation was discontinued for 1
week and phenobarbital given to stop the seizures. Although the spontaneous seizures stopped, hypersexuality in response to various treatments did not develop. The lack of sexuality could have been due to
postictal depression of the system subsequent to the prolonged and
recurring spontaneous discharges and the phenobarbital.[7]

DISCUSSION

Testosterone Graded Effects on Postictal Hypersexuality. Although
seizure induced postictal hypersexuality is androgen dependent, it is not
an "all-or-none" response. In the castrated male cat, the behavioral
level of postictal hypersexuality can be graded. Increasing the dose of
testosterone will increase the level of response. A low level postictal

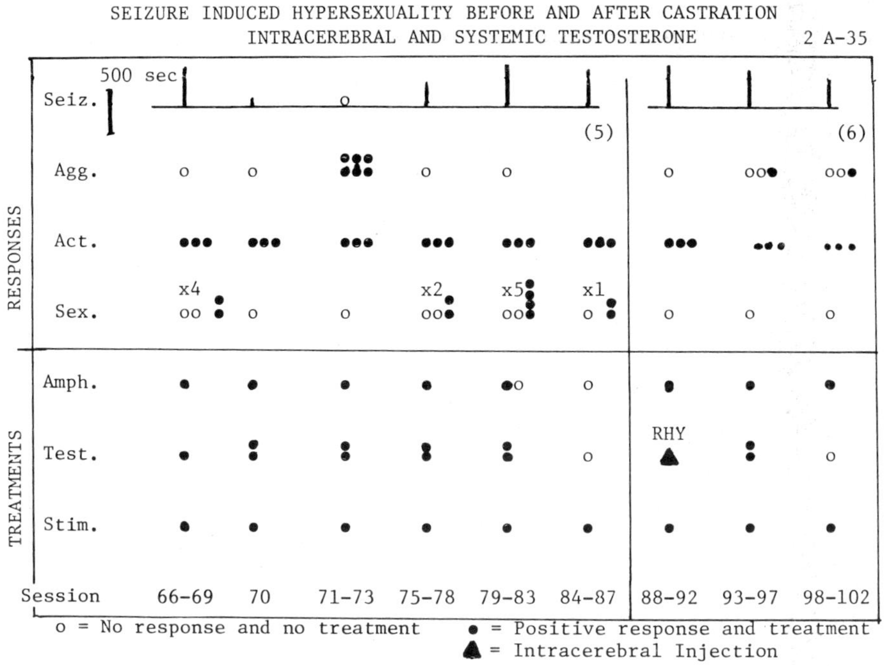

SEIZURE INDUCED HYPERSEXUALITY BEFORE AND AFTER CASTRATION
INTRACEREBRAL AND SYSTEMIC TESTOSTERONE   2 A-35

Seiz. 500 sec	┃	┃ ᴵ	o	┃	┃	┃ (5)	┃	┃	┃ (6)

RESPONSES

	66-69	70	71-73	75-78	79-83	84-87	88-92	93-97	98-102
Agg.	o	o	●●● ●●●	o	o		o	oo●	oo●
Act.	●●●	●●●	●●●	●●●	●●●	●●●	●●●	●●●●	●●●
Sex.	x4 oo ●	o	o	x2 oo●	x5 oo●	x1 o ●	o	o	o

TREATMENTS

Amph.	●	●	●	●	●o	o	●	●	●
Test.	●	●●	●●	●●	●●	o	RHY ▲	●●	o
Stim.	●	●	●	●	●	●	●	●	●

Session   66-69   70   71-73   75-78   79-83   84-87   88-92   93-97   98-102

o = No response and no treatment   ● = Positive response and treatment
                                        ▲ = Intracerebral Injection

Fig. 6. Subject A-35. This figure is a continuation of fig. 5. Note
that the 4 plus sexual response was elicited in each of 5 sessions
(sessions 79-83). However, following injection of testosterone in the
posterior hypothalamus, the response was blocked (session 93-97).

response to testosterone also can be changed to a higher level response
by adding a catecholamine agonist, such as amphetamine or apomorphine.
The dopaminergic facilitation of the testosterone effects is in agreement
with previous observations[2,7].

    Theoretical Mechanisms Underlying Postictal Sexual Changes.

    Testosterone and Postictal Hypersexuality. The limbic after-discharge
in part, identifies the hypersexual system in addition to other
behavioral systems and leaves them in a state of postictal hyperexit-
ability. Since several systems are similarly affected they tend to
remain in a balanced functional interrelationship to one another, and no
specific behavioral system predominates over the other. However, the
sexual system can specifically be further activated by testosterone
injections. This will tilt the balance in favor of the androgen labelled
system and hypersexuality will emerge as the predominant activity.

Catecholamine, although not considered specific for the system, can further potentiate the testosterone triggered behavior. Under these circumstances, hypersexuality will become the dominating postictal behavior in spite of the discharge having also implicated other behavioral systems. On the other hand, reducing the available androgen may reduce sexuality and simultaneously permit another behavioral system to become surfaced.

Testosterone and Postictal Hyposexuality . Excessive activity in the sexual system, as reflected by the occurrence of spontaneous hypersexuality, makes the system vulnerable to being postictally depressed by repeated seizures. This statement, which is an apparent contradiction to the one in the preceeding paragraph necessitates further amplification. Hypersexuality behavior is more likely to occur in the early stages of seizure evolution in both the cat[1] and human[8,9] and hypersexuality is more likely to occur in the later stages of seizure evolution as also demonstrated in both the cat[1] and human[9, 11, 12, 13]. This evolved change in sexuality associated with the evolution of limbic seizures was identified as the "hypersexual growth and decay curve"[1]. The late hypersexual effects may in part be due to involvement of serotonergic inhibitory mechanisms.[1] Recurrent interictal seizures also leave the system in a depressed or hypersexual state as observed in subject A-41. This also is in agreement with previous observation[1, 14]. Administration of testosterone in this instance does not counteract the seizure induced postictal depression (fig. 4, insert 3).

Testosterone and Posterolateral Hypothalamic Inhibition of Sexuality. The inhibitory effects associated with the posterolateral hypothalamic injection of testosterone may be due to the activation of posterior hypothalamic inhibitory mechanisms. That a sexual inhibitory system may be activated through the posterior hypothalamus is also suggested from human and animal lesions in that area[15, 16, 17]. In contrast, a facilitatory system for sexual activity exists in the anterior hypothalamus-preoptic-septal area as suggested by the loss of sexual potency and activity following lesions[15, 16] and facilitation of sexual behaviors following stimulation in these areas[19, 20]. The question remains as to what is the underlying neurophysiologic and anatomic mechanism for the testosterone induce inhibition when injected into the posterior hypothalamus. One speculation is that the serotonergic mesencephalic inhibitory system (fig. 7) is secondarily activated by way of the mammillotegmental tract which sends fiber projections to the dorsal and ventral tegmental

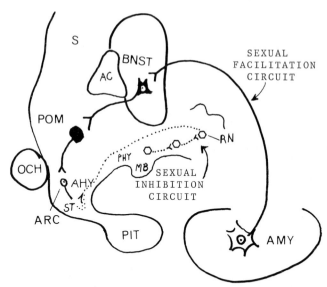

Fig. 7. Diagram atic respresentation of limbic and mesencephalic sexual facilitatory and inhibitory circuits (theoretical). Anterior commissure (AC), amygdala (AMY), anterior hypothalamus (AHY), arcuate nucleus (ARC), mammillary body (MB), bed nucleus of stri terminalis (BNST), posterior hypothalamus (PHY), pituitary gland (PIT), medial preoptic area (POM), raphe nuclei (RN), septum (S), and serotonergic terminals (ST).

nuclei the mesencephalic reticular nuclei and interpeduncular nucleus. This projection may both directly and indirectly implicate the inhibitory serotonergic neurons of the mesencephalic raphe nucleus. The projected serotonergic terminals in the anterior hypothalamus releases the monoamine.

SUMMARY

1. Postictal hypersexual behavior is testosterone dependent in the male cat.

2. The testosterone effect is not an all-or-none phenomenon. The magnitude of the sexual response is in part dose dependent.

3. The testosterone effect is potentiated during the first 24 to 48 hours following castration. This may be a rebound phenomenon due to sudden endogenous androgen deprivation and/or post operative stress released catecholamines.

4. Seizure characteristics 24 hrs. after castration displayed either an increased duration or increased frequency of occurrence.

5. The testosterone dependent postictal hypersexual state is
    potentiated by catecholamine agonists and attenuated by
    catecholamine antagonists.

6. Spontaneously existing interictal hypersexuality can be abolished
    by the same limbic discharges which were responsible for its
    development.

7. The amygdala was the optimum anatomical site for testosterone in
    order to activate postictal hypersexual behavior. Testosterone
    injection in the basal ganglia, thalamus and hypothalamus did not
    activate postictal hypersexuality.

8. Posterolateral hypothalamic-injected testosterone abolished
    postictal hypersexual behavior which had been previously activated
    by either systemic or intracerebral (amygdala) injected test-
    osterone.

9. Theoretical facilitatory and inhibitory mechanisms underlying
    postictal hypersexuality and hyposexuality in relation to test-
    osterone were discussed.

REFERENCES

1. Andy, O. J., (1977) Hypersexuality and limbic system seizures,
    Pav. J. Biol. Sci., V 12 N4, pp. 187-228.

2. Andy, O. J. and Velamati,(1978) Temporal lobe seizures and
    hypersexuality (Dopaminergic Effects) J. of Applied Neurophysical.

3. Blumer, D. and Walker A. (1975) The neural basis of sexual
    behavior, Ch. 11, Psychiatric Aspects of Neurologic Disease
    Ed Benson, D. F. and Blumer D., Grune Stratton.

4. Beach FA: (1940) Effects of cortical lesions upon the copulatory
    behavior of male rats, J. Comp Psychol 29: pp. 193-239.

5. Beach FA: (1943) Effects of injury to the cerebral cortex upon
    the display of masculine and feminine mating behavior by female
    rats, J. Comp Psychol 36: pp. 169-199.

6. Andy and Velamati, (1978) presented at the Am. Assc. of Neurol.
    Surgeons, New Orleans, LA.

7. Resan T. K., (1972) Shahida, NT, Korst, D. R., The effect of
    phenobarbital on testosterone induced erythropoiesis, J. Lab,
    Clin. Med., 79: p. 187.

8. Gessa, G. and Tagliamonee, A. (1974) Role of brain monoamies in
    male sexual behavior, Life Sciences, 14: pp. 425-426.

9. Gastaut, H. and Callomb, H. (1954) Etude the comportement
    sexual chez les Epileptiques Psychomoteurs, Ann Med. Psychol, 112:
    pp. 657-696.

10. Peters, U. H., (1971) Sexualstortungen bei psychomotorischer
    Epilepsie, J. Neurol. Transm. Suppl X: pp 491-497.

for instance, all referrals concerned indicate subjectively
sexual drive as high, so that they have a certain motivation for
the operation. After the intervention, patients understate the
strength of sexual drive to document the success of the procedure
and to have an argument for their release and this should be
taken into consideration.

The table shows the subjective statements about strength of
sexual drive and the frequency of masturbation reported by the
patients and by observations of the prison guards. Other explanations such as frequently changing contacts or heterosexual
experience are not acceptable since patients were in custody.
Instead of this, visual excitability was taken as a criterion. This
means sexual excitability when looking at stimulating objects,
no matter where and when. The visual stimulation was especially
high in patients sentenced to prison for rapes.

For all patients the strength of postoperative sexual drive
was reported as reduced (Table 4). The frequency of masturbation
and the visual excitability were almost always reduced. The
patients also reported that the preoperative highly intensive
thoughts of sexual ideas and sexual phantasies were reduced
substantially. This resulted in a better concentration because
of freedom from sexual thoughts. The frequency of masturbation

Table 4

Postoperative Sexual Excitability of Sexual Delinquents

	Reduced	Unchanged
Strength of Sexual Drive (n = 11)	11	-
Frequency of Masturbation (n = 10)	9	1
Visual Excitability (n = 9)	8	1

is only reported in 10 patients because one of the 11 patients denied masturbatory activity before operation. The visual excitability is reproted only in 9 patients because it was not investigated in the first 2 patients.

The majority of the patients reported preoperatively an extreme sexual restlessness. In this state they were looking for sexually stimulating objects with increasing intensity. This led to a walking and driving around for hours. If such an object was found, a pursuit of the same duration followed. This extreme sexual restlessness was reported by 8 patients preoperatively especially the rape delinquents; postoperatively it disappeared (Table 5).

Table 5

Extreme Sexual Restlessness and Aggressiveness in Sexual Delinquents

Extreme Sexual Restlessness (n = 11)		Aggressiveness (n = 9)	
preop.	postop.	preop.	postop.
8	-	7	1

Aggressiveness upon denial or during sexual intercourse existed preoperatively among all 11 patients to varying degrees. Post-operatively patient 10 and 11 cannot be judged, because they are not released yet. Among the other 9 patients 7 showed this aggressiveness preoperatively, but only one patient postoperatively showed an aggressiveness upon denial but not during intercourse. This judgement was based on the statements of the intimate partners.

A high sexual drive and a high sexual excitability, an extreme sexual restlessness and the sexual aggressiveness were the deciding criteria for the indication of a stereotactic hypothala-motomy.

Table 6 shows the family relations before and after the operation. The marriage of 3 patients lasted even through a long confinement so that it could be continued after release. After release, another patient married the woman he was divorced from 10 years

Table 6

Family Status in Sexual Delinquents

Name		Preoperative	Postoperative
1) A.I.	(ped.)	married	married
2) G.H.	(ped.)	unmarried	married
3) G.J.	(rape)	divorced	married
4) J.K.	(ped.)	married	married
5) R.S.	(rape)	unmarried	intimate partnership
6) P.B.	(arson)	divorced	married
7) K.F.	(rape)	married (1 child)	married (2 Children)
8) J.P.	(rape)	unmarried	unmarried
9) H.S.	(ped.)	unmarried	unmarried
10) K.M.	(ped.)	unmarried	
11) C.K-B.	(ped.)	unmarried	

ago. 2 other men married for the first time after the operation and another one lives unmarried in an intimate partnership.

Concerning the question of sexual reorientation from homosexual to heterosexual interests, it can be stated in general, that in our pedophilic patients the homosexual interests were not eliminated but fewer pedophilic acts occurred and they were able to control their behaviour better. In these cases a marriage occurred for reasons of family care and some reported heterosexual intercourse. In the case of primarily existing heterosexuality, especially so-called "hypersexuality", the former is reduced but not extinguished.

Table 7 shows the development in profession after the operation. Here we can only refer to 9 patients, because the other 2 are still imprisoned. 2 patients, No. 2 and 7, showed remarkable professional advancement; another 4 patients show stabilization in the acquired profession. Patient No. 8 reveals the only deteriorated case; he was an unskilled worker preoperatively, became unemployed postoperatively, became neglected because there were no family relations, became an alcoholic and is now in prison again for warehouse-theft. He had already been prosecuted for the same offence preoperatively. Patient No. 4

Table 7

Development in Profession of Sexual Delinquents

		Preoperative	Recent State
1)	A.I.	Waiter	Head Waiter
2)	G.H.	Engineer	Vice-President
3)	G.J.	Unskilled Worker	Skilled Worker
4)	J.K.	Trucker	Unemployed
5)	R.S.	Welding Operator	Welding Operator
6)	P.B.	Labourer	Foreman
7)	K.F.	Trucker	Storekeeper
8)	J.P.	Unskilled Worker	Unemployed
9)	H.S.	Mason Apprentice	Chief Mason

pre- and postoperatively worked as a trucker but became unemployed
due to a disease of his knee-joint and there is no causal relation
between unemployment and operation. Concerning the rehabilitation
in profession one has to remember that the operative intervention
and the subsequent release in most cases took place after a long
period of detention. Such a history is no recommendation for
re-employment in the old profession or new employment in another
profession. From this point of view the rehabilitation in
profession of our patients, with the exception of patient No. 8,
should be considered as good.

In the complex results of the psychological tests we found a
decrease in the intensity of sexual needs, a change in reaction
to colours and changes of recognition in the subject field of
experience. In most patients a previously existing disturbing
egocentrism was diminished and patients seemed to be more stable.
With one exception they lived in a serious social system. The
tendency of the integration in profession or stabilization up
to promotion is clear. The reduction of the sexual drive and the
configuration of sexuality during normal daily life are two
experiences which are obviously caused by the organic intervention.

There were no other side-effects from unilateral anterior
hypothalamotomy. About half of the patients showed a strong
feeling of hunger and consequently gained weight postoperatively
for 2 or 3 years, although this was controllable to a certain
extent. Other side-effects (Dieckmann and Hassler 1975, 1977)
were transient.

CONCLUSION

Although the investigations are incomplete they reveal
that anterior hypothalamotomy has a specific influence on
sexual behaviour, substantially reducing sexual excitability,
aggressiveness and extreme sexual restlessness so that the sexual
behaviour can be adapted to the normal conditions necessary in
society. From a psychological point of view a different situation
is created by the organic intervention in which the patients are
able to solve their problems in a better way, corresponding to
their plans and attitudes as well as their wants, so achieving
better motivation. The changed interior situation post-operatively
reflects the beginning of further development supported by psychotherapy which is the aim of the operation.

ABSTRACT

The present study deals with the long-term results of unilateral
anterior hypothalamotomy in the treatment of sexual violence in
11 patients. The results on sexuality, social outcome and
personal development of these patients are reported after their
release from imprisonment.

REFERENCES

1. Dieckmann, G. and Hassler, R. (1975) Confin. Neurol. 37,
   pp. 177-186.

2. Dieckmann, G. and Hassler, R. (1977) in Neurosurgical Treatment
   in Psychiatry, Pain, and Epilepsy, Sweet, W.H., Obrador, S.
   and Martin-Rodriguez, J.G. eds., University Park Press, Baltimore, London, Tokyo, pp. 451-462.

3. Roeder, D. (1966) Confin. Neurol. 27, pp. 162-163.

© 1979 Elsevier/North-Holland Biomedical Press
Modern Concepts in Psychiatric Surgery
E.R. Hitchcock, H.T. Ballantine, Jr. and B.A. Meyerson, eds.

LONG-TERM FOLLOW-UP RESULTS OF THE POSTEROMEDIAL HYPOTHALAMOTOMY

YOSHIAKI MAYANAGI and KEIJI SANO
Department of Neurosurgery, University of Tokyo,
7-3-1, Hongo, Bunkyo-ku, Tokyo (Japan)

ABSTRACT

Stereotactic surgery to the posteromedial hypothalamus gave satisfactory results for controlling violent or aggressive behavioral disorders in the long-term follow-up for 2 to 16 years. From the endocrinological point of view, this procedure activated the hypothalamic-pituitary axis only temporarily, without causing any serious dysfunctions. Postoperative physical development in childhood cases was normal. The follow-up results showed effect of this procedure for controlling epileptic seizures.

INTRODUCTION

In order to ameliorate behavioral disorders, particularly those of violent or aggressive nature, a small lesion was made stereotactically in the postero-medial hypothalamus, which is actually a continuation of the central periaqued-uctal grey matter. Since the first operation in 1962, for the treatment of this condition, 60 cases have been accumulated, 44 males and 16 females, includ-ing 29 childhood cases. These patients have been followed for more than two years, with 58 cases for as long as 5 to 16 years. This paper deals with long-term follow-up results of these cases, concerning not only behavioral, but also endocrinological, developmental and epileptic conditions.

OPERATIVE PROCEDURE

After demonstration of the third ventricle, a fine concentric bipolar needle electrode was stereotactically inserted through a frontal burr hole into the target point. The coordinate of the target point, at present, is 2 mm below the midcommissural point and 2 mm lateral from the wall of the third ventricle.

Responses caused by high frequency stimulation of this point can be summar-ized as follows:

1) Autonomic responses, mainly sympathetic

   Elevation of blood pressure

   Increase of pulse rate

   Respiratory arrest followed by hyperpnea or tachypnea

   Mydriasis

   Flushing of the face

2) Somatomotor responses

   Inward and downward movement of the eye ball on the stimulated side

   Lateral flexion of the neck toward the stimulated side

3) EEG responses

   Diffuse slow waves of 2-3 Hz (under light general anesthesia)

   Diffuse desynchronization (in awake state)

4) Endocrinological responses

   Elevation of plasma value of pituitary hormones

   Elevation of plasma value of catecholamines

   Elevation of plasma value of nonesterified fatty acids

The area, where good sympathetic responses could be obtained, forms a small "ergotropic triangle" in the posterior hypothalamus, surrounded by lines connecting the midcommissural point, the mammillary body and the posterior commissure. On the frontal plane, it occupies from 2 to 5 mm lateral from the third ventricle wall. Electrocoagulation with high frequensy current (one mega Hz, 2-3 Watts for one minute) was performed usually in the area where the elevation of blood pressure was most prominent. The operation on the other side was carried out in the same manner after one to three weeks.

The lesion in the autopsied cases was less than 4 mm in diameter. The details of the operative procedure and the results of stimulation have been described in our previous publications.[1-6]

BEHAVIORAL DISORDERS

Among 60 cases, there were 2 reoperations and one operative death. In the postoperative follow-up period, 7 cases died of various causes: suicide 2, status epilepticus 2, hepatitis, pneumonia and accidental drowning one case each.

In 38 cases, the effect of the operation on the behavioral disorders and present status of the patients could be assessed (Table 1). 19 cases (50%) showed excellent results: no rage attacks, the patients became so cooperative

Results	Total No	%	Home Empl.	Home Unempl.	Centers handicapped	Psych. Instit.
Excellent	19	50.0	4	10	5	0
Good	13	34.2	0	7	4	2
Fair	4	10.5	0	0	3	1
Unchanged	2	5.3	0	1	0	1
Total	38	100.0	4	18	12	4
				22		

Table 1. Follow-up assessment (2 to 16 years)

that social and familial adaptation has been possible. It is encouraging that 4 patients have been since employed. However, 10 cases stay home, economically dependent and 5 cases have been accepted to centers for handicapped people. 13 cases(34.2%) showed good results: no rage attacks, but still easily excited. In this group, 7 cases live at home, 4 in centers and 2 cases are in psychiatric institutions, due to preoperatively existing and still persisting mental retardation. In 4 cases(10.5%) the results were fair: showing still rage attacks, although less frequently and less intensively. Their social adaptation is not satisfactory. In 2 cases(5.3%) the operation was unsuccessful. In summary, this procedure is considered to have been effective in 95% of these 38 cases. Satisfactory results were obtained in 84%.

Intelligence was not impaired by this procedure. Amelioration of I.Q. was noted in about a half of the cases examined.

ENDOCRINOLOGICAL FINDINGS

The location of the surgical intervention in this procedure is close to the endocrine center of the hypothalamic-pituitary axis. Therefore, the plasma value of various pituitary hormones were estimated in recent operations.[6] Although the stimulation and coagulation of the target point resulted in a temporary elevation of various pituitary hormones, particularly prolactin and luteinizing hormone, no significant findings which were common for all cases could be attributed to these results (Fig. 1).

In follow-up period, no clinical manifestations of serious endocrine disturbances were found. Although several cases showed relatively low values of urine cortisols, no substitutional treatment was necessary.

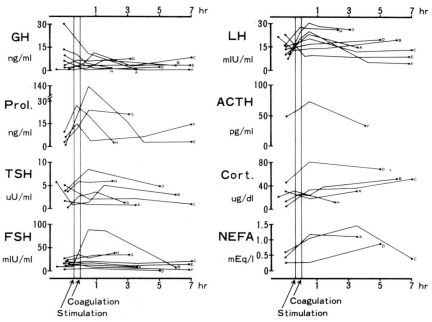

Fig. 1. Changes in plasma value of pituitary hormones, cortisols and nonesterified fatty acids, following the posteromedial hypothalamotomy for behavioral
disorders and intractable pain. Alphabet indicates different operations.

In 4 cases, follow-up stimulation
tests of pituitary hormones (Insulin
test, TRH test and LHRH test) were
performed. The results were normal
for all 4 cases, showing the regulat-
ory systems of these pituitary hormones
are functioning well even after the
bilateral operations (Fig. 2).

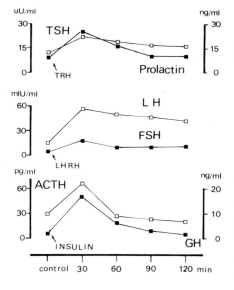

Fig. 2. Follow-up stimulation test of
pituitary hormones. The patient (S.H.
31 years old male) had bilateral
posteromedial hypothalamotomy 7 years
ago.

PHYSICAL DEVELOPMENT

The physical development curves of
10 patients, who were operated upon
in childhood, could be made. Although
a few cases showed a tendency to gain
weight after the operation, there was
no significant retardation found in
these cases (Fig. 3).

The timing of development of
secondary sexual characteristics were
within normal limits. Menstruation
in girls began between 10 to 13 years.

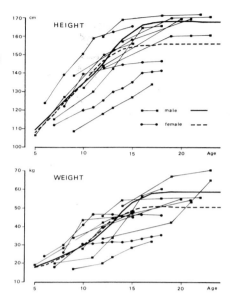

Fig. 3. Physical development curve.
Values of the youngest age for each
case are those at the time of operation.

EPILEPTIC SEIZURES

Most of these patients had epileptic seizures and mental retardation as well,
besides the chief problem of behavioral disorders. Types of seizures encountered in 60 cases of this series were analyzed (Table 2).

Types of seizures	No	%
Gen. conv. seizure	29	48.3
Gen. conv. seiz. + minor seiz.	10	16.7
Minor seizures	8	13.3
Psychomotor seizure	4	6.7
Focal motor seizure	3	5.0
No seizure	6	10.0
Total	60	100.0

Table 2. Types of seizures in the cases of behavioral disorders.

About 65% of the cases had generalized convulsive seizures, in which 10
cases had minor seizures combined. Minor seizures of various types were seen

in 13%. There were several cases of psychomotor seizures and focal motor seizures. In total, combination of epileptic seizures and behavioral disorders in
this series reached to 90%.

Before the time of operation, the seizures in 15 cases had been completely
controlled with antiepileptic drugs. However, 29 cases still had episodes of
seizures, frequently or occasionally. In these 29 cases, frequency and intensity of seizures and necessary amount of drugs were compared. In this study,
some effect of the operation for controlling epileptic seizures was assessed
in 12 cases (41%). Frequency of seizures markedly reduced in 8 cases, intensity of seizures reduced in 2 cases and in other 2 cases only a small dosis of
antiepileptic drugs became enough to control seizures (Table 3).

In relation to the types of seizures, minor seizures, which were mainly
seen in childhood cases, seemed to show the most effect, then generalized
convulsive seizures with or without minor seizures, and psychomotor seizures
seemed to be least influenced. However, a definitive conclusion may be difficult, because of too few cases for each group.

Types of seizures	Effect		Total
	Yes	No	
Gen. conv. seizure	3	6	9
G.c.s. + Minor seiz.	4	5	9
Minor seizures	4	3	7
Psychomotor seizure	1	3	4
Total	12(41.4%)	17(58.6%)	29(100%)

Table 3. Effect of the posteromedial hypothalamotomy on epileptic seizure.

DISCUSSION

The present study confirmed the results of our previous follow-up studies
on the effect of the posteromedial hypothalamotomy for controlling behavioral
disorders.[3,4,5] Recently the results of other series have been reported.[7,8,9]
There seems a general agreement among these reports that satisfactory results
can be expected over 80%.

Although indication of such a procedure in childhood is still controversial,
our experiences with 29 children seems to support an early surgical intervention. The most advantage of an early operation is to bring these children with
behavioral disorders out of necessary isolation and to provide them possibility
to recieve special and intensive education in schools or in handicapped centers.

From the endocrinological point of view, the procedure activates the hypothalamic-pituitary axis only temporarily, without causing any serious dysfunction. It is reasonable, because the surgical intervention is limited in the
posterior portion of the hypothalamus, without including various hypothalamic
nuclei in the anterior hypothalamus.

The mechanism of effect on epileptic seizures is not clear yet. The stimulation of the posteromedial hypothalamus sometimes elicited epileptic spikes
on EEG, which in several occasions resulted in seizures. This fact implies
the possibility of a favorable effect for controlling epileptic seizures in
this procedure. The surgical lesion in a part of the diffuse projecting system may give an indirect influence on the activities of epileptic foci, which
may situate mostly in the neocortex. This operation, however, has not been
indicated as yet for epilepsies per se.

In several early cases of this series, in which a lesion may have been made
more anteriorly, mild memory disturbance occured, probably due to an influence
on the mammillothalamic tract. It was, however, rarely observed in late cases
with the present target point. The anatomical structure, which was stimulated
and electrocauterized, probably corresponds to the rostral end of the central
periaqueductal grey matter and the dorsal longitudinal fasciculus of Schültz,
which is said to contain strong sympathetic fibers. The greatest advantage
of this procedure is that sympathetic responses caused by stimulation are available as a good indicator to find the most effective place for surgical intervention and also to estimate its outcome. Thus, with the aid of physiological
study, a discreet operation is possible. The mechanism of ameliorating behavioral disorders is probably explained by normalizing effect on the balance
of the ergotropic and trophotropic functions, by means of decreasing the ergotropic one, which may parallel the sympathetic circuit.

REFERENCES

1. Sano, K. (1962) Neurol. medicochirur. 4, 112-142.

2. Sano, K., Yoshioka, M., Ogashiwa, M., Ishijima, B., Ohye, C., Sekino, H.
   and Mayanagi, Y. (1967) Confin. neurol. 29, 257-261.

3. Sano, K., Mayanagi, Y., Sekino, H., Ogashiwa, M. and Ishijima, B. (1970)
   J. Neurosurg. 33, 689-707.

4. Sano, K., Sekino, H. and Mayanagi, Y. (1972) in Psychosurgery, Hitchcock,
   E., Laitinen, L. and Vaernet, K. eds., Charles C Thomas, Springfield, pp.
   57-75.

5. Sano, K. (1974) in Recent progress in neurological surgery, Sano, K. and
   Ishii, S. eds., Excerpta med. pp. 210-218.

204

6. Mayanagi, Y. and Sano, K. (1978) Appl. neurophysiol. (in press).

7. Balasubramaniam, V. and Kanaka, T.S. (1975) Confin. neurol. 37, 195-201.

8. Rubio, E., Arjona, V. and Rodriguez-Burgos, F. (1977) in Neurosurgical treatment in psychiatry, pain and epilepsy, Sweet, W., Obrador, S. and Martin-Rodriguez, J.G. eds., Univ. park press, Baltimore, pp.439-444.

9. Schvarcz, J.R. (1977) in Neurosurgical treatment in psychiatry, pain and epilepsy, Sweet, W., Obrador, S. and Martin-Rodriguez, J.G. eds., Univ. park press, Baltimore, pp. 429-438.

© 1979 Elsevier/North-Holland Biomedical Press
Modern Concepts in Psychiatric Surgery
E.R. Hitchcock, H.T. Ballantine, Jr. and B.A. Meyerson, eds.

RESULTS OF SEPARATE VERSUS COMBINED AMYGDALOTOMY AND HYPOTHALAMOTOMY FOR BEHAVIOUR DISORDERS

JORGE R. SCHVARCZ

Institute of Neurosurgery, School of Medicine, University of Buenos Aires, Buenos Aires, Argentina

Functional neurosurgery has a definite place in the treatment of patients with a long-standing history of severe, uncontrolled, violent behaviour disorders, provided that all contemporary conservative therapies have been unsuccessful.

In these cases of abnormal, aggressive, restless and/or destructive behaviour, whether it is directed against others or toward themselves, and whether it is presummably associated or not to focal brain damage, psychosurgical procedures are aimed at, and can succeed in, inducing a less detrimetal behaviour without untoward side-effects, somehow restoring their ability to react like normal human beings do. Classic open operations which preclude such results are therefore unacceptable.

There is, for the time being, a clear trend **toward** two types of stereotactic procedures, lesioning either the amygdaloid complex or the posterior hypothalamic area. Both structures are, however, related to the central mechanisms involved in emotional behaviour. Furthermore, both show a complex functional relation-ship. Two interesting questions therefore arise: first, is there any critical case selection criterion as regards aetiology and target election; second, is there any added effect when both structures are destroyed, i.e. what results are to be expected

from a subsequent, additional procedure when one of them has
already failed.

Twenty-one such cases, with successive, combined amygdaloid
and hypothalamic lesions, are reported.

MATERIAL AND METHODS

The technique has already been reported and will not be
further elaborated here[1,2,3]. However, the definite placement of
the lesion was always based on physiological parameters, namely,
the site of maximum cardio-vascular sympathetic response to
electrical stimulation for the posterior hypothalamus, and the
recording of both spontaneous and olfatorily-evoked activity as
well as the respiratory changes induced by electrical stimulation,
for the amygdala.

These patients had, without exception, a long-standing history
of uncontrolled, aggressive behaviour, which was often associated
with hyperactivity and destructiveness. They were episodically or
chronically violent and assaultive, having severe social
maladjustment. Institutionalization had been required or was
already impending for all of them.

They had all been seen by at least two different psychiatrists
before referral, and all had had extensive but unsuccessful
conservative treatment.

Patients who already had a different psychosurgical procedure
performed elsewhere as well as those cases with less than one
year follow-up, have not been considered for this report. The
posterior hypothalamus was selected as the primary target, except

in cases with evidence of focal temporal lobe damage, which were therefore selected for amygdalotomy. However, if either of these primary, bilateral operations failed, the remaining opposite procedure was subsequently performed. Thus, 21 cases underwent such successive, combined lesions, viz. 9 following unsuccessful hypothalamotomy and 12 following unsuccessful amygdalotomy.

Seventeen of these patients were mentally subnormal, 12 of whom were erethics. These hyperactive cases were often severely auto- as well as hetero-aggressive. Destructiveness was usually a conspicuous associated feature. These constantly agitated patients had fluctuations in the intensity of their violence rather than separate episodes, without displaying a normal behaviour in between. 19 cases were epileptics.

A marked reduction in, or abolition of, violently aggressive, restless and/or destructive behaviour was obtained in 4 patients who underwent bilateral amygdalotomy after failure of bilateral hypothalamotomy, and in 5 patients who underwent bilateral hypothalamotomy after failure of bilateral amygdalotomy. I.e., 42.8 % of the cases overall were significantly improved by a second, complementary procedure, without deterrent side-effects.

There was no obvious difference as to which procedure was performed first. The average interval between each set of lesions was 9 months. The follow-up period ranged from 1 to 10 years.

Most of the failures, however, corresponded to the severely agitated, idiocy group.

DISCUSSION

Selected cases with otherwise uncontrollable aggressive, restless and/or destructive behaviour have benefited from accurate stereotactic procedures which usually involved either the amigdaloid complex or the posterior hypothalamic area. Both structures have, however, a complex functional relationship [1,2].

In 1958, Narabayashi introduced stereotactic amygdalotomy for behaviour disturbances such as rebellious, explosive aggressiveness, destructiveness, and erethistic feeble-mindedness. Both aggression and hyperkinesis were markedly reduced in 48 % and moderately reduced in 36 % of the cases[4], although further long-term assessment showed a slightly decreased success rate [5,6]. The crucial target, according to Narabayashi and Shima[7], seems to be the lateral part of the corticomedial nuclei, probably involving also the stria terminalis, with its strong projection to the hypothalamus, i.e. the region which shows the highest content of monoamine oxidase. Similar long-term results have also been reported by Heimburger et al.[8], Hitchcock and Cairns[9], Ramamurthi[10], and Siegfried[11].

Sano[12] proposed the placement of lesions within the so-called ergotropic circuit at the posterio-medial hypothalamus in cases of abnormal, aggressive and/or hyperkinetic behaviour. Long-term assessment showed excellent results in 38 % and good results in 56 % of the cases[13]. The critical area seems to be the caudal part of the posterior hypothalamic area, involving also the dorsal longitudinal fasciculus, but posterior to the mammillo-thalamic tract[12,14,1]. Similar long-term results have been reported by

Kalyanaraman[15], Ramamurthi[10] and, for oligophrenia erethica, by Arjona[16] and Rubio et al.[17].

The author has obtained long-term, marked improvement in 47 % and moderate improvement in 25 % of the cases after bilateral single stage hypothalamotomy[1,2]; and long-term, marked improvement in 37 % and moderate improvement in 34 % of the cases after bilateral single stage amygdalotomy[3]. However, patients who have undergone either of these procedures without ameloration of their behaviour disorders were offered a second operation directed at the remaining, opposite target. In 43 % of the cases, violent, rebellious hetero- as well as auto-aggressive episodes were significantly improved, and frustation tolerance was increased. Erratic, wandering tendencies and hyperkinesis were reduced, and destructive crises were alleviated. Atention and concentration span were increased.

Comparable results were also obtained by Siegfried[18] following failure of amygdalotomy.

Thus, near half of the patients who already had an unsuccessful bilateral operation may expect protracted benefit from successive, combined amigdaloid and hypothalamic lesions, seemingly regard-less to the order in which they are performed.

REFERENCES

1. Schvarcz, J.R. (1977) in Neurosurgical Treatment in Psychiatry, Pain, and Epilepsy, Sweet, W., Obrador, S. and Martin, J. eds., University Park Press, Baltimore, pp. 429-438.
2. Schvarcz, J.R. (1978) in Neurological Surgery, with Emphasis on Non-invasive Methods of Diagnosis and Treatment, Carrea, R.

    ed., Excepta Medica, Amsterdam, pp. 325-328.

3. Schvarcz, J.R. (1977) Bol. Asoc. argent. Neurocir., 22,46.

4. Narabayashi, H., Nagao, T., Saito, Y., Yoshida, M. and
   Nagahata, M. (1963) Arch. Neurol., 9, 11-26.

5. Narabayashi, H. and Uno, M. (1966) Confin. neurol., 27,168-171.

6. Narabayashi, H. (1972) in Neurobiology of the Amygdala,
   Eleftheriou, B. ed., Plenum Press, New York, pp. 459-483.

7. Narabayashi, H. and Shima, F. (1973) in Surgical Approaches
   in Psychiatry, Laitinen, L. and Livingston, K. eds., Medical
   and Technical Publishing Co., Lancaster, pp. 129-134.

8. Heimburger, R., Whitlock, C., and Kalsbeck, J. (1966) J.amer.
   med. Ass., 198, 741-745.

9. Hitchcock, E. and Cairns, V. (1973) Postgrad. med. J., 49,
   894-904.

10. Ramamurthi, B. (1975) Confin. neurol., 37, 384-398.

11. Siegfried, J. (1973) in Surgical Approaches in Psychiatry,
    Laitinen, L. and Livingston, K. eds., Medical and Technical
    Publishing Co., Lancaster, pp. 138-141.

12. Sano, K. (1966) in Progress in Brain Research, vol. 21 B,
    Tokizane, T. and Shadé, J. eds., Elsevier, Amsterdam,pp.350-372

13. Sano, K. (1974) in Recent Progress in Neurological Surgery,
    Sano, K. and Ishii, S. eds., Excerpta Medica, Amsterdam,
    pp. 210-218.

14. Sano, K., Sekino, H. and Mayanagi, Y. (1972) in Psychosurgery,
    Hitchcock, E., Laitinen, L. and Vaernet, K. eds.,Charles
    Thomas, Springfield, pp. 57-75.

15. Kalyanaraman, S. (1975) Confin neurol., 37, 189-192.

16. Arjona, V. (1974) Acta neurochir., Suppl. 21, 185-191.

17. Rubio, E., Arjona, V. and Rodriguez, F. (1977) in Neurosurgical
    Treatment in Psychiatry, Pain, and Epilepsy, Sweet, W.,
    Obrador, S. and Martin, J. eds., University Park Press,
    Baltimore, pp. 439-444.

18. Siegfried, J. (1977) Personal communication.

TARGET, MANAGEMENT AND ASSESSMENT STUDIES

© 1979 Elsevier/North-Holland Biomedical Press
Modern Concepts in Psychiatric Surgery
E.R. Hitchcock, H.T. Ballantine, Jr. and B.A. Meyerson, eds.

STEREOTACTIC GAMMACAPSULOTOMY

LARS LEKSELL M.D. and ERIK-OLOF BACKLUND M.D.
Department of Neurosurgery, Karolinska sjukhuset and Sophiahemmet Hospital, Stockholm (Sweden)

INTRODUCTION

This preliminary report describes a psychosurgical method using radiation lesions in the anterior part of the internal capsule without opening the skull.

Stereotactic technique was first developed and used for making radiofrequency heat lesions in the internal capsule and then applied to an extensive series of psychiatric cases[1]. In 1977, Bingley and co-workers reported the long-term results from stereotactic RF-capsulotomy[2].

The first radiosurgical capsulotomy was carried out in 1953, with 300 kV X-rays[3]. Later, proton beam experiments in Uppsala[4] led to the development of the present radiosurgical technique[5] using the stereotactic gamma radiation unit in Sophiahemmet. The clinical results from a pilot series of 16 patients with obsessive-compulsive neurosis and severe anxiety will be reported by Rylander[6].

METHOD

The technique of stereotactic radiosurgery has been described previously[5,7]. The gamma unit, shown in Fig.1, irradiates the target area in the internal capsule by cross-firing 179 narrow beams of ^{60}Co gamma radiation. Small, disc-shaped, oval lesions are produced with an estimated size of 8 by 10 mm.

The target areas were localized by lumbar pneumo-encephalography except in four cases when CT-scanning was used[8,9] (Fig. 2). The targets lie 10 mm in front of the anterior commissure, 8 mm above the inter-commissural line and on average 17 mm lateral to the mid-plane. The radiation dose on each side varied between 14 and 18 krads which for the present cobalt source activity requires about two hours irradiation. General anaesthesia is not needed, and the patients receive only a slight premedication.

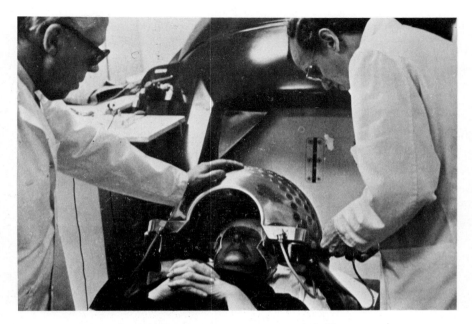

Fig. 1. Placement of patient in the collimator helmet.

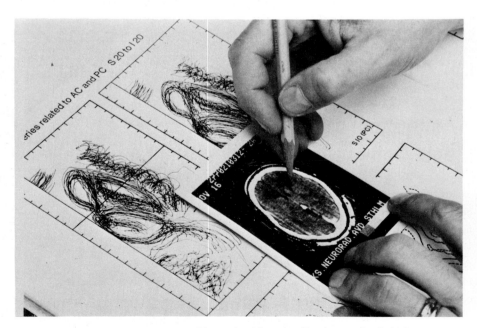

Fig. 2. Target determination: Stereotactic coordinates calculated by
computer tomography.

DISCUSSION

The final psychiatric results with this radiosurgical technique will probably be the same as those from conventional open stereotactic capsulotomy (see Rylander[6]). The radiolesions are not fully developed until two or three weeks after radiosurgery but an initial pronounced relief of symptoms is usually observed during the first four or five postoperative days. Slight cellular changes in the area irradiated may explain this finding; recent experiments with neural cells in tissue culture, for example, have shown early but transient cellular changes after similar, heavy single dose irradiation[10].

So far we have not been able to study these gamma lesions in white matter, but lesions in the thalamus have been thoroughly examined in cases of intractable cancer pain[11,12,13]. We do not know yet whether the lesions in the internal capsule differ significantly as regards size and shape from those in the grey matter but in animal experiments they seem similar.

All patients have been regularly checked by CT-scan and as a rule there are no observable changes. In some cases, however, an area of low attenuation at the site of irradiation was found.

In conclusion, we have today at our disposal a closed operative method for psychiatric surgery, stereotactic gamma-capsulotomy, which is bloodless, painless, and without the risks inherent in open surgical methods. With computed tomography, the localization of the lesions can be made with sufficient accuracy and, if desired, the whole procedure can be performed on an out-patient basis.

Psychiatric surgery is still controversial. At the present level of development, our indications for capsulotomy are restricted to intractable obsessive-compulsive states and severe anxiety.

REFERENCES

1. Herner, T.(1961) Treatment of mental disorders with frontal stereotaxic thermolesions, Acta Psychiatr. Scand.36, Suppl.158, pp. 1-140.

2. Bingley, T., Leksell, L., Meyerson, B. and Rylander, G.(1977) in Neurosurgical Treatment in Psychiatry, Pain and Epilepsy, Sweet, W., Obrador, S. and Martin-Rodriguez, J. eds., University Park Press, Baltimore, pp. 287-299.

3. Leksell, L., Herner, T. and Lidén, K.(1955) Kungl. Fysiogr. Sällsk. Lund Förhandl., 25, pp. 1-10.

4. Larsson, B., Leksell, L. and Rexed, B.(1963) Acta Chir. Scand., 125, pp. 1-7.

216

5. Leksell, L.(1971) Stereotaxis and radiosurgery - an operative system, Ch. C. Thomas, Springfield, Ill., pp. 1-69.

6. Rylander, G.(1978) in This Volume.

7. Leksell, L. and Backlund, E. O.(1978) Läkartidningen, 75, pp. 547-549.

8. Bergström, M. and Greitz, T.(1976) Am. J. Roentgenol., 127, pp. 167-170.

9. Meyerson, B.(1978) in This Volume.

10. Anniko, M.(1978) Personal communication.

11. Leksell, L.(1968) Acta Chir. Scand., 134, pp. 585-595.

12. Dahlin, H., Larsson, B., Leksell, L., Rosander, K., Sarby, B. and Steiner, L.(1975) Acta Radiol.(Ther.Phys.Biol.), 14, pp. 139-144.

13. Wennerstrand, J. and Ungerstedt, U.(1970) Acta Chir. Scand., 136, pp. 133-137.

© 1979 Elsevier/North-Holland Biomedical Press
Modern Concepts in Psychiatric Surgery
E.R. Hitchcock, H.T. Ballantine, Jr. and B.A. Meyerson, eds.

217

TARGET LOCALIZATION IN STEREOTACTIC CAPSULOTOMY WITH THE AID OF COMPUTED
TOMOGRAPHY

B.A.MEYERSON, M.BERGSTRÖM, T.GREITZ

Departments of Neurosurgery and Neuroradiology, Karolinska sjukhuset,
S-104 01 Stockholm, Sweden

INTRODUCTION

In psychiatric stereotactic surgery the anatomical structures that
constitute the region of interest for lesioning, electrode implantation
or other procedures are rarely visible targets. That is to say that they
can not be directly visualized with the use of conventional radiological
methods. Instead, stereotactic localization has to be made with the help
of reference structures demonstrated with the aid of encephalography with
positiv or negativ contrast, angiography or plain skull X-ray. The spatial relationship between the target and the reference structures is given by stereotactic atlases which have been worked out on brains considered to represent normal anatomy. Hence, in a particular patient deviation from the normal can seldom be accounted for with accurancy although
most atlases also contain data on variability. Stereotactic atlases are
primarely devoted to diencephalic structures whereas the frontal lobes
and rhinencephalic structures, being the prime regions of interest for
psychiatric surgery, are not delt with in detail. The problem of individual variability in the relative location of various regions is negligible when structures used as reference are close to the target region.
Conversely, when the reference structure is situated remotely from the
target, individual variability may cause considerable errors in localization. This is the case in stereotactic capsulotomy. However, with the
aid of computor tomography (CT) the targets in this operation, the internal capsules, can be directly visualized. The technique for the transfer of the targets demonstrated in CT to the stereotactic operative system is described in the present report.

METHODS

In stereotactic capsulotomy the target region, the anterior part of
the internal capsule, is remote from the reference points, i.e. the midline, the tip of the frontal horns and the anterior commissure,

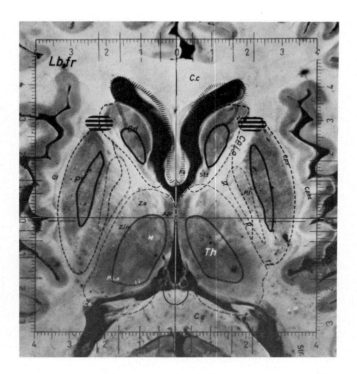

Fig. 1. Horizontal brain section from the stereotactic atlas of Schalten-brand and Bailey[4]. The targets in stereotactic capsulotomy, located in the anterior portions of the internal capsules, are marked as hatched ovals. The dotted lines denote the range of variability in the extent of the different parts of the basal ganglia.

visualized with the aid of pneumoencephalography[1].The shape and the size of the ventricles may vary considerably even in a normal material. It is conceivable that variations in the width of the frontal horns influence the location of the internal capsule relative to the midline, similarly to what has been demonstrated for the thalamocapsular border,the location of which is correlated to the width of the third ventricle[2]. There is nothing to suggest a constant anatomical relationship between the tip of the horns, the anterior commissure and the internal capsule.There is a considerable distance between the targets and these reference points,and, for instance, in the coronal plane the target in the internal capsule is located no less than two cm from the midline. Thus, it is obvious that the determination of the stereotactic coordinates of the targets in this operation is influenced in a way that has no constant relationship to the real location of the capsule. The variability of the relative location of the internal capsule has been clearly demonstrated in stereotactic atlases [3,4]. In fig. 1. is shown a stereotactic horizontal section corresponding to the level of the targets, marked as hatched ovals. It is obvious that unless the variability of the location of the capsules relative to neighbouring structures can be accounted for there is a considerable risk that at least part of the lesion will encroach on the head of the caudate nucleus or the putamen.

Of particular importance in this context is the fact that localization in capsulotomy is generally performed with the aid of pneumoencephalography. The presence of air in the ventricles causes a considerable

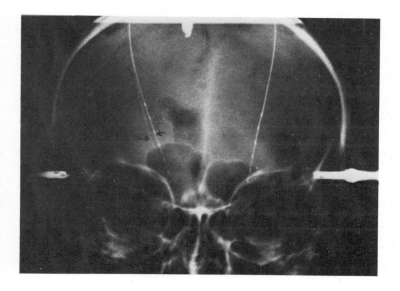

Fig. 2. Effect of intraventricular air on the location of the targets in stereotactic capsulotomy. Two superimposed stereotactic skull radiographs, one taken before and the other after lumbar air injection. The electrodes had been implanted in the target region with the aid of CT localization. Air is present only in the right lateral ventricle and on that side the electrode has been displaced in lateral direction.

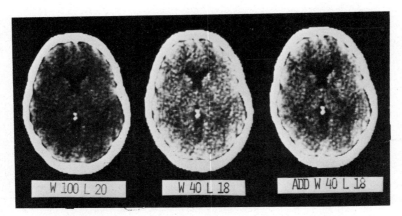

Fig. 3. To improve the visibility of the internal capsules as targets for stereotactic capsulotomy attenuation differences between grey and white matter can be increased by varying the window widths (W) and the level of the grey scale (L). The third image was obtained after repeated scanning of one and the same cut.

dilatation, and occasionally even a collapse of the lateral ventricle[5], which tends to influence significantly the location of the internal capsules. If one compares CT scans obtained with and without intraventricular air the distance between the targets regions in the internal capsules may differ with a distance of no less than about 10mm [6]. The effects of ventricular dilatation due to the presence of air is illustrated in fig.2. In this patient temporary depth electrodes had been implanted in order to be able to study the effect of electrical stimulation in the target area. Prior to the actual operation a pneumoencephalography was performed. A stereotactic skull radiograph has been superimposed on a radiograph taken with air in one of the frontal horns, and it can be seen that on that side the lateral dislocation of the electrode is considerable, amounting to about 4mm. The electrode on the other side is not influenced.

With the aid of computer tomography it is now possible to visualize directly intracerebral structures and the high contrast resolution also enables differentiation between grey and white matter. This had been utilized for localization of the internal capsule as a visible target for capsulotomy. Several methods are available to enhance attenuation differences in CT scans. The most common is to use intravenous contrast media but this does not significantly increase the attenuation differences between grey and white matter, and hence the visibility of the internal capsule. As illustrated in fig. 3. it is often helpful to vary the window widths and to ajust the level. The third image illustrates the result of repeating several times the scanning of one and the same cut. The addition of such repeated examinations decreases the noice level provided that there is no movement of the head. This method of decreasing the noice level is similar to the averaging technique used for the study of evoked potentials. It is also possible to add partly overlapping cuts, which is made by successively moving the collimator one or two mm.

Computer tomography for localization in stereotaxis was originally developed by Bergström & Greitz[7] and has been used mainly in connection with stereotactic biopsis of tumors[8]. This technique has now been applied also for functional stereotaxis. The location of a target in a scanner image may be defined by the coordinates of the position of the corresponding elements. These coordinates can be determined on the print-out but in practice it is simpler to use the polaroid picture. The X and Z coordinates are calculated by measuring the distance from the edge of the matrix to the target. These values are fed into the computer and the resulting location of the corresponding element is shown in the oscilloscop display (fig. 4.). It is then possible to check the location of the target and to make corrections of the measurements.

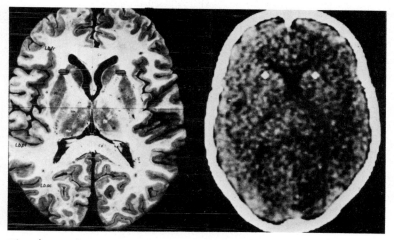

Fig. 4. Horizontal brain section from Schaltenbrand & Bailey´s atlas[+]. (Cf. fig. 1.) and the corresponding CT scan with indications of target sites for stereotactic capsulotomy.

The Y coordinate is defined by the tomographic cut intersecting the
target point. It is also possible to further improve the accuracy in determining the Y coordinate with the aid of a reconstruction in the orthogonal plane using additive or partly overlapping cuts[9]. When applied to
capsulotomy reconstruction only in the frontal plane is of interest.After
specifying the location of the frontal projection, the size of the area
to be reconstructed and the number of slizes, the computer chooses a few
evenly distributed cuts through the area and puts the reconstructed cuts
in a picture for further processing or viewing. The computer time is
about 1 min. In fig. 5. is shown an example of frontal reconstruction
for the use in capsulotomy. Although the resolution in the reconstructed
cuts is much less than in the horizontal one the ventricles can be easily
identified.

The crucial point in the transfer of data obtained with the computer
tomograph to the therapeutic stereotactic system is the fixation of the
head. A fixation device, originally developed for radiosurgery, has been

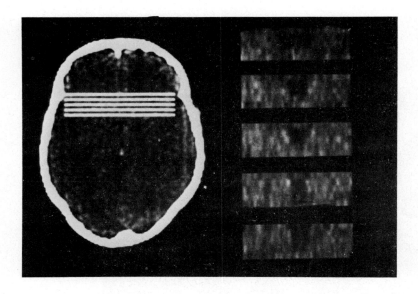

Fig. 5. CT scan with lines indicating the planes of frontal orthogonal reconstruction of the region of interest for stereotactic capsulotomy (left),
and the resulting reconstructions showing the frontal horns of the lateral
ventricles (right).

adopted[10]. A band of thermoplast is firmly applied around the patient head. Brackets are attached to support a ring which is then secured to the opening of the scanner. This same ring is then used to support the stereotactic frame, thus ensuring a constant spatial relationship between the scanner cuts and the stereotactic coordinate system.

A computer program is available for the transfer of the target coordinates in the diagnotic system, i.e. the computer tomograph, to coordinates in the therapeutic system, the stereotactic frame. The numerical values of these coordinates to be used on the stereotactic instrument are printed out by the computer. The frame is secured to the ring that has been used for fixation of the head to the scanner opening. This implies that the fixation between the head and the frame depends on the plastic bandage and the frame burrs are not used. The bandage, it must be admitted, is to be regarded as a prototype, and as it is firmly wrapped around the head of the patient it causes some pain and headache. Work is in progress to develop a more convenient and reliable method of fixation[8].

For open stereotactic operations the ring, supporting the frame, is secured to the operating table. For radiosurgical procedures bearings are attached to the plastic bandage in a position corresponding to the X and Y coordinates of the target (Leksell and Backlund, this volume).

COMMENTS

With the aid of computer tomography a non-visible target, which may otherwise be localized only in terms of its postulated relationship to reference structures, can now be directly visualized. This has largely improved the precision of stereotactic operations. This method of localization has hitherto been applied only to capsulotomy but will certainly also prove to be of value in other types of stereotactic procedures. It should be emphasized that CT target localization has been developed using a machine of the first generation (EMI Mark I). With the access to more advanced equipment a higher degree of sensitivity resolution is possible and thereby the accuracy of target localization may be further improved. This, of course, is indispensable when small lesions are to be produced in critical regions. The possibility to obtain primary CT cuts in all three dimensions will add to the versability of the method.

REFERENCES

1. Bingley, T., Leksell, L., Meyerson, B.A. and Rylander, G. (1977) Neurosurgical Treatment in Psychiatry, Pain and Epilepsy, Sweet,W., Obrador, S. and Martin-Rodriguez, J. eds., University Park Press, Baltimore, pp. 287-299

2. Hawrylyshyn, P.A., Tasker, R.R. and Organ, L.W. (1976/77) Appl. Neurophysiol. 39, 34-42.

3. Van Buren, J.M. and Borke, R.C. (1972) Variations and Connections of the Human Thalamus, Springer, Berlin and New York.

4. Schaltenbrand, G. and Bailey, P. (1959) Introduction to stereotaxis with an atlas of the human brain. Thieme, Stuttgart.

5. Probst, F.P. (1972) Rapid changes in the volume of the lateral ventricles at encephalography. Acta Radiol. Diagnosis. 12, 757-768.

6. Meyerson, B.A. (1977) International Congress Series No. 433. Neurological Surgery. Excerpta Medica, Amsterdam-Oxford, Raúl Carrea, ed. pp 307-312.

7. Bergström, M. and Greitz, R. (1976) Am J Roentgenol, 167-170.

8. Bergström, M., Boëthius, J., Collins, V.P., Edner, G., Lewander, R. and Willems, J. (1977) International Congress Series No. 433. Neurological Surgery. Excerpta Medica, Amsterdam-Oxford, Raúl Carrea, pp 45-50.

9. Bergström, M. and Sundman, R. (1976) Am J Roentgenol 127, 17-21.

10. Leksell, L. (1971) Stereotaxis and Radiosurgery, Charles C. Thomas, Springfield, Ill.

Part of this study has been supported by agrant from the Swedish Cancer Society.

© 1979 Elsevier/North-Holland Biomedical Press
Modern Concepts in Psychiatric Surgery
E.R. Hitchcock, H.T. Ballantine, Jr. and B.A. Meyerson, eds.

PSYCHIATRIC PROCESS ANALYSIS OF OBSESSIVE COMPULSIVE BEHAVIOR MODIFICATION
BY PSYCHIATRIC SURGERY.

PAUL COSYNS[x] and JAN GYBELS[xx]

[x]Psychiatric Clinic Kortenberg, B-3070 Kortenberg and Free University
Brussels (Belgium).
[xx]Department of Neurology and Neurosurgery, University of Leuven, B-3000
Leuven (Belgium)

For the psychiatrist and behavioral scientist a great deal of the literature on psychiatric surgery is unconvincing for several reasons. We wish
to stress briefly two of them. Firstly, most authors utilize the conventional patient group averaging approach, also known as the extensive model.
Group averages of psychological testing "before" and several months "after"
are perhaps interesting but will never contribute to a better understanding
of the produced behavior change in each individual case. A result can be
statistically significant, and at the same time clinically not relevant.
A significant mean figure is not transferable to the individual case,
learns nothing about the studied characteristic as far as each member of
the group is considered.

Secondly, the literature reveals a flagrant lack of precise data and
facts about the patients, their post-operative behavior, and above all
the meaning of their psychopathological behavior. Psychiatrists are more
interested in understanding and demonstrating the process of the therapeutic effect, rather than a mere evaluation of the result. They try to investigate the meaning of patterns of conduct from the point of view of
the patient and their change by psychiatric surgical procedures. The
generally utilized group approach makes this impossible because here one
looks for systematically similar characteristics and this implies that
individual characteristics are not relevant. But even looking only at
obsessive compulsive patients, we can not stress enough the fact for each
patient even a same problem behavior has a different meaning and is controlled by different variables, familial, cultural, cognitive, educational..

We can not consider these patients as being a group since the differences amoung them are more striking than their similarities. They are at
best a collection of individuals displaying to an outside observer an

analoguous kind of behavioral problem.

It is not the place here to fully criticize the much employed extensive research model, applied to psychopathological problems. Others have been done such a critic, as Chassan and Bellak (1), Shapiro (2) and De Waele (3). We want only to stress that the clinical study of the individual case, i.e. the intensive design, is at very last a much needed complementary approach. Each patient is treated apart, serves as his own control and is continuously assessed during several months by a combination of observational and experimental methods and of focussed interviews. The focus must lie upon an analysis of variation of responses within the individual patient. We try to learn and to extract the maximum information for each individual case taking advantage of its own particularities.

The highly individualized and problem centered assessment procedures include several aspects:

1. Quantification of several defined Target Behaviors, mainly with the visual analogue scale (V.A.S.), as described and validated by Aitken (4, 5) and Luria (6). The patient and the therapist separately rate daily or more on 10 cm lines the intensity of the defined target behaviors.

2. Direct continuous observation by trained nurses of behavior patterns in various social and daily life settings extending over a long time period.

3. Quantification of all-round ward behavior by standardized rating scales.

4. Interviews focussed on the several verbally expressed statements or displayed behaviors of the studied patient. This will enable us to construct a functional analysis showing how several variables influence the problem behavior, and to disclose meanings of patterns of conduct.

5. Brain stimulation and recording of physiological variables during surgery.

6. Psychological tests to assess organic deterioration.

CASE STUDIES

During a five year study period 65 hospitalized psychiatric patients were diagnosed as obsessive compulsive neurotics according to D.S.M. II (300.3). Of these 65 patients ten (i.e. 15 %) were found by the psychiatric therapeutic team suitable for psychiatric surgery. Following criteria

have been proved useful for referal:
- failure of current psychiatric therapeutic methods, including drugs,
  E.C.T., verbal psychotherapy and behavior therapy. This implies already an illness duration of several years.
- complete invalidation of the patient who spends the whole day ruminating or performing rituals or avoidance behaviors.
- the absence of clear-cut delusional systems of hallucinations.
- the symptoms must exist on themselves and not being significantly
  manipulated by the patient in a relational-manipulative context.
  We avoid to propose this therapy to patients who display a too pronounced hysterical personality structure or acting out tendencies.

These ten cases were also reviewed by the neurosurgeon and an independent (non Hospital bound) specialized committee which safeguards the
scientific and ethical aspects. If that committee agrees we give full
explanation to the patient and his family or life partner and we try to
gain their informed consent.

Five patients and their family agreed and were operated, while five
others were not for several reasons. Space limitations do not allow us
to go into further details. Only one case will be discussed in some extent
and a summary of our observations in the other cases will be presented.

W. Irène: A 30 year old woman displaying since 4 years (during her thirth
pregnancy) severe washing and cleaning rituals evoked by an obsessive
phobic fear of the "cancer microbe". The symptoms disappeared completely
after surgery (subcaudate tractotomy of Knight (7)) and further psychiatric
treatment (mainly behavior therapy), but this cure provoked new problems.
Her husband asked a divorce and we can not stress enough in our experience
that even after psychiatric surgery patients need further psychiatric
therapy. After 4 years follow-up she remains symptom free, as far as compulsive washing rituals are concerned.

X. Elise: Is a 32 years old unmarried intelligent woman displaying since
nine years severe obsessional thoughts around sexual and religious matters.
She appeared later on to be a schizophrenic patient. The surgery improved
a little her obsessive thinking but did not at all influence the schizophrenic process. She worsened further: more and more withdrawn, bizarre,

blunting of affects and catatonic symptoms.

<u>S. Karine</u>: A married woman of 49 presenting since 20 years severe washing and cleaning rituals elicited by everywhere present dust. Three years after surgery she is less anxious but as obsessional. This patient refused psychiatric therapy (mainly behavior therapy) after surgery.

<u>M. David</u>: A man of 57 years displaying severe obsessive thinking. This case is too recently operated to be discussed.

<u>B. Stephane</u>:

B. Stephane is a sturdy 50 years old married man displaying a severe impulsion phobia. He is continuously panic-stricken by the ego dystonic impulsion he has to strangle his wife. He is an intellectually deficient unskilled worker. After a psychiatric hospitalization of 11 months and a sham operation followed by a stereotactic subcaudate tractotomy of Knight, he was discharged and remained obsession free at a follow-up of more than one year and half notwithstanding the presence of other temporary side effects.

Stephane is the only son of overprotecting parents. The parental educational style failed to develop any sense of autonomy in this already borderline mental retardated boy. Mother provided everything and father was very severe maintaining discipline by physical means, striking and smaching. Stephane was very submissive, passive and dull. He never expressed any aggressive feelings, but as hobby he boxes. After a school period where he performed poorly, he started working but could never bring it beyond the level of an unskilled worker.

Thirty years ago he developed for the first time obsessional symptoms following a severe somatic illness of his father. It involved obsessive counting and impulsive phobic symptoms about committing suicide or harming one self. This symptomatology can be interpreted as a tentative way to reduce anxiety evoked by, first the unacceptable aggressive feeling towards his father and secondly the threatening danger of being abandoned. The anticipation of loosing a parent elicits unbearable anxiety in this dependant man (table I).

TABLE 1

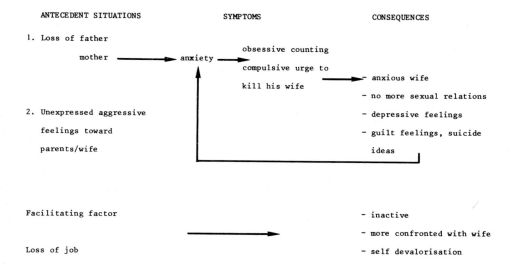

ANTECEDENT SITUATIONS   SYMPTOMS   CONSEQUENCES

1. Loss of father

        mother ————————▶ anxiety

                                    obsessive counting

                                    compulsive urge to

                                    kill his wife   ▶ — anxious wife

                                                                       — no more sexual relations

2. Unexpressed aggressive   — depressive feelings

    feelings toward   — guilt feelings, suicide

    parents/wife   ideas

Facilitating factor   — inactive

                                                                       — more confronted with wife

Loss of job   — self devalorisation

B. Stephane: functional analysis of complaints

When father died 21 years ago he married immediately (at 29) a more
intelligent and dynamic woman, who takes over fathers role.

When it appeared that their marriage would remain childness the impulsion fobia about killing his wife started but notwithstanding the
anxiety provoked by it he could manage the situation.

Two years ago he changed his job to earn more but was unable to perform
it correctly and so he became jobless. The inactivity and daily confron-
tation with his wife worsened his state.

When his mother died he denied the decease and refused to take leave
of his mother by not placing a flower on the coffin. His wife did and
since then he feared to lose control upon his more and more intense urge
about killing his wife. He slept separately and he was urging for medical

help. He had also various obsessional sexual sadistic fantasies about
his mother, felt guilty about it and became more depressive and had suicidal ideas.

A tentative verbal therapeutic approach failed. E.C.T. and drugs had
no lasting effects. We tried to cope with his unexpressed aggressivity
by non verbal means. Patient was engaged to express physical aggressivity
in role playing sessions with a behavioral therapist and in boxing sessions
with a psychomotor therapist. This also failed partly because patient
had heard of psychiatric surgery and expected a cure only from such a
procedure.

He was very surgery seeking and all the other therapies were only
time loosing in his eyes. So we decided to make first the burrholes
under general anesthesia without making lesions and to send patient back
to the psychiatric hospital.

This sham operation remained without any effect on his symptomatology
(fig. 1). He over and again was ruminating and talking about his "bad ideas".

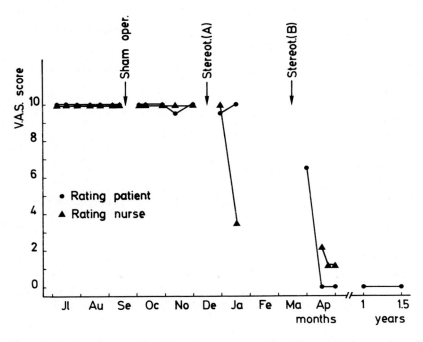

Fig. 1: B. Stephane. Visual Analogue Scale (0-10) of his impulsion fobia
rated by the patient and the nurse. (Fear of killing wife)

Two months later bilateral medial-baso-frontal lesions were placed. Initially he worsened, being more apathic, untidy and neglecting elementary personal hygiene. Drug withdrawal and starting of an operant program improved very well his all-round ward behavior.

Patient was after. the operation more sensitive to sedative and anxiolytic drugs which had to be removed.

According to his wife, nurses and for an outsider he was clearly improving, being more active, friendly; less anxious and less talking about his impulsive ideas. But subjectively according to the patient, they were always present and he felt hopeless about it. He went home and had for the first time sex with his wife since 3 years. Little transient obsessional rituals were observed, such as controlling over and again the taps, the crease of his pyjama.

Three months later the lesions were laterally enlarged and we saw an improvement of his compulsive phobic ideas who disappeared after six weeks and never came again during the one and half year follow-up.

Other psyhological changes were seen after the second operation:
- patient was transiently for the first time openly aggressive, verbally defiant and even physically;
- he was regressive and totally relying upon his wife (she had even to shave him);
- patient showed some memory deficits and organic symptoms during several months but they improved gradually.

On the somatic level we notice a greater sensitivity to alcohol and and one epileptic fit after a slight alcoholic excess (1 year after stereotaxis B). He also complained during the first months of miction troubles, even unintentional urine voiding.

The organic symptoms improved gradually and disappeared after 6 months. All the other symptoms such as apathy, overdependence on his wife and regressive tendencies disappeared during marital therapy via the establishment of an operant program and therapeutic contracts.

SUMMARY OF OUR OBSERVATIONS AND DISCUSSION

1. In five patients with obsessive compulsive neurosis lesions were placed bilaterally in the medial-baso-frontal regions (from 10 to 20 mm from midline) using the stereotactic coordinates of G. Knight. We never explored other areas such as the cingulum because the until now obtained results were satisfactory enough.

2. The lesions had to be expanded laterally to 23 mm from the midline during a second intervention. It is our opinion that lesions must be placed bilaterally and that a certain amount of tissue has to be destroyed, under which no effect can be expected.

3. Stimulation of the target area of the awake patient during the operation gave little information. Subjective responses were never recorded. Occasionally vegetative responses as a change of respiratory rhythm or a psycho-galvanic skin response were observed, but even when the patient was very collaborative, very little valuable information could be obtained in the operating room.

4. A beneficial effect on depressive mood and anxiety feelings was seen prior to any improvement of obsessive compulsive complaints. We never noticed any immediate effect of surgery on this performative aspect of behavior.

5. Several patients were immediately after surgery more sensitive to psychopharmacological drugs. They could no longer tolerate their previous medication.

6. Unsuccessful psychiatric therapies before surgery became successful after it. Patients were more able to manage the anxiety elicited by the behavior therapy, mainly flooding in vivo and response prevention. Their improvement seems to be secondary to a decrease of tension and anxiety.

7. A sham operation was performed without any success.

8. Even after successful surgery and post-operative treatment the patient does not automatically feel happier. Several problems remain to be solved. For example, how will the patient fill all the time coming free by the shortening of the time consuming rituals. Therapeutic programs to develop alternative behavior are necessary. We would now refuse to operate if the patient refuses to follow simultaneously an appropriate psychiatric therapy.

9. In a schizophrenic patient the surgery improved after several months a little her obsessive doubts, but did not at all influence the further bad evolution of the schizophrenic process.

10. Minor personality changes (sometimes transient) could be observed in all the cases. They are not always seen on psychometric tests, but quite obvious to everyone, observer or relative, who know the patient before the operation. Some features are:

- being more aggressive, W. Irène, B. Stephane and S. Karine,
- being more impulsive, W. Irène, S. Karine,
- being more apathic, withdrawn and regressive, B. Stephane,
- no blunting of affects was seen. Operated patients remain able to react emotionally to interpersonal situations.

11. Undesirable somatic side effects were noted:

- transient. urinary problems, W. Irène, B. Stephane and X. Elise,
- epileptic fits, one B. Stephane, one W. Irène.

AKNOWLEDGEMENTS

We are grateful to the Staff of St. Lukas ward (Psychiatrische St. Jozef Kliniek) for the cooperation, to Mrs. Feytons-Heeren and Mr. P. De Sutter for their skillful technical assistance, and to Monique Van Humbeek and Marthe Naegels for the typing work.

REFERENCES

1. Chassan, J.B. and Bellak, L. (1966) In Methods of research in psycho-therapy, Gottschalk and Auerbach, eds., Century Crofts, Appleton, New York.

2. Shapiro, M.B. (1964) Brit. J. Med. Psychol., 34, 255-262.

3. De Waele, J.P.: Personal communication.

4. Aitken, R.B.C. (1969) Proceedings of the Royal Society of Medicine, 62, 989-993.

5. Aitken, R.B.C. (1970) Psychother. Psychosom., 18, 74-79.

6. Luria, R.E. (1975) J. Psychiat. Res., 12, 51-57.

7. Knight, G (1969) Postgrad. Med. J., 45, 1-13.

© 1979 Elsevier/North-Holland Biomedical Press
Modern Concepts in Psychiatric Surgery
E.R. Hitchcock, H.T. Ballantine, Jr. and B.A. Meyerson, eds.

STEREOTACTIC RADIOSURGERY IN ANXIETY AND OBSESSIVE-COMPULSIVE STATES:
PSYCHIATRIC ASPECTS

GÖSTA RYLANDER   Professor Dr Med.
Karolinska Hospital, 104 01 Stockholm, Sweden.

In 1970, a team at the Neurosurgical Department of Karolinska Hospital began to perform small bilateral radiofrequency heat or thermo
lesions in the anterior part of the internal capsule of patients suffering from obsessive-compulsive states and chronic anxiety. The team consisted of two neurosurgeons (Lars Leksell and Björn Meyerson) and two
psychiatrists(Torsten Bingley and I).

The technique and the results of the operation were reported at the
international congresses in Cambridge(1972), in Madrid(1975), and last
summer at the International Congress of Neurosurgery in Sao Paulo.

Today I would like to start with some words about the heat lesions in
the internal capsule as a background to my account of the gamma lesions
in approximately the same place. Also, this makes a comparison possible
between the two methods. Our series of heat operations now consists of
38 patients (22 women and 16 men). They all suffered from obsessive-
compulsive states with severe anxiety. Before the operation they had
been subjected to all available psychiatric therapy, psychotropic drugs,
ECT, Insulin treatment, individual psychiatric therapy, group therapy,
hypnosis and, in some cases, year-long psychoanalysis with no effect. The
age ranges from 22 to 49 years. The duration of the illness before the
operation ranged from 2 to 30 years with a mean value of 16.5 years.These
figures demonstrate the chronic nature of the illness in these patients.
The length of the follow-up for the whole material varied from 21 months
to eight years. Of 38 patients operated, one half of them (19), are free
from symptoms and 8 are much improved. This means 71% which I think is a
satisfactory result, considering that these patients were quite hopeless
from a therapeutic point of view. Of the remaining 11, ten were slightly improved, and one unchanged. I will add that no intellectual changes
and no undesirable personality manifestations occurred.

Doctor Leksell and I thought that it should be of no importance whether
the lesion in the internal capsule was caused by heating the tissue (as
in the cases just described) or by gamma rays. This method is possible
with the gamma unit constructed by Leksell which doctor Backlund just has
described. It has a great advantage in that it is bloodless. Using com-

236

puted tomography for determining the reference points, the whole procedure is mild. Backlund, who heads the Stereotactic Unit of the Neurosurgical Department, joined Leksell and me in January 1976 when we started
the radiosurgical treatment of compulsive-obsessive states with severe
anxiety. Last year (1977) Sten Levander, psychiatrist with special experience in psychophysiological concomitants to anxiety, joined our team.

Table 1 shows the whole gamma series of 14 cases with 9 women and 5
men, diagnoses, duration of illness, time of follow-up and results.

TABLE 1 GAMMA-CAPSULOTOMY IN ANXIETY AND OBSESSIVE-COMPULSIVE STATES

CASE NO.	SEX	AGE	DOMINANT SYMPTOMS IN ADDITION TO CHRONIC ANXIETY	DURATION OF ILLNESS (YRS)	FOLLOW-UP (MONTHS)	RESULTS +
1	F	37	Phobias, Compulsive Thoughts	12	23	A
2	F	42	Phobias, Compulsive Thoughts & Rituals	13	23	B
3	F	36	Phobias	8	10	D
4	M	31	Phobias	6	26	B
5	F	32	Phobias	11	25	A
6	F	32	Phobias, Compulsive Thoughts	15	23	A
7	M	39	Phobias	13	18	A
8	F	67	Compulsive Thoughts & Rituals	49	12	D
9	F	55	Compulsive Thoughts & Rituals	30	21	C
10	M	43	Phobias, Compulsive Thoughts	6	17	B
11	M	24	Phobias, Compulsive Thoughts	4	18	C
12	M	33	Phobias	11	16	B
13	F	47	Phobias	26	9	A
14	F	37	Phobias	23	9	A

+ RESULTS: A = Free from symtoms, B = Much improved, C = Slightly improved,
D = Unchanged

The radiosurgical clientele is of the same type as in our series of
heat lesion, i.e., they suffered from chronic illnesses and they were resistant to all other forms of therapy. In addition, they were socially
disabled. Their age ranges from 24 to 67 years, with a mean of 35 years
(Table 2). The duration of the preoperative illnesses varied from 4 to
49 years and the follow-up time from 9 months to two years and two months.

TABLE 2. SOME CHARACTERISTICS OF CAPSULOTOMIA ANTERIOR

TYPE OF OPERATION	NO. OF CASES	AGE		DURATION OF ILLNESS (YEARS)		FOLLOW-UP TIME (YEARS)	
		Range	Mean	Range	Mean	Range	Mean
Thermo lesion	38	22-59	40	2-30	16.5	1.3-8	3.5
Gamma lesion	14	24-67	35	4-49	16.2	0.75-2.2	1.5

Some further characteristics of these two series, thermo and gamma lesions, are demonstrated in table 2. I have already mentioned that both series consist of chronic cases, who had been given every available kind of psychiatric treatment. The table shows that they are rather alike also in other respects. The mean age is 40 years, respectively 35. The mean duration of the illness is nearly the same, 16.5 respectively 16.2 years. Furthermore, I can mention that there is an accumulation of cases between 30 to 40 years in both series.

Before speaking about the therapeutic results I will describe what happens immediately after the radiosurgical intervention, as compared with the reactions in the heat lesion series.

During the first two to four days after the heat lesion operation, about half of the patients became moderately confused and disoriented. These symptoms disappear within a few days. However, there are two other symptoms which all patients show, namely, an increased tendency to tiredness and reduction initiative.

I emphasize that these symptoms in heat lesion patients are temporary. They fade away after some weeks or months. The increased tendency to tiredness generally lasts longer than the reduction of initiative.

Let us now have a look at the gamma cases. No confusion and no disorientation occur. There is only a slight indication of reduction of initiative and of increased tendency to tiredness. Sometimes these symptoms do not appear at all. I have just mentioned that gammacapsulotomy is a very mild intervention from neurosurgical point of view. The same can be said in psychiatric respects. The gamma patients feel more or less better immediately after the intervention. During the following days their improvement continues so they can be classified as much better or

restored. This immediate positive reaction is temporary; it lasts from
a couple of days to two weeks in the cases I have studied. Then the symptoms reappear without being so marked and painful as before the operation.
The relapse varies in length from some weeks to several months. However,
in one case it lasted a little more than a year. After this phase the
patients again feel better if the operation has been successful, and they
advance to the symptom-free group or to the groups "much improved" or
"slightly improved".

Typically their condition changès during the relapse. For some days
or weeks they may feel worse and at other periods better. It is necessary to treat them with anxiolytic drugs in a flexible way, increasing the
dose when they feel worse and reducing it as soon as they are getting
better. In most patients these drugs have a much better effect now than
before the operation.

Thus, allt the patients, with one exeption, have shown an immediate
symptom-reduction after the operation, followed by a relapse and, in
successful cases, complete recovery or improvement. The only exception
from this pattern is a 30-year old woman with severe anxiety and phobia.
She did not get a relapse. After the operation she felt much better and
was soon restored and remaind restored.

An interesting point is, I think, that the pattern is quite the same
as after gamma treatment for pain, in spite of the fact that concerning
pain, brain cells are destroyed, but in our cases white matter, i.e. nerve
paths. Concerning the follow-ups, I think I have performed these examinations rather thoroughly. Personally, I have seen the patients up to 12
times since they left the hospital. The mean of the number of follow-up
examinations is 6. I have also interviewed the patient's relatives. In
this way I have been able to follow my patients very closely, noticing
all changes which can be caused by exogenous and endogenous stress factors. No patient has lost the so important psychophysiological function
of anxiety which only has been reduced to more normal proportions. Relap-
ses in quite restored patients have occurred after, for instance, severe
attacks of influenza or pneumonia or serious psychic traumata. These re-
lapses pass soon over after treatment with anxiolytica and antidepressiva.
This pattern follows quite what mcy happen in heat lesion if they are exposed to severe stress. The same psychometric tests have been applied
before and 5 to 28 months after operation as used in heat lesion series,
examining memory functions, concentration ability, abstract thought functions, and intellectual level (Wechsler-Bellevuescale). No intellectual

reduction has been observed on the contrary, there is a tendency to achieve better results in several tests after operation. We noticed the same tendency in the heat series. This is understandable, considering that the patients have been freed from their anxiety of had it reduced.

Two personality tests were applied, namely, Eysenck´s personality inventory and an anxiety scale, The multi-compound anxiety inventory. The last mentioned test showed significant reduction of anxiety both psychic and somatic as well as muscle tension. Thus, a more objective measure verifies the clinical judgement and the opinion of the patients that their anxiety has been reduced or disappeared. Concerning Eysenck´s inventory no significant differences were observed in neuroticism. Extraversion showed an increase which was marginally significant.

Through psychophysiological measures Sten Levander is trying to get a more objective quantification of some of the anxiety concommitants, i.e. the level of autonomic arousal. Continuous recording of skin conductance, heart rate and respiratory pattern are obtained during rest and repeated tone stimulation. This work is going on.

Now the results. I want to stress that the results shown in table 3 must be looked upon as preliminary and with great care considering the small series involved and the limited periods of observation. After this reservation I would like to tell you that 6 of our patients are symptom-free, 4 are much improved, 2 slightly improved, and 2 unchanged. In percentage, for sake of comparison, this would mean that 71% of the gamma

TABLE 3. RESULTS OF GAMMA-CAPSULOTOMY

NO. OF CASES	EFFECT OF OPERATION
6	(A) Free from symptoms; all working
4	(B) Much improved; all working
2	(C) Slightly improved; one working
2	(D) Unchanged

cases show satisfactory results, or the same percentage as in the heat lesion series. From a social point of view it should be emphasized that, as you can see from table 3, 11 patients are working, namely, all in the groups A and B and one patient in group C. Before the operation they were unable to work. There are many other things to take up, for example, the normalizing effect of the operation on sexual life. Most patients suffer from disturbances, because of anxiety, obsessive-compulsive troubles or overdosage of medicine. After the operation the sex function became normal or at least improved.

Another observation is that several of the patients and their relatives think that their personalities have improved. Before the illness they showed psychasthenic traits with shyness, sensitiveness, tendencies to inferiority feelings and difficulties in making contact with other people. After the operation their shyness has been reduced or disappeared. It was easier for them to contact others; they were more self-confident and less disposed to self-reproaches.

REFERENCES
1. Bingley T., Leksell L., Meyerson B.A. and Rylander G. (1973): In:Surgical Approaches in Psychiatry, p. 160. eds. L.Laitinen and K.E.Livingston. University Park Press, Baltimore.
2. Bingley T., Leksell L., Meyerson B.A. and Rylander G., (1977): In: Neurosurgical Treatment in Psychiatry, Pain and Epilepsy, p.287, eds. W.Sweet, S.Obrador and J. Martin-Rodriguez, University Park Press, Baltimore.
3. Bingley T., and Person A. (1978): Electroenceph. clin. Neurophysiol.

4. Meyerson B.A.(1977): In: Neurological Surgery Proceedings of the Sixth International Congress, Sao Paulo, eds Raúl Carrea. p 307.

© 1979 Elsevier/North-Holland Biomedical Press
Modern Concepts in Psychiatric Surgery
E.R. Hitchcock, H.T. Ballantine, Jr. and B.A. Meyerson, eds.

STEREOTACTIC SUBCAUDATE TRACTOTOMY:LONG-TERM RESULTS AND MEASURING OF EFFECTS
ON PSYCHIATRIC SYMPTOMS.

JAIME BROSETA,JUAN LUIS BARCIA-SALORIO,PEDRO ROLDAN and JOSE BARBERA.

Departamento de Neurocirugia.Hospital Clinico Universitario.Valencia.Spain.

Different criteria in the selection of target and the surgical indications
are of the most outstanding problems that psychiatric surgery is confronted with
today.However,there is general agreement as to the efficacy of subcaudate tractotomy in certain mental disorders.Many authors using this technique had excellent results in chronic depression and anxiety states,some improvement in obsessional neurosis and a little change in schizophrenia[1,2,3,4,5].

Psychiatric surgery in general is applied to main psychiatric diagnoses,often
disregarding other less florid accompanying symptoms.In such cases,the surgical
results offer scant information.Furthermore,the psychosurgical indication has an
eminently empiric base,largely due to the non parametric character of psychia-
try.The latter leads to the lack of uniformity in psychiatric information and to
the imposibility of quantifying treatment of same.A universal standardization of
terminology and a common system of measuring would facilitate the comparison between the results obtained by the same surgical technique,aiding a better selection of candidates for psychiatric surgery.

Along these lines,this study serves a double purpose.On the one hand,to analyze and attempt to quantify the effect that subcaudate tractotomy has on different psychiatric syndromes,but considering these changes symptom by symptom,in-
dependent of the main diagnosis.On the other hand,a computarized mathematical
model,grounded on the Bayesian theory of decision,has been formulated,in order
to predict in new cases the utility of the operation and the probability of improvement of each symptom.

CLINICAL MATERIAL AND METHODS

Between 1968 and 1975,in our Department,stereotactic subcaudate tractotomy
(SST) was carried out on 43 patients with different mental illnesses (19 obsessional neurosis,11 chronic depressions and 13 schizophrenics).As a retrospective study,some difficulties appeared in the attempt to adapt all previous psychiatric information to the present quantitative method.Therefore,in only 15 of
the 43 patients was it possible to transfer this in a reliable way.

Table I shows the details of age,sex,duration of illness and prior diagnosis of this sample.Psychiatrists from different schools and criteria referred the patients,attending mainly to the chronic resistence of mental process to any therapy.But in all cases our own Department of Psychiatry indicated the operation.As shown,diagnoses which finally determined the operation were always framed within the main classical categories.

To analyze the surgical results,the standardized system described by WING et al.[6] was followed.All psychiatric information was adapted to the Present State Examination (PSE),preoperatively by transfering the past history to this questionary,assisted by the patient and relatives;postoperatively by personal interview.The 140 items of the PSE were grouped into 38 syndromes: nuclear syndrome (NS),catatonic syndrome (CS),incoherent speech (IS),residual syndrome (RS),depressive delusion and hallucination (DD),simple depression (SD),obsessional neurosis (ON),general anxiety (GA),situational anxiety (SA),hysteria (HT),affective flattening (AF),hypomania (HM),auditory hallucinations (AH),delusions of persecution (PE),delusions of reference (RE),grandiose and religious delusion (GR), sexual and fantastic delusions (SF),visual hallucinations (VH),olfactory hallucinations (OH),overactivity (OV),slowness (SL),non specific psychosis (NP),depersonalisation (DE),special features of depression (ED),agitation (AG),self neglect (NG),ideas of reference (IR),tension (TE),lack of energy (LE),worry (WO) irritability (IT),social unease (SU),loss of interest and concentration (IC),hypochondriasis (HY),other symptoms of depression (OD),organic impairment (OR),subcultural delusions or hallucinations (SC),and doubtful interview (DI).This Syndrome Check List (SCL) and its code are used throughout this study.The value of each syndrome was obtained from the sum of the individual constituent scores.

Table II shows the preoperative scores of the SCL and the preoperative state of the 15 patients.The analysis of the frequency of appearance and the intensity of each syndrome showed that those that appear more frequently tally with the more severe ones:SD,ON,GA,SA,TE,LE,AG,WO,SU and IC.

From SCL,the psychiatric descriptive categories of each patient can be obtained.Table I (1 and 2) compares the prior psychiatric diagnosis with the preoperative descriptive category,showing a discordance in 26 % of cases,demonstrating the possible inconsistency of psychiatric diagnosis when done in broad terms.

In all cases a pre and postoperative psychometric study was done.The Wechsler Adult Intelligence Scale (WAIS) was used to assess the changes in intellectual output and organic impairment.The Rorschach test was used to evaluate variations in the personality structure.By means of personal and family interview,the

C	Age/Sex	Duration of illness	Previous diagnosis[1]	Pre DC[2]		Post DC[3]		Follow-up
1	24/f	4 years	Schizophrenia	N	++			5 years
				S	+			
				M	?			
2	20/m	1 year	Schizophrenia	N	++			7 years
3	28/f	10 years	Obsessional neuros.	N	+	N	+	8 years
4	33/m	10 years	Schizophrenia	S	++	S	++	3 years
				N	?	N	?	
5	30/m	16 years	Obsessional neuros.	N	++	N	++	4 years
				S	?	S	?	
6	17/m	7 years	Obsessional neuros.	N	+	N	+	4 years
				U	?	U	?	
7	37/m	11 years	Depression	N	++	N	++	3 years
				D	+	D	+	
8	23/m	6 years	Schizophrenia	N	++	N	+	8 years
				D	++	D	+	
				M	+	M	?	
				S	?	S	?	
9	50/m	4 years	Depression	N	++			4 years
10	18/f	2 years	Obsessional neuros.	N	++	N	++	5 years
				M	?			
				D	?			
11	30/f	5 years	Schizophrenia	N	++	N	++	6 years
				S	+	S	+	
				D	?			
12	42/f	10 years	Obsessional neuros.	N	++	N	++	6 years
13	17/f	4 years	Schizophrenia	S	+	S	++	8 years
				N	?	N	++	
				M	?			
14	51/m	11 years	Depression	N	++	N	++	4 years
				M	++	M	++	
15	34/f	4 years	Obsessional neuros.	N	++	N	++	9 years

Table I.- General data and comparison between the previous psychiatric diagnosis (1) and the preoperative (2) and postoperative (3) descriptive categories (DC) in each of the 15 cases.Descriptive categories,after WING et al:S,schizophrenic type; D,psychotic depressive type; M,manic type; U,non specific psychosis type; N,neurotic type (depressive,anxiety,obsessional and residual neurosis).Degree of certainty: ++,high present; +,present; ?,partially present.

effect of operation on the socioeconomic and occupational enviroment of the patient and relatives,was also studied.

Stereotactic subcaudate tractotomy was performed under general anaesthesia. Our own multipurpose stereoencephalotome was used.An air-ventriculography was

SCL	Cases															F	Score (%)
	1	2	3	4	5	6	7	8	9	10	11	12	13	14	15		
NS	1	0	0	5	0	0	0	0	0	0	4	0	0	0	0	3	4.2
DD	0	0	0	0	0	0	2	4	0	0	0	0	0	0	0	2	4.4
SD	8	9	2	3	6	0	7	2	6	0	7	4	3	4	5	13	40.0
ON	1	2	2	0	6	0	0	0	0	5	6	2	0	0	6	8	33.3
GA	3	4	2	2	3	2	4	6	3	3	3	0	0	2	5	13	50.0
SA	4	3	0	1	0	1	5	3	3	1	2	0	2	1	5	12	34.4
AF	0	0	0	1	0	0	0	0	0	0	2	0	0	0	0	2	10.0
HM	3	0	0	0	0	0	0	0	0	1	0	0	0	3	0	3	4.7
PE	0	0	0	1	0	0	0	0	0	0	2	0	2	0	0	3	16.7
RE	1	0	0	2	0	0	0	0	0	0	4	0	2	0	0	4	15.0
GR	0	0	0	0	0	0	0	1	0	0	0	0	2	0	0	2	3.3
SF	3	0	0	2	2	0	0	3	0	0	4	0	2	0	0	6	4.8
OV	0	0	0	0	0	0	0	6	0	0	0	0	1	0	0	2	10.0
SL	2	0	0	0	0	0	0	0	2	1	4	0	0	0	0	4	7.5
NP	1	0	0	0	0	2	0	1	0	0	2	0	0	0	0	4	1.0
DE	2	0	0	2	0	0	0	1	0	0	1	0	0	0	0	4	10.0
ED	2	5	0	2	2	1	0	0	2	1	3	1	0	0	0	9	12.7
AG	0	0	0	0	0	2	0	2	2	0	2	0	2	0	1	6	56.7
NG	0	0	0	0	0	0	0	0	0	0	2	0	0	0	0	1	6.7
IR	0	2	0	0	1	1	0	2	1	0	2	0	2	0	0	7	36.7
TE	2	1	0	2	4	1	2	1	5	1	5	0	2	0	2	12	31.1
LE	1	1	1	2	2	0	2	0	2	1	2	1	0	0	0	10	50.0
WO	7	7	7	7	10	2	10	1	5	2	4	6	2	5	7	15	54.7
IT	1	1	1	2	0	1	2	1	0	0	2	1	3	1	0	11	21.3
SU	5	5	0	1	2	2	2	5	4	0	4	0	3	2	5	12	44.4
IC	2	2	2	0	3	0	4	2	2	0	1	4	0	0	4	10	43.3
HY	0	0	0	0	0	0	2	0	1	0	1	0	0	0	0	3	13.3
OD	2	1	1	0	1	0	3	1	4	0	1	5	3	5	4	12	23.0

Table II.- Preoperative frequency and intensity scores of each syndrome in the 15 patients of the sample (lines).Preoperative psychiatric state of each patient (columns).For SCL code see text.CS,IS,RS,HT,AH,VH,OH,OR,SC, and DI were not present in any patient.

carried out to visualize the ventricular system and the cerebral midline.It was possible to obtain the caudatum outline by means of stereotactic angiopneumotomography,assisted by a computarized laplacian trasformation that corrected individual anatomic variations,so to avoid corpus striatum damage[7].The SST target was placed on a line 1 cm. above and parallel to the orbital roof at 1 cm. from the anterior clinoid process and 16 mm. from the midline.In previously diagnosed cases of obsessional neurosis,a second target was established,localized 3 mm. above the former one.Through bicoronal burr-holes,the electrode was introduced under fluoroscopic control.Radiofrequency was used to produce a thermolesion,raising the temperature to 75°C during 120 sec.With these parameters a spherical lesion of 6 mm. in each target was assumed.The operation was always performed bilaterally.

RESULTS

Measurement of effects of SST on psychiatric symptoms

Inmediately after the operation 80 % of the cases showed a marked alleviation of symptomatology during approximately 1 year,after which the good results deteriorated.

Table III shows the postoperative SCL psychiatric state in the 15 patients of the sample at the end of the follow-up time,which varied from 3 to 10 years with an average of 6.3 years.

SCL	1	2	3	4	5	6	7	8	9	10	11	12	13	14	15	F	Score (%)
NS	0	0	0	5	0	0	0	0	0	0	6	0	0	0	0	2	4.6
CS	0	0	0	0	0	0	0	0	0	0	0	0	4	0	0	1	6.7
IS	0	0	0	0	0	0	0	0	0	0	0	0	2	0	0	1	3.3
DD	0	0	0	0	0	0	2	1	0	0	0	0	0	0	0	2	2.2
SD	0	0	2	3	3	0	2	0	0	0	3	7	9	4	0	8	20.0
ON	0	0	2	0	0	0	0	1	0	3	3	3	0	0	2	6	15.5
GA	0	0	0	3	0	1	1	0	0	0	0	2	2	1	0	6	11.1
SA	0	0	0	2	0	0	2	0	0	0	1	0	6	1	0	5	13.3
AF	0	0	0	1	0	0	0	0	0	0	0	1	2	0	0	3	13.3
HM	0	0	0	0	0	0	0	3	0	0	0	0	0	1	0	2	2.7
PE	0	0	0	2	0	0	0	0	0	0	0	0	2	0	0	2	13.3
RE	0	0	0	2	0	0	0	0	0	0	2	0	2	0	0	3	10.0
GR	0	0	0	0	0	0	0	0	0	0	0	0	0	0	0	0	0.0
SF	0	0	0	2	2	0	0	1	0	0	1	0	4	0	0	5	3.0
OV	0	0	0	0	0	0	0	2	0	0	0	0	4	0	0	2	6.7
SL	0	0	0	0	0	0	0	0	0	0	1	1	6	0	0	3	6.7
NP	0	0	0	0	0	1	0	0	0	0	0	1	4	0	0	3	1.2
DE	0	0	0	1	0	0	0	0	0	0	0	0	0	0	0	1	1.7
ED	0	0	0	2	1	0	1	0	0	0	2	1	2	0	0	6	6.0
AG	0	0	0	0	0	1	0	1	0	0	0	1	2	0	0	4	16.7
NG	0	0	0	0	0	0	0	0	0	0	0	0	2	0	0	1	6.7
IR	0	0	0	0	1	0	0	1	0	0	1	0	0	0	0	3	10.0
TE	0	0	0	2	2	0	2	1	0	0	1	4	2	0	0	7	15.5
LE	0	0	1	2	1	0	1	0	0	0	2	2	2	0	0	7	36.7
WO	0	0	7	7	5	2	5	0	1	0	4	4	6	5	2	11	32.0
IT	0	0	1	2	2	0	1	2	0	0	2	1	5	1	0	9	22.7
SU	0	0	0	1	1	0	3	0	0	0	1	0	6	2	1	7	18.2
IC	0	0	2	0	2	0	1	0	0	0	1	4	4	0	2	7	26.7
HY	0	0	0	0	0	0	2	0	0	0	1	0	0	0	0	2	10.0
OD	0	0	1	0	1	0	3	0	0	0	0	3	5	4	1	7	20.0

Table III.- Postoperative frequency and intensity scores of each syndrome in the 15 patients of the sample (lines).Postoperative psychiatric state of each case (columns).For SCL code see text.RS,HT,AH,VH,OH,OR,SC and DI do not appear in any patient.

Figure 1 establishes a comparison between the pre and postoperative states of the SCL,offering the percentage of improvement of each syndrome.The certainty of

246

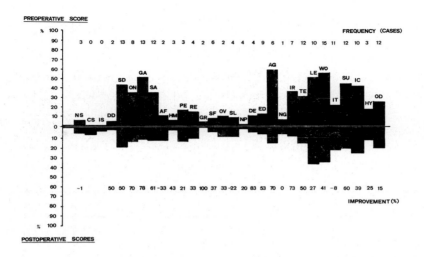

Figure 1.- This histogram establishes a comparison between the pre and postoperative intensity of the SCL,offering the mean improvement percentage related to the preoperative frequency of each syndrome.

the results are directly related to the preoperative frequency of appearance of each syndrome.

Considering the more intense and frequent preoperative syndromes,the following results were obtained:simple depression (SD) disappeared in 39 % of cases with a reduction of preoperative intensity of 50 %;obsessional neurosis (ON) ceased in 25 % of patients with a decrease in intensity of 53 %;general and situational anxiety (GA)(SA) were abolished in 54 % and 58 % of cases with an attenuation of 78 % and 61 % respectively;agitation (AG) was annuled in 32 % and decreased its preoperative intensity in 70 %;ideas of reference (IR) ceased in 60 % of cases with a reduction in intensity of 73 %;tension (TE) disappeared in 41 % of patients and was attenuated in 50 %;lack of energy (LE) was abolished in 30 % of the cases with an intensity decrease of 27 %;worry (WO) disappeared in 27 % reducing its intensity in 41 %;social unease (SU) ceased in 34 % of patients and reduced in 60 % its intensity;and loss of interest and concentration (IC) was

annuled in 30 % of cases with an attenuation of 38 %.Results obtained in less
frequent preoperative syndromes were only taken as orientative,because in the
case of their being considered as significant can lead to spurious conclusions
due to the brief sample.This is noted in the schizophrenic component syndromes,
where grandiose and religious delusions (GR) and depersonalisation (DE) were the
most improved syndromes,with 100 % and 83 % of improvement respectively,but on
the base of 2 and patients.In certain syndromes,slight postoperative impairment
was noted (NS,AF,NP and IT),but also this deterioration was found in preoperative low frequent syndromes,so the results are not conclusive either.

Table IV illustrates the same results on SCL according to a 5-point scale
stated by PIPPARD[8],where the former data are reconfirmed.

Concluding,the best results were observed in the neurotic type syndromes,whe-
re anxiety states were the most improved.The alleviation observed in obsessional
neurosis was greatly dependent on this last factor,because ceremonial and ritual
component only seldom disappeared,but when the patients were relieved of the anxiety load,they felt very amielorated.Analyzing the changes gained in all syndromes that measure depression (DD,SD,ED,OD) an average reduction of previous intensity of 45 % was showed,with a more marked improvement in depressive neurosis.
Suicidal attempts were abolished in all cases of the sample.

WAIS test showed that SST does not produce or increase organic impairment.In-
tellectual output was not altered in any patient.An IQ decrease was never observed and,occasionally,slight increase of IQ levels was noted.Postoperative Rorschach test continued to show an emotional disorder in 80 % of the cases,showing
the same preoperative disturbance.The latter was confirmed in the comparative
study between the pre and postoperative psychiatric categories (Table I,2 and 3)
where as many as 80 % of cases still presented the same combination of descriptive categories in both states.This suggests that SST do not modify the pathological structure of personality but decrease the intensity of its manifestations.

In 50 % of patients,the operation allowed a total occupational reintegration,
with a decrease of 60 % of the previous incapacity.After treatment,social and family life was notably improved in 50 % of cases.Following SST,of the 15 patients
2 got married,3 of them increased the family,and 2 became engaged,with no unusual problems.Operation reduced the effect of mental illness on different concepts of the family members (interfamilial relations,health,economy,occupational
duties and social and recreational activities) in 64 % as average.

There was no mortality due to the surgical procedure.The postoperative adverse effects were limited to transitory disturbances such as confusion,lethargia
and desinhibition.In 2 cases,previously diagnosed as schizophrenics,SST did not

SCL	Improvement scale					Cases	SCL	Improvement scale					Cases
	I	II	III	IV	V			I	II	III	IV	V	
NS	1	0	0	1	1	3	SL	3	1	0	0	2	6
CS	0	0	0	0	1	1	NP	2	0	1	0	2	5
IS	0	0	0	0	1	1	DE	3	0	1	0	0	4
DD	0	1	0	1	0	2	ED	5	0	2	2	2	11
SD	5	2	1	3	2	13	AG	3	1	1	1	1	7
ON	3	1	2	1	2	9	NG	1	0	0	0	1	2
GA	9	3	0	0	3	15	IR	4	0	2	1	0	7
SA	7	1	1	1	2	12	TE	6	1	1	4	1	13
AF	1	0	0	1	2	4	LE	4	0	2	3	2	11
HM	2	1	0	0	1	4	WO	4	2	3	5	1	15
PE	1	0	0	1	1	3	IT	3	0	1	5	3	12
RE	1	0	1	2	0	4	SU	4	2	2	2	2	12
GR	2	0	0	0	0	2	IC	4	0	3	3	1	11
SF	1	2	0	2	1	6	HY	1	0	0	2	0	3
OV	0	1	0	0	1	2	OD	4	1	2	3	1	11

Table IV.- Surgical results on SCL according to the 5-point scale of improvement stated by PIPPARD[8]: I,symptom free; II,much improved; III,improved; IV,unchanged; V,worse.For SCL code see text.

only modify the preoperative situation but postoperatively certain syndromes priorly absent (CS,IS) appeared.This phenomenon was interpreted as caused by the operation or,more probably,as previously masked symptoms that became more evident by the natural course of the illness,more so in the absence of the syndromes removed by SST.In an other 2 cases,certain impulse and acting out disturbances appeared in excess or defect.

Predictive assessment

Recently,reliable automatic processes of decision have been introduced in the field of medical diagnosis and treatment [9,10] .Our purpose was to design a mathematical model capable of predicting the advantages that SST could offer to a new candidate,proffering the probability of improvement of each symptom and the feasable utility of the operation.

This model must be based on the conduct that SST followed in the cases of the sample.In this analysis,the first stage was to conceptually uniform and quantify the psychiatric information,which was reached by means of the WING et al system[6]. The second stage was to study the mechanism by which the patients had passed from the preoperative situation to the postoperative one.To this aim,the Bayesian theory of decision was applied.

To determine the utility (u) of the operation in a psychiatric case supposes a risk.Therefore,a linear system of evaluation is being developed.But,at the moment,to quantify the utility of SST,an operative method was followed.As all syndromes do not have the same clinical importance within the psychiatric picture, the present SCL syndromes in the sample were assembled into 3 groups,according to a decreasing order of significance: Group A.- NS,CS,IS,DD,SD,ON,HM,PE,RE,GR, SF,NP and DE; Group B.- GA,SA,OV,AF,ED,IR and SU; Group C.- SL,AG,NG,IT,TE,LE, IC,HY,WO and OD,where A>B>C.In this classification the criterion of the psychiatrist,neurosurgeon and social worker have intervened.The percentage of improvement in the three groups were calculated in each patient.These percentages were transfered to a 5-point scale: 1,symptom free; 2,improvement higher than 50 %; 3,improvement equal or lower than 50 %; 4,unchanged; 5,worse.In this way,a 3 digits number was obtained (triad),where the ordinal sequence corresponded to the order of clinical importance of the groups.A utility for SST was establish in each possible variation of the triads,according to a 5 to 0 decreasing scale.Table V illustrates the percentages of improvement in each group of clinical importance,the triads and the utility index for each patient of the sample.

Once the utility of SST in the sample was observed with this system,to find out the surgical utility in a new case (j) the following logical tree can be applied:

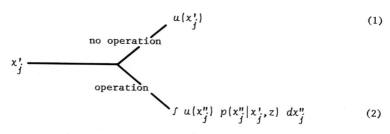

$$u(x_j')\tag{1}$$

$$\int u(x_j'')\ p(x_j''|x_j',z)\ dx_j''\tag{2}$$

where x' is the preoperative situation of the new patient,x'' is the unknown situation of same,and z are all possible pairs of data from the sample of this study.It is assumed that without operating on the patient,the postoperative state is similar to an unchanged result with operation.Operating on the patient the utility the utility will be dependent on (2),calculated according to a probabilistic judgement.Once the surgical utility in both possibilities is known,when that resulting from (2) be higher than that obtained in (1) SST will be indicated,although its application is dependent on the amplitude of the differences between them.

To calculate the prior probabilistic distribution it was supposed that between x' and x'' existed a probabilistic relation of the type $p(x''|x') = N(x''|x' +d,H)$ where the latter function represented a multivariant normal model

Case	Improvement (%) Group A	Group B	Group C	Triad	Utility of SST
1	100	100	100	111	5
2	100	100	100	111	5
3	0	100	0	414	1
4	–	–	0	554	0
5	77	51	34	223	5
6	50	88	55	322	3
7	53	40	39	233	4
8	81	49	33	233	4
9	100	100	100	111	5
10	47	100	100	311	4
11	61	73	53	222	5
12	–	–	–	555	0
13	–	–	–	555	0
14	30	20	10	333	3
15	77	100	73	212	5

Table V.- Percentages of improvement in each SCL group, triads and the utility of SST in each patient of the study.

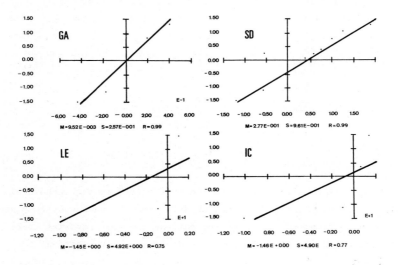

Figure 2.- The highest and lowest accomodation of the pre/postoperative varia – tions of the SCL to the multivariant normal model (r_{GA}=0.99; r_{SD}=0.99; r_{LE}=0.75; r_{IC}=0.77).

with unknown $x' + d$ and H precision matrix, estimated from data. In a new patient (j) the probability of improvement of each syndrome was estimated by means of a probabilistic argument between x''_j and x', according to the function $p(x''|x',z)$[11].

All SCL syndromes presented in more than 5 cases with different scores were tested in semilogarithmic paper according to this model,demonstrating their accomodation to the multivariant normal type (Figure 2).By means of multivariant t-Student test,the posterior probabilistic distribution of syndromes was obtained,offering the probability of improvement of same.

DISCUSSION

SST selectively produces a lesion in the area between the corpus striatum and the orbital cortex.This surgical region supposes a pathway network,which interconnects the dorsomedial nucleus of the thalamus with the orbital cortex,the gyrus cinguli and orbital cortex with hypothalamic nuclei,and the amigdalopiriform complex with the preoptic-pituitary region.In cats and rabbits,the anterior nucleus of the thalamus pathways to gyrus cinguli pass through this area.In man, the latter projections mainly travel by the anterior part of the internal capsula,being near to the frontal lower medial quadrant,where SST target is placed. KNIGHT[4] reported good results in depression by means of SST,but had encountered certain resistence in the remission of obsessional neurosis.BINGLEY et al.[12] reported much improved results in obsessional neurosis with the anterior capsulotomy.Following the former considerations,in those patients of this study previously diagnosed as chronic depressives or schizophrenics,the target was chosen according to KNIGHT[4],with slight modifications due to the use of radiofrequency lesioning system.In cases diagnosed as obsessional neurosis,the size of the former lesion was superiorly extended by means of a second lesion that tried to include the more anterior cingulothalamic connections.

The results obtained with SST by other authors[2,3] improved chronic depression in 70 % of patients,varying in obsessional neurosis cases from 50 to 66 %.These results agree with those presented in this study.The improvement percentage gained in anxiety states are slight higher here than those of the former authors.

On the basis of these long-term results,SST has proved to be a safe technique in our experience,that allowed good improvement levels in anxiety states,mixed rebel neurosis,depression and even in obsessional neurosis.

Since results are difficult to compare,it would be better to adopt standardized methods of quantification in universal psychosurgical environs.Furthermore, while the base to improve results would be the better selection of candidates, bearing in mind all limitations that these automatic models of decision can have,the future collaboration of such methods in assisting human decision appears atractive.

252

ACKNOWLEDGEMENTS

The authors are much indebted to F.Iglesias.M.D.,C.Leal.M.D.,I.Montero.M.D. and I.Tomas.M.D. for their valuable criticism and assessment in psychiatric concepts;to J.M.Bernardo,Sc.D.,for his help in the mathematical treatment of the model of decision;and to Mr.K.Martin for his unestimable assistence in English language.

REFERENCES

1.Bartlett.J.R. and Bridges.P.K. (1977) The extended subcaudate tractotomy lesion.In Neurosurgical Treatment in Psychiatry,Pain and Epilepsy.Sweet.W.H., Obrador.S. and Martin-Rodriguez.J.G.,eds.University Park Press,Baltimore.pp. 387-398.

2.Goktepe.E.O.,Young.L.B. and Bridges.P.K. (1975) a further review of the results of stereotactic subcaudate tractotomy.Brit.J.Psychiat,126,270-280.

3.Bridges.P.K.,Goktepe.E.O.,Maratos.J.,Browne.A. and Young.L. (1973) A comparative review of patients with obsessional neurosis and depression treated by psychosurgery.Brit.J.Psychiat.,123,663-674.

4.Knight.G.G. (1972) Bifrontal stereotactic tractotomy in the substancia innominate.A experience of 450 cases.In Psychosurgery.Hitchcock.E.,Laitinen.L. and Vaernet.K.,eds.Charles.C.Thomas,Springfield.pp.267-277.

5.Strom-Olsen.R. and Carlisle.S. (1972) Bifrontal stereotactic tractotomy.A follow-up study.In Psychosurgery.Hitchcock.E.,Laitinen.L. and Vaernet.K.,eds. Charles.C.Thomas,Springfield.pp.278-288.

6.Wing.J.K.,Cooper.J.E. and Sartorius.N. (1974) Measurement and classification of psychiatric symptoms.Cambridge University Press,London.

7.Barcia-Salorio.J.L.,Barbera.J.,Broseta.J. and Soler.F. (1977) Tomography in stereotaxis.A new stereoencephalotome designed for this purpose.Acta Neurochirurgica.Suppl.24,77-83.

8.Pippard.J. (1955) Rostral leucotomy:A report on 240 cases personally followed up after 1½ to 5 years.J.Ment.Sci.,101,756-773.

9.Gorry.G.A. (1973) Computer-assisted clinical decision-making.Methods.Inf.Med, 12,45-51.

10.Betaque.N.E. and Gorry.G.A. (1971) Automatic judgemental decision making for serious medical problem. Manag.Sci.,17,421-434.

11.Bernardo.J.M. (1977) Metodos bayesianos y diagnosis clinica.Estadistica Esp., 72/73,34-51.

12.Bingley.T.,Leksell.L.,Meyerson.B.A. and Rylander.G. (1973) Stereotactic anterior capsulotomy in anxiety and obsessive-compulsive states.In Surgical Approaches in Psychiatry.Laitinen.L. and Livingston.K.,eds.MTP Co.Ltd,Lancaster.pp.159-164.

© 1979 Elsevier/North-Holland Biomedical Press
Modern Concepts in Psychiatric Surgery
E.R. Hitchcock, H.T. Ballantine, Jr. and B.A. Meyerson, eds.

SAFETY AND EFFICACY OF CINGULOTOMY FOR PAIN AND PSYCHIATRIC DISORDER

SUZANNE CORKIN, THOMAS E. TWITCHELL, and EDITH V. SULLIVAN
Department of Psychology and Clinical Research Center
Massachusetts Institute of Technology, Cambridge, Massachusetts, 02139

ABSTRACT

A prospective study of therapeutic outcome, neurologic status, and behavioral test performance was carried out with 57 patients who received bilateral stereotactic anterior cingulotomy for the relief of intractable pain or psychiatric disorder. The therapeutic outcome of 34 patients was evaluated at two times about a year apart; the incidence of improvement was 64 percent at the first assessment and 71 percent at the second, suggesting that their postoperative conditions were relatively stable. When the total group of 57 patients was subdivided according to diagnosis, the incidence of improvement was high in patients with persistent pain and also in those with depression, but low in those with a diagnosis of schizophrenia or obsessive-compulsive neurosis. A comparison of preoperative and postoperative behavioral test scores revealed significant gains in the Wechsler I.Q. rating and, for patients under 30 years of age, in a nonverbal fluency task. In the early postoperative period, patients over 30 years of age showed significant losses on an embedded figures task and in copying a complex drawing, while men, but not women, showed a decline on two tapping tasks. Follow-up studies are now underway to determine the course of these changes. There is currently no evidence of lasting neurologic or behavioral deficits after cingulotomy.

INTRODUCTION

An investigation of therapeutic outcome, neurologic status, and behavioral test performance in patients who have undergone bilateral stereotactic anterior cingulotomy[1] for the relief of persistent pain or for the alleviation of severe psychiatric disease has been in progress since the latter part of 1973. The results for Phase I of the study, carried out between 1973 and June, 1976, suggested that some patients were markedly improved following the surgical procedure, whereas others were not helped at all[2,3]. Regardless of therapeutic outcome, however, there were no lasting neurologic or behavioral deficits attributable to the brain operation per se. Phase II of the study, to be reported here, covered the period from June 1976 through November 1977. This continuation and extension of the earlier study included a qualitative reassessment of therapeutic outcome in the 34 patients who participated in Phase I, and the addition of 23 new cases to the sample for preoperative and postoperative interview and examination.

PATIENTS

This report is based upon the results obtained with 57 patients, 21 men and 36 women, who have undergone cingulotomy for the relief of chronic, non-neoplastic pain, which was usually coupled with depression, or for the alleviation of severe psychiatric disorders that had been refractory to alternative forms of treatment (Table 1). Of the 57 patients, 41 were consecutive cases examined both before and after operation, and 16 were evaluated after operation only. Patients who were operated upon for pain differed from the other cases in that the pain and concomitant depression had begun later in life and was of shorter duration than the other disorders (Table 2). The pain cases were also older at the time of operation and testing, but there was no difference between the two main diagnostic groups in overall intellectual capacity.

TABLE 1.   PREOPERATIVE DIAGNOSIS OF 57 CINGULOTOMY PATIENTS

Group	No. of Cases	
	M	F
Pain (N = 15)		
Back or leg pain	3	7
Abdominal pain	1	2
Thalamic syndrome	0	1
Amputation stump	1	0
Psychiatric (N = 42)[a]		
Depression or probable depresssion	7	13
Schizophrenia	4	6
Obsessive-compulsive neurosis	2	5
Anxiety neurosis or probable anxiety neurosis	3	0
Other conditions	0	2

[a] For diagnostic criteria see Woodruff, Goodwin & Guze[4]

The bilateral radiofrequency lesions, confirmed by CT scan in many cases, typically included the anterior portion of the cingulate gyrus and bundle and the underlying corpus callosum. The lesion in each hemisphere was intended to come within 5 mm of the midline and was approximately 2 cm along the greatest axis and 1/2 to 1 1/2 cm perpendicular to the greatest axis. The lesions were placed 1 - 4 cm posterior to the anterior tip of the lateral ventricle[5,6].

TABLE 2. AGE AND I.Q. DATA FOR 57 CINGULOTOMY PATIENTS: MEANS AND RANGES

Diagnosis	Age at Onset of Illness or Complaint (Years)	Preop. Duration of Illness or Complaint (Years)	Age at First Cingulotomy (Years)	Age at Time of Present Study (Years)	Wechsler I.Q. at Time of Operation
Pain (N = 6M, 11F)	36.8 (18-59)	11.3 (3-38)	48.1 (28-76)	50.1 (28-76)	103.2 (76-121)
Psychiatric Disease (N = 15M, 25F)	22.9 (4-55)	15.7 (2-40)	38.5 (20-63)	39.6 (20-65)	99.5 (77-127)

METHOD

Evaluation of therapeutic outcome

On the basis of information obtained in a review of the patient records, case histories provided by patients and their relatives, written communications from patients, and telephone conversations with them, it was possible to document each individual's preoperative condition as well as his or her status at various times after operation. The analysis of therapeutic effect relied heavily upon tape-recorded interviews with the patient and a close relative, in which each one, in separate sessions, recounted the patient's history from before the onset of illness to the present. These interviews were directed toward obtaining an account of previous treatments and their effectiveness, employment and participation in household tasks, the quality of relationships with close relatives and friends, hobbies, travel, sleep, sexual behavior, and consumption of food, alcoholic beverages, and drugs. From all available information each patient was rated postoperatively as showing marked, moderate, slight, or no improvement; no patient was deemed worse after cingulotomy.

Neurological examination

The neurological examination included the standard procedures for evaluation of cranial nerve function, motor function (strength, tendon reflexes,

plantar responses, resistance to passive movement, presence or absence of involuntary movements, etc.), coordination, sensation (pinprick, light touch,
position and vibration), and gait and station. Additional tests were used
that have been found to detect more subtle abnormalities of posture and movement. These included procedures to assess the ability to dissociate head and
eye movements, both on command to look in a certain direction and on tracking
a moving target, to purse the lips, puff out the cheeks both together and separately, and to move the tongue to right and left and up and down. Any alteration in posture of the hand or fingers when the patient sat with arms out-
stretched and eyes closed was noted. Particular attention was given to any
fragment of a grasp reflex or avoiding response elicited by contact stimulation of the hand, and even the slightest degree was recorded if detected[7].
For testing hand and finger dexterity, a series of alternating pronation-supin-
ation of the hand and flexion-extension of the fingers of increasing difficulty
and emphasizing each hand alone and simultaneously with the other hand were
used. The ability to rapidly oppose the thumb to each finger was also assessed.
Any synkinetic movements or postures induced by these movements were recorded.
Finally, in addition to noting the gait and the ability to tandem walk, each
subject was asked to walk on toes or heels to bring out any abnormal dystonic
posture of the upper extremities.

Behavioral tasks

In order to assess the possible effects of bilateral lesions of the cingulate gyrus and bundle, tasks were chosen to sample behaviors thought to be dependent upon the integrity of the cortical and subcortical areas that are
interconnected through this region. It has been known for some time that
there is a fronto-limbic connection in monkey[8,9,10,11], which originates in
frontal granular cortex and is distributed via the cingulum bundle to the gyrus fornicatus (composed of the gyrus cinguli, retrosplenial cortex, and
parahippocampal gyrus). This system connects in turn with the circuitry of
the temporal lobe (Pandya & Domesick, unpublished data)[12], which receives
additional afferents from various subcortical limbic structures[12,13,14,15].
Thus, it seemed profitable to search for signs ordinarily associated with
frontal-lobe or temporal-lobe dysfunction in man, and to look for the kind of
impairment found in monkey or man after lesions of the cingulate cortex and
other limbic structures. Test items that sampled overall intelligence or
personality were also included. All measures were quantitative, permitting an
objective description of any changes that might have been revealed.

For most of the tasks in the extensive battery of cognitive, sensory, and

motor tests[2] there were no significant changes after operation. The procedures to be described below were the exceptions: the few measures on which
there were significant alterations in behavior after cingulotomy. These tasks
were given both before and after operation so that each patient could serve
as his or her own control. This aspect of the experimental design was crucial
to an accurate interpretation of postoperative performance, because it had
previously been found that some candidates for cingulotomy showed deficits before operation when their scores were compared with those of normal control
subjects[2,3].

Wechsler Adult Intelligence Scale (WAIS) and Wechsler-Bellevue Intelligence
Scale, Form II. The WAIS[16] was administered preoperatively, whenever possible,
to patients undergoing cingulotomy. When these scores were available for patients in the present series, they were compared with postoperative I.Q. ratings obtained in connection with the present study, when patients were given
Form II of the Wechsler-Bellevue Intelligence Scale[17]. This instrument is
considered to be an alternate form of the WAIS.

Nonverbal Fluency Test. A task was devised in which the patient was given
a number of colored plastic cylinders and squares that could be fit together.
The patient was then told to construct as many different structures as possible
in 5 minutes, using four pieces in each structure. The idea for this test
originated with the finding that patients with left frontal-lobe lesions do
poorly on a verbal fluency test[18], and it was hoped that the task described
here would be a nonverbal analogue.

Hidden Figures Test. Gottschaldt's[19,20] embedded figures were used in a
timed pencil and paper task in which the subject tried to detect and trace
simple geometric figures that were hidden in larger, more complex figures[21]
(Fig. 1). The five parts of the test were usually completed in about 20 minutes. Since previous studies had found this task to be a general sign of
cerebral dysfunction, poor performance having been seen with lesions in any
lobe of either hemisphere[22,23], it was hypothesized that the placing of lesions in the cingulate region bilaterally would result in poorer scores post-
operatively than preoperatively.

Rey-Osterrieth-Taylor Complex Figure Test. Subjects were given unlimited
time to copy a complex line drawing, and then 1 hour later, without having
been warned, were asked to draw it again from memory. The Taylor figure[24]
was given preoperatively and the Rey-Osterrieth figure[25,26] was given postoperatively (Fig. 2). Both the copy and the delayed recall were scored quantitatively, according to a system devised by Rey and refined by Taylor. This
procedure permitted a comparison of visuo-spatial capacities not dependent upon

258

recent memory, with those that were.

PART IV

Look at the two adjacent figures.
One of them is contained in each of
the drawings below.

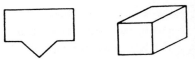

In each of the following drawings, mark
that part which is the same as one of the
adjacent figures. Mark only one figure
in each drawing.

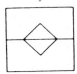 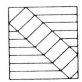 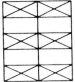 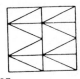

Fig. 1. Sample of the Hidden Figures Test (reproduced from Corkin[27]).

Tapping. Two tapping tests were given. One measured the patients' maximum
rate when tapping for 10 seconds with each index finger alone and with the two
tapping simultaneously. The other test, devised by Thurstone[21] required the
patient to tap four adjacent targets in sequence with a stylus for 30 seconds
per trial, both unimanually and bimanually, the movement sequences in the latter condition being different for each hand (Fig. 3).

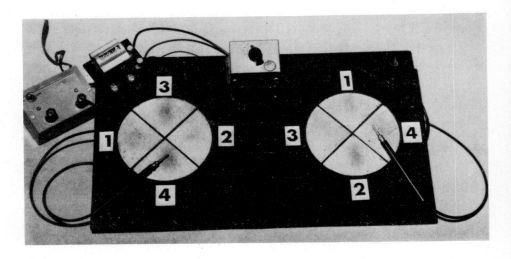

Fig. 3. Thurstone Tapping apparatus (reproduced from Corkin[27]).

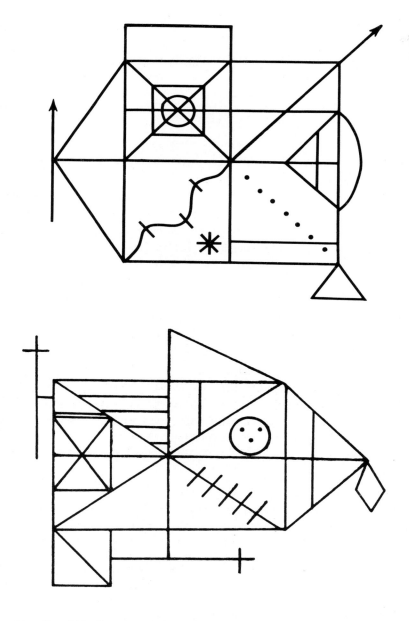

Fig. 2. Stimulus materials for Rey-Taylor Complex Figure Test. Top: Taylor figure[24] given preoperatively. Bottom: Rey[25,26] figure given postoperatively. (Reprinted with permission of L.B. Taylor).

Using tapping tasks somewhat similar to the two described here, other investigations have revealed deficits following bilateral lesions of the cingulum bundle or cingulate cortex in patients with intractable pain or severe emotional disturbance[28,29].

RESULTS
Evaluation of therapeutic outcome

These results present (1) a re-evaluation of therapeutic effect in the 34 Phase I patients, and (2) a description of the relationship between preoperative diagnosis and therapeutic result in the total group of 57.

The 34 cingulotomy patients whose therapeutic outcomes were described in the Phase I report[2,3] were re-evaluated in 1977. It was therefore possible to compare the incidence of improvement and ratings of improvement for the two time periods, and thereby to say something about the reliability of the qualitative evaluation. In this comparison, patients were assigned to the same diagnostic group as in the earlier report. These were pain, depression, obsessive-compulsive neurosis, and other psychiatric conditions (Table 3). The patient's preoperative condition was used as the baseline of comparison for both postoperative periods. The incidence of improvement for the group as a whole was 64 percent in 1975-1976 and 71 percent in 1977, this improvement being marked in 39 and 42 percent of the cases, respectively. In both time periods, the pain cases stood out as showing the greatest therapeutic success. Those with obsessive-compulsive neurosis were the least impressive in this respect, and patients with depression or other psychiatric conditions were intermediate. During the time interval between the two evaluations, 5 of the 34 patients underwent a second cingulotomy, which was followed by improvement in 2 cases but not in the other 3.

Having determined that estimates of the success of cingulotomy as a therapeutic tool held up over time, the next task was to specify more precisely which diagnostic groups benefited most from the surgical procedure. This further analysis could only be done satisfactorily with a larger number of cases; the 34 Phase I patients were combined with the 23 Phase II patients for this purpose.

It seemed desirable to subdivide patients not only on the basis of diagnosis[4] but also according to the number of cingulotomies they had undergone (Table 4). The incidence of improvement was impressive in patients whose primary complaint was persistent pain (94 percent) and in those with depression or probable depression (78 percent). In contrast, the majority of schizo-

TABLE 3. THERAPEUTIC OUTCOME AT TWO TIME PERIODS IN 34 CINGULOTOMY PATIENTS
OPERATED UPON BETWEEN 1964 and 1976 (PHASE I PATIENTS)

Diagnosis	1975 - May 1976		Sept. - Nov. 1977	
	Incidence of Improvement	Rating of Improvement	Incidence of Improvement	Rating of Improvement
Persistent Pain (N = 11)	9 (82%)	8 marked 1 moderate	10 (91%)	7 marked 2 moderate 1 slight
Depression (N = 7)	5 (71%)	3 marked 2 moderate	4 (57%)	3 marked 1 moderate
Obsessive-Compulsive Neurosis (N = 4)	1 (25%)	1 slight	2 (50%)	2 slight
Other Condidions (N = 12)	6 (55%)	2 marked 3 moderate 1 transient	6 (67%)	3 marked 2 moderate 1 slight

[a] 1 undetermined   [b] 3 undetermined

TABLE 4. RELATIONSHIP BETWEEN DIAGNOSIS AND RATING OF IMPROVEMENT IN 57
CINGULOTOMY PATIENTS

Diagnosis	N	Number of Cingulotomies		
		1	2	3
Pain	16	9 marked 3 moderate 3 slight	1 none	
Depression or Probable Depression	19	5 marked 3 moderate 2 slight 1 none	2 marked 1 moderate 1 slight 2 none 1 undetermined	1 none
Schizophrenia	10	1 slight 4 none	1 marked 2 none	1 marked 1 none
Obsessive-Compulsive	7	2 none	1 moderate 2 slight 1 none	1 none
Anxiety Neurosis or Probable Anxiety Neurosis	3	2 moderate 1 undetermined		
Other Conditions	2	1 marked 1 undetermined		

262

phrenics and obsessive-compulsives who had cingulotomies did not benefit from
the procedure. Of the 3 men whose diagnosis was anxiety neurosis or probable
anxiety neurosis, 2 gave evidence of moderate improvement. The third could not
be contacted. The two cases that fell into the remaining category, other conditions, included one woman with temporal-lobe epilepsy, who had marked improvement in her psychiatric disorder after cingulotomy, and another whose diagnosis
and present status could not be resolved.

Of the 57 patients, 15 (26 percent) were thought to require a second cingulotomy and 4 of them (7 percent) a third. The overall success rate declined
with each successive brain operation; it was 81 percent after the first, 57
percent after the second, and 25 percent after the third (Table 4).

Neurological examination

Many patients had prior evidence of neurologic illness. In the sample of
57 patients, 21 had a past history of disease affecting the brain (Table 5).
This included 13 cases of closed head injury, 5 of seizures, 1 of neurosyphilis,
1 of hepatic encephalopathy, and 1 of stroke.

TABLE 5.   INCIDENCE OF PRIOR CEREBRAL DISORDER IN 57 CINGULOTOMY PATIENTS

Disorder	No. of Cases
None	36 (63.2%)
Head Injury	13 (22.8%)
Seizures	5 (8.8%)
Neurosyphilis	1 (1.7%)
Hepatic Encephalopathy	1 (1.7%)
Stroke	1 (1.7%)

The results of the neurological examinations after cingulotomy showed that
21 patients had completely normal neurologic status (Table 6). In 19 patients
the neurologic abnormalities were those of drug-induced parkinsonism or dys-
kinesiae. All of these patients had been on various combinations of psychotropic drugs over a long period. In 13 patients the only abnormalities were
related to the primary disease that led up to the eventual cingulotomy. All
of these patients were in the pain group, and the neurologic deficits were primarily those of root or nerve dysfunction. Of the other patients who showed
postoperative neurologic abnormalities, 2 were known to have had prior cerebral
disease, and in 2 others, who were not examined before operation, the etiology
could not be unequivocally ascertained. However, in those patients examined

neurologically both before and after cingulotomy, there were no changes in neurologic status or new abnormal signs detected. There were 2 patients, without an antecedent history of seizures or head injury, who experienced isolated seizures after cingulotomy. In 1 of these cases the seizure followed the abrupt withdrawal of excessive quantities of medication on two occasions.

TABLE 6. NEUROLOGICAL EXAMINATION AFTER CINGULOTOMY (N = 57)

Abnormality	No. of Cases
None	21 (36.8%)
Side Effects of Psychotropic Drugs	19 (33.3%)
Related to Primary Disease	13 (22.8%)
Related to Prior Cerebral Disease	2 (3.5%)
Etiology Unclear	2 (3.5%)

Behavioral Tasks

The data to be presented here are for tests given to cingulotomy patients both before and after operation, on which there were statistically significant changes in test scores after operation. It is too soon to determine if these effects are transient or lasting, because the postoperative testing in most cases was done less than 5 months after operation. In order to answer this question, these patients are now being retested in follow-up study, and the results will be reported in future publication.

Wechsler Adult Intelligence Scale (WAIS) and Wechsler-Bellevue Intelligence Scale, Form II. Preoperative Wechsler I.Q. ratings were available for 4 of the 16 patients who underwent cingulotomy before the present study began and, therefore, participated in this investigation only after operation. As a result, for this test it was possible to compare preoperative scores with postoperative data obtained more than 4 months after operation. Table 7 illustrates the relationship between changes in overall intelligence at the time of test for 22 patients. Those who were examined before operation and then retested in the early postoperative period showed no change from their preoperative ratings. In contrast, patients who were given their second test more than 4 months after operation showed significant rises in Full Scale (t = 3.90, $P <$ 0.01), Verbal (t = 3.56, $P <$ 0.01) and Performance (t = 2.78, $P <$ 0.02) I.Q. ratings.

TABLE 7   MEAN I.Q. RATINGS (AND RANGES) FOR 22 PATIENTS TESTED BEFORE AND
AFTER CINGULOTOMY

No. of Patients	Time of Test	Wechsler I.Q. Rating		
		Full Scale	Verbal	Performance
10	Preoperative	103.1 (89-117)	105.3 (91-121)	99.8 (88-110)
	Fewer than 4 mo. Postoperative	104.5 (99-115)	106.1 (94-118)	103.2 (88-111)
12	Preoperative	96.8 (73-114)	101.8 (79-122)	91.2 (73-115)
	4 to 18 mo. Postoperative	105.3 (88-124)	108.8 (89-125)	100.5 (72-122)

Nonverbal Fluency Test. The results for this task, the Hidden Figures Test,
and for the Rey-Osterrieth-Taylor Complex Figure Test were related to the patient's age at the time of cingulotomy. On the Nonverbal Fluency Test, patients
under 30 years of age produced significantly more structures after operation
than they had before operation (t = 3.00, $P < 0.05$) (Table 8). The achievement
of patients over 30 was the same after operation as it had been before operation. This absence of a postoperative gain in the older patients indicated a
subtle impairment in that group. To date there is no evidence, however, that
this is a lasting deficit.

TABLE 8.   NONVERBAL FLUENCY TEST: RELATIONSHIP BETWEEN AGE AND ACHIEVEMENT
BEFORE AND AFTER CINGULOTOMY

Group	N	Before Operation		Fewer than 5 mo. After Operation	
		Mean	Range	Mean	Range
Under 30 years old	5	8.7	0-13	15.4	8-33
Over 30 years old	16	9.1	4-22	10.0	5-16

Hidden Figures Test. The results of retesting fewer than 5 months after
operation were again a function of the patient's age (Table 9). Statistical
comparisons were carried out using the Wilcoxon Signed-Ranks Test[30]. Those
under 30 years of age, as a group, showed no change in the ability to detect

hidden figures ($\underline{T} = 8$, n.s.), whereas patients over 30 showed a significant drop in performance ($\underline{T} = 16$, N = 23, $\underline{P} < 0.01$). A clearer picture of Hidden Figures Test performance in cingulotomy patients over 30 years of age is found in the results for 7 such patients who were examined at all three testing periods (before operation, fewer than 5 months after operation, and later in follow-up study) (Fig. 4). A comparison of their preoperative with their early postoperative scores revealed a slight, non-significant drop in mean number correct, fewer than 5 months after operation. However, the difference between the early and later postoperative results indicated a significant increase in achievement at the time of follow-up examination ($\underline{T} = 1$, N = 7, $\underline{P} = 0.032$) to a level significantly above that obtained before operation ($\underline{T} = 0$, $P < 0.02$).

TABLE 9. HIDDEN FIGURES TEST: RELATIONSHIP BETWEEN AGE AND MEAN NUMBER CORRECT BEFORE AND AFTER CINGULOTOMY

Group	N	Before Operation		Fewer than 5 mo. After Operation	
		Mean	Range	Mean	Range
Under 30 years old	9	19.9	2-33	22.6	10-40
Over 30 years old	25	13.9	1-34	10.6	0-30

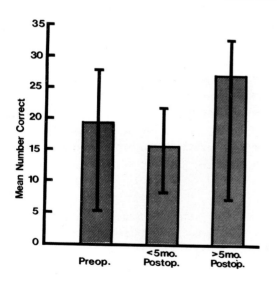

Fig. 4. Hidden Figures Test scores of 7 cingulotomy patients over 30 years of age who were tested three times (Reproduced from Corkin[27]).

Rey-Osterrieth-Taylor Complex Figure Test. Cingulotomy was associated with a
change in performance on the copying part of this task but not in the capacity
to recall the drawing after a 1-hour delay (Table 10). Patients over 30 years
of age copied the complex figure more accurately before operation than they
did after operation (t = 2.99, P < 0.01), whereas patients under 30 showed no
change in the accuracy of their copies.

TABLE 10. REY-OSTERRIETH-TAYLOR COMPLEX FIGURE TEST: RELATIONSHIP BETWEEN
AGE AND MEAN SCORES BEFORE AND AFTER CINGULOTOMY (MAXIMUM SCORE = 36)

Group	N	Before Operation		Fewer than 5 mo. After Operation	
		Copy (Range)	Delayed Recall (Range)	Copy (Range)	Delayed Recall (Range)
Under 30 years old	5	29.6 (20.5-34.0)	12.0 (4.5-22)	29.2 (22.0-33.5)	12.2 (5.5-18)
Over 30 years old	19	27.3 (19.5-35.0)	12.0 (4.5-24)	24.9 (13.0-35.0)	11.1 (2-31)

Tapping. The data obtained with the two tapping tasks were analyzed separately for men and women, because of the apparent sex differences in the performance of these tasks. The results for the 7 women showed no change in tapping score after operation. In contrast, the 8 men performed more poorly after
cingulotomy than they had before (Tables 11 and 12). Specifically, there were
two unimanual conditions in which there was a statistically significant decline
in output after operation (tapping rate: t = 2.86, P < 0.05; Thurstone tapping:
t = 2.94, P < 0.05). These changes in tapping performance were not accompanied
by decreases in grip strength. The hint of a sensorimotor loss in the early
postoperative period will be pursued by retesting the 8 men a year or more
after operation and by adding new cases to the sample.

DISCUSSION

It is not clear why cingulotomy benefits patients whose primary complaint
is chronic pain or depression or why it does not help those diagnosed as having
obsessive-compulsive neurosis or schizophrenia. Such factors as placebo effect,
spontaneous remission, or major changes in the patient's life situation may
contribute to the high incidence of improvement seen in the pain and depression
groups. Most candidates for cingulotomy and their relatives are convinced that

TABLE 11. TAPPING RATE BEFORE AND AFTER CINGULOTOMY (N = 8 MEN)

	Before Operation				Fewer than 5 mo. After Operation			
	Left Hand		Right Hand		Left Hand		Right Hand	
Condition	Mean	Range	Mean	Range	Mean	Range	Mean	Range
Unimanual	42.7	26.0-80.8	47.3	42.0-59.0	45.1	30.5-46.0	41.9[a]	26.5-59.0
Bimanual	37.2	16.5-52.0	45.1	34.5-57.0	38.0	26.5-49.5	43.1	36.5-56.5

[a] Significant difference between these preoperative and postoperative scores (t = 2.86, $P \leq 0.05$).

TABLE 12. THURSTONE TAPPING TEST BEFORE AND AFTER CINGULOTOMY (N = 8 MEN)

	Before Operation				Fewer than 5 mo. After Operation			
	Left Hand		Right Hand		Left Hand		Right Hand	
Condition	Mean	Range	Mean	Range	Mean	Range	Mean	Range
Unimanual								
First Trial	96.0[a]	53-142	105.9	64-137	84.4[a]	40-124	98.5	57-142
Second Trial	92.0	53-125	99.9	56-144	81.5	29-108	88.4	40-111

	Before Operation		Fewer than 5 mo. After Operation	
	Mean	Range	Mean	Range
Bimanual[b]				
First Trial	19.3	12-42	17.8	10-36
Second Trial	12.4	5-18	12.9	4-19

[a] Significant difference between these preoperative and postoperative scores (t = 2.94, $P \leq 0.05$).
[b] There is only one score for the bimanual condition, representing the coordinated response of the two hands.

the brain operation represents the patients' last chance of being helped, and as a result there is great anticipation of improvement. Such factors can presumably influence the results of any treatment, perhaps even more in the treatment of pain. It is normally impossible to deal with the question of placebo effect because of ethical restraints against performing sham operations. The operation in one patient in this series, however, was terminated before the lesions were made, because her brain anatomy was found to be so distorted that the surgeon could not locate the lesion targets. Postoperatively, she was told merely that the procedure had gone well, but had been modified. She did appear to be less disabled by her thoracic pain for several months after operation, but this relief was only transient.

Other evidence of a possible placebo effect with psychiatric surgery comes from a recent study by Mirsky and Orzack[31], who examined patients after they had undergone ultrasonic irradiation aimed at the white matter of the prefrontal lobes. Of the 10 patients studied several years postoperatively, 4 were judged to have a very favorable outcome, even though such sonic treatment is not intended to destroy brain tissue (Lindstrom, 1978, personal communication to Orzack). It is difficult to explain the lasting therapeutic effect of this procedure without considering the role of suggestion.

Another explanation of the therapeutic successes that have been seen in some psychiatric patients is a physiologic one. The possibility exists that cingulotomy produces biochemical changes in the brain that have long-lasting sequelae. These neurochemical events could take place at the site of the cingulate lesion or at some distance from it. Serotonergic and dopaminergic pathways begin in the midbrain and terminate in the region of the cingulotomy (Fig. 5). These or other neuroregulatory systems with which they interact could have been altered as a result of the brain operation. Biochemical mechanisms have been implicated in several psychiatric disorders, particularly schizophrenia, in which it is hypothesized that brain dopamine metabolism or activity is excessive[34]. In depression as well, norepinephrin and serotonin are thought to be underactive or deficient[35]. Although the relationships between neuroregulators and mental disease are poorly understood, there is at least a theoretical basis for implicating biochemical changes in the therapeutic mechanism of the cingulate surgery.

There is also a theoretical framework suggesting that the therapeutic effect of the cingulotomy in the treatment of chronic pain is related to the action of chemical substances in the brain. The recently discovered opiate receptors and endogenous opiates, or endorphins, are concentrated in brain regions in-

volved in pain transmission and emotion, namely, in central grey substances
of the midbrain and in the limbic system, in particular, the amygdala[36].
Thus, the internal opiates are ideally situated to influence the central sub-
strata of normal or pathological pain, but the physiological mechanisms by
which their role in behavior is exerted, normally or following cingulotomy, is
unknown.

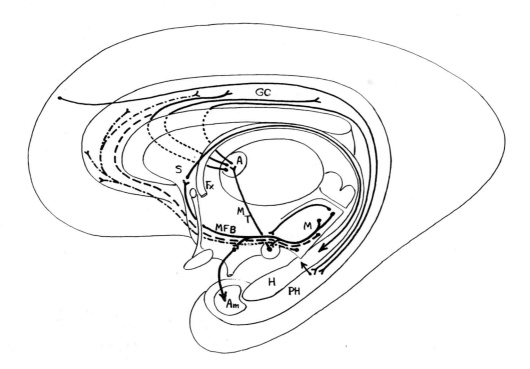

Fig. 5.   Diagram of some components of the fasciculus cinguli that are likely
to be interrupted by cingulotomy. Quantitatively the most prominent of these
pathways is the projection from the anterior nucleus of the thalamus (A)· note
the initially rostral orientation of this thalamo-cingulate fiber system[32], a
disposition suggesting that lesions in the rostral part of the fasciculus may
disconnect from the thalamus most or all of the cingulo-parahippocampal cortex
caudal to the lesion. The same holds true for the monoaminergic mesocortical
systems: the serotonin system (broken line) originating from the mesencephalic raphe nuclei, and the dopamine system (dot-dash line) arising in cell
group A10 of the nigral complex. Also indicated in the diagram is the fronto-
limbic association system extending caudally as far as the parahippocampal gyrus (PH). Other abbreviations: Am: amygdala; Fx: fornix bundle; GC: gyrus
cinguli; H: hippocampus; M: midbrain; MFB: medial forebrain bundle; MT:
Mamillo-thalamic tract; S: septum. (Adapted from Nauta, 1973[33]by Dr. Nauta,
and reproduced with his permission.)

SUMMARY

It can tentatively be said that cingulotomy, as performed in these patients, seems to have a better success rate in the treatment of certain types of chronic, non-neoplastic pain than do most alternative medical or surgical interventions[37]. Patients with depression also have a reasonably good chance of being helped by cingulotomy, whereas obsessive-compulsives and schizophrenics do not. Regardless of therapeutic outcome, however, there is no evidence of new neurologic signs or lasting behavioral deficits that can be linked to the brain operation. The evaluation of these and subsequent cases will be expanded in the next several years in order to determine the long-term effects of cingulotomy.

ACKNOWLEDGEMENT

We are grateful to Dr. H. Thomas Ballantine, Jr. for allowing us to study his patients, and to his staff, especially Mrs. Ida Giriunas, for help in scheduling them. Dr. W.J.H. Nauta kindly modified a brain diagram from an earlier paper of his for use in the present report. We also thank our statistician, Loretta Clement, and our secretary, Mark Hagerty. This work was supported by N.I.H. Contract No. N01-NS-62116A, and by grants from N.I.M.H. (MH 24433-04) and from the General Clinical Research Centers Program of the Division of Research and Resources, N.I.H. (RR-00088).

REFERENCES

1. Ballantine, H.T., Cassidy, W.L., Flanagan, N.B., and Marino, R. (1967) J. Neurosurg., 26, 488-495.

2. Teuber, H.-L., Corkin, S., and Twitchell, T.E. (1977) in Neurosurgical Treatment in Psychiatry, Pain, and Epilepsy, Sweet, W.H., Obrador, S. and Martin-Rodriguez, J.G. eds., Baltimore, University Park Press, pp. 333-353.

3. Teuber, H.-L, Corkin, S., and Twitchell, T.E. (1977) in Appendix: Psychosurgery, National Commission for the Protection of Human Subjects of Biomedical and Behavioral Research (DHEW Publication No. [OS]77-0002), Washington, D.C., U.S. Government Printing Office.

4. Woodruff, R.A., Goodwin, D.W., and Guze, S.B. (1974) Psychiatric Diagnosis, New York, Oxford University Press.

5. Ballantine, H.T., Jr., Levy, B.S., Dagi, T.F., and Giriunas, I.B. (1977) in Neurosurgical Treatment in Psychiatry, Pain, and Epilepsy, Sweet, W.H., Obrador, S., and Martin-Rodriguez, J.G. eds., Baltimore, University Park Press, pp. 333-353.

6. Laitinen, L.V. and Vilkki, J. (1973) in Surgical Approaches in Psychiatry, Laitinen, L.V. and Livingston, K.E., eds., Lancaster, Medical and Technical Publishing Co., pp. 74-80.

7. Twitchell, T.E., Lecours, A.R., Rudel, R.G., and Teuber, H.-L. (1966) Trans. Am Neurol. Ass., 91, 353-335.

8. Adey, W.R. and Meyer, M. (1952) J. Anat., 86, 58-74.

9. Nauta, W.J.H. (1964) in The Frontal Granular Cortex and Behavior, Warren, J.M., and Akert, K., eds., New York, McGraw-Hill, pp. 397-409.

10. Pandya, D.N., Dye, P., and Butters, N. (1971) Brain Res., 31, 35-46.

11. Pandya, D.N., Van Hoesen, G.W., and Domesick, V.B. (1973) Brain Res., 61, 369-373.

12. Anden, N.-E., Dahlstrom, A., Fuxe, K., Larsson, K., Olson, L., and Ungerstedt, U. (1966) Acta Physiol. Scand., 67, 313-326.

13. Conrad, L.C.A., Leonard, C.M., and Pfaff, D.W. (1974) J. comp. Neurol., 156, 179-206.

14. Domesick, V.B. (1972) Brain Behav. Evolut., 6, 457-483.

15. Hedreen, J.C. and Chalmers, J.P. (1972) Brain Res., 47, 1-36.

16. Wechsler, D. (1955) Manual for the Wechsler Adult Intelligence Scale, New York, Psychological Corporation.

17. Wechsler, C. (1946) Wechsler-Bellevue Intelligence Scale, Form II, New York, Psychological Corporation.

18. Milner, B. (1964) in The Frontal Granular Cortex and Behavior, Warren, J.M., and Akert, K., eds., New York, McGraw-Hill, pp. 313-334.

19. Gottschaldt, K. (1926) Psychol. Forsch., 8, 261-317.

20. Gottschaldt, K. (1929) Psychol. Forsch., 12, 1-87.

21. Thurstone, L.L. (1944) A Factorial Study of Perception, Chicago, University of Chicago Press.

22. Teuber, H.-L., Battersby, W.S., and Bender, M.B. (1951) J. nerv. ment. Dis., 114, 413-429.

23. Teuber, H.-L., and Weinstein, S. (1956) Arch. Neurol. Psychiat., 76, 369-379.

24. Taylor, L.B. (1969) Clin. Neurosurg., 16, 269-287.

25. Rey, A. (1942) Archs. Neurol., Paris, 28, 286-340.

26. Osterrieth, P. and Rey, A. (1944) Archs. Neurol., Paris, 30, 205-356.

27. Corkin, S. (1979), Neuropsychologia, 17, in press.

28. Faillace, L.A., Allen, R.P., McQueen, J.D., and Northrup, B. (1971), Dis. nerv. Sys., 32, 171-175.

29. Long, C.J., Pueschel, K., and Hunter, S.E. (1978) J. Neurosurg., 49, 264-271.

30. Siegel, S. (1956) Nonparametric Statistics for the Behavioral Sciences, New York, McGraw-Hill.

31. Mirsky, A.F. and Orzack, M.H. (1977) in Appendix: Psychosurgery, National Commission for the Protection of Human Subjects of Biomedical and Behavioral Research (DHEW Publication No. [OS]77-0002), Washington, D.C., U.S. Government Printing Office.

32. Domesick, V.B. (1969), Brain Res., 20, 19-32.

33. Nauta, W.J.H. (1973) in Surgical Approaches in Psychiatry, Laitinen, L.V. and Livingston, K.E., eds., Lancaster, Medical and Technical Publishing Co., 303-315.

34. Berger, P.A., Elliot, G.R., and Barchas, J.D. (1978) in Psychopharmacology: A Generation of Progress, Lipton, M.A., DiMascio, A., and Killam, K.F, eds., New York, Raven Press, pp. 1071-1082.

35. Schildkraut, J.J. (1978) in Psychopharmacology: A Generation of Progress, Lipton, M.A., DiMascio, A., and Killam, K.F., eds., New York, Raven Press, pp. 1223-1234.

36. Snyder, S.H. and Mathysse, S. (1975) Neurosciences Res. Prog. Bull., 13.

37. Bonica, J.J. and Albe-Fessard, D.G., eds., (1976) Advances in Pain Research and Therapy (Vol.1), New York, Raven Press.

© 1979 Elsevier/North-Holland Biomedical Press
Modern Concepts in Psychiatric Surgery
E.R. Hitchcock, H.T. Ballantine, Jr. and B.A. Meyerson, eds.

TREATMENT OF DEPRESSION AFTER CINGULOTOMY

FRANK WINSTON

6402 Odana Road, Madison, Wisconsin 53719, United States of America.

ABSTRACT

The development of the biogenic amine hypotheses has led to increasing sophistication in the administration of antidepressant medication. Nevertheless a small proportion of depressed patients either respond poorly to these agents or become non-responsive with time. Stereotactic psychiatric surgery may, however, induce striking changes in responses to psychopharmacological treatment.

This paper compares the pre and post operative treatment histories of seven chronically depressedpatients referred for cingulotomy over a three year period. Responses to pharmacotherapy before and after surgery are examined. Six of the patients showed an excellent response to electrotherapy prior to surgery but consistently relapsed within a short while. This relapse was at first delayed by the use of combined antidepressants but these patients eventually became non-responsive to this form of treatment and required increasingly frequent electrotherapy. After surgery only two patients have required electrotherapy and two patients, who became totally unresponsive to combined antidepressants, showed an excellent response to a single antidepressant when they tended to relapse. Three patients were on no medication a year after surgery.

Significant relief of symptoms following stereotactic cingulotomy for refractory depression can be expected in approximately 60% of patients (1). However, results reported by the same surgeon may range from 40% to 65% significant improvement (2) and there is some evidence that attainment of results in the higher range is dependent on the quality of psychiatric care following operation as well as on accuracy of patient selection (2).

Table "A" classifies depression according to treatment response. Depressions in the last four categories can properly be termed refractory depressions. It is, of course, patients in the last two categories who are likely to be candidates for psychiatric surgery.

While the various forms of the biogenic amine hypotheses have not been proved, evidence is very strong that depression is in some way dependent on the levels of biogenic amines at crucial receptor sites (3). Therefore, when treating depression from theory one first tries to increase levels of amines at receptor sites by use of tricyclic antidepressants or increase the total brain concentration of amines by use of M.A.O. inhibitors. Alternatively one can attempt to influence levels of amines by precursor therapy (4) and it has been suggested that receptor sensitivity may be increased by means of electrotherapy (5). If all these manoeuvres fail singly, they may then be tried in combination (6) and Table "B" suggests a rational treatment protocol that should (in the absence of other clinical contraindications) be carried out before referral for psychiatric surgery is considered. Unless all possible treatments are tried serious mistakes in referral may be made. In 1967 one of my patients, who appeared to be in Category 8, was given L-tryptophan following Coppen's report (4) and made a complete recovery. Fortunately this was before the publication of other reports showing

TABLE "A".

CLASSIFICATION OF DEPRESSION ACCORDING TO TREATMENT RESPONSE

Category 1. Remits and no treatment required.

2. Responds adequately to tricyclic antidepressant, M.A.O. inhibitor or L-tryptophan.

3. Responds adequately to antidepressant medication but requires indefinite maintenance therapy with antidepressants or lithium.

4. Responds only to electrotherapy.

5. Responds to electrotherapy but requires indefinite maintenance with antidepressants or lithium.

6. Responds only to combination of tricyclic anti-depressant and M.A.O. inhibitor.

7. Responds only to electrotherapy but requires maintenance with combined tricyclic and M.A.O. inhibitor therapy.

8. Responds only to electrotherapy but remission transient and return of symptoms cannot be prevented by combined antidepressants.

9. Responds to no treatment at all.

TABLE "B"

PROTOCOL FOR TREATMENT OF REFRACTORY DEPRESSION

1. Tricyclic antidepressant to maximum tolerance – e.g. Amitriptyline 400 mg. daily for 30 days.

2. Electrotherapy.

3. Tranylcypromine to 60 mg. daily if tolerated for 30 days.

4. L-tryptophan 2G. t.i.d. for 30 days (may be combined with 3.)

5. Amitriptyline plus Tranylcypromine in gradually increasing dosage (up to 150 mg. Amitriptyline and 30 mg. Tranylcypromine). May be combined with further electrotherapy.

that L-tryptophan was ineffective (7,8). Assuming the patient is found to be in Category 8 or 9 and is referred for psychiatric surgery - what next?

There is a great deal in the literature regarding indications for psychiatric surgery but very little concerning postoperative treatment. While we do not know how psychiatric surgery works, we do know that following operation patients often respond to treatments that were ineffective preoperatively (1,9). More recently Kelly (10) has pointed out that "following stereotactic procedures symptoms often clear very gradually and it is essential that patients are aware of this fact preoperatively or premature disappointment will result. Depressions generally do not need a specialised programme for the relief of symptoms but mood swings, which are invariably present, usually require treatment during the first two months when they are most common. The contribution of rehabilitation to the eventual postoperative outcome is difficult to assess, but certain key events like getting a job, embarking upon new social activities or moving away from home need to be achieved within the first year."

The importance of continuity of pharmacotherapy cannot be overemphasized since the effect of the operation is often to change the patient's treatment category in a favorable direction. Patients will respond to treatments previously ineffective and as the patient's treatment category changes it is important to see that necessary medication is given appropriate to the change.

Some of these points are illustrated by the post treatment histories of seven patients referred for cingulotomy during the period July, 1975 to February, 1978.

Table "C" summarizes the pre and post treatment histories of these patients. Two patients are asymptomatic and on no medication. One is asymptomatic but still on medication. Two are much improved but still need medication and two at 6 and 8 months postoperatively remain unchanged.

The first patient made an almost complete recovery within one month but continued to need 150 mg. Amitriptyline h.s. and any attempt to lower the dose was met by a return of depression. However, on this dose of medication there was a complete change in her life. She rapidly obtained a new job, a promotion, a husband and a child and is expecting a second child in October. She has, of course, changed to Category 3.

The second patient, who had been stabilized for several years on combined antidepressants, eventually became nonresponsive. After surgery she changed to category 3 and a year after surgery was taking only 50 mg. Amitriptyline daily. However, some symptoms began to return and three years later she seems fairly stable on lithium and combined antidepressants (Category 6).

Patient 3 with only 18 months history with many hospitalizations and suicidal attempts reverted after surgery to Category 6. She was symptom free on Tranylcypromine and Amitriptyline, relapsing when Amitriptyline was reduced and responding to increase in dosage. However, a year later she improved to Category 1 and has been symptom free and off medication for 8 months.

The fourth patient, who was in Category 9, remained unchanged for 2½ months postoperatively and then suddenly developed hypomania which responded to lithium. Unfortunately she stopped taking her lithium and is subject to frequent mood changes. She appears to be in Category 3 but refuses psychiatric follow-up.

The fifth patient ten years before operation had an attack of depression lasting three years and required 150 electrotherapies before depression remitted. She was nonresponsive to any medication. Her second attack of depression ten years later followed the same pattern but this time she was referred for cingulotomy after thirty electrotherapies. She immediately reverted to Category 1 and eight months following surgery is asymptomatic on no medication.

The sixth and seventh patients eight and six months after surgery have shown no change. They still respond well to electrotherapy, but transiently. They remain in Category 8.

Patient No.6 who had suffered from hypertension for many years was the only one who developed organic confusion following surgery, which fortunately cleared up after a few weeks. Patient No. 7 will be referred for a second operation if there is no improvement by the end of the year. It might be added that, though these patients still required electrotherapy after operation, there does seem to be a better quality of remission after each treatment but relapse occurs within two or three weeks. No medication prevents relapse and in the case of Patient No.7 all medication has been stopped since she made a suicidal attempt by means of an overdose about two months after surgery.

To sum up, one can hardly do better than to quote Sargent and Slater (11): "It is sometimes difficult to judge the eventual success of the operation by the results seen in the first three months. Some of the patients do well from the beginning and never look back. Others begin as apparently complete success but later develop some undesirable symptoms. And yet others only begin to improve some months after operation and continue to do so steadily during the ensuing years..........the patient's constitution has been changed. One is so to speak back to square one, with avenues, previously closed, opening again on all sides."

TABLE "C"	SUMMARY OF TREATMENT HISTORIES OF PATIENTS REFERRED FOR ANTERIOR CINGULOTOMY		
AGE & SEX	1. 28.F.	2. 50.F.	3. 28.F.
Duration of treatment prior to surgery.	7 yrs.	14 yrs.	18 mths.
Previous treatment	Psychotherapy	Psychotherapy (8 yrs.) Elavil Tofranil Marplan Electrotherapy	----
First seen	Nov., 1968.	Nov., 1970.	Aug., 1975.
Diagnosis	Manic depressive disease (unipolar)	Manic depressive disease (unipolar)	Manic depressive disease (unipolar)
Treatment	Chlorpromazine Electrotherapy Megavitamins Elavil & Parnate Elavil & Reserpine Demerol & Dexedrine L-tryptophan Lithium	Parnate Elavil Lithium Ritalin L-tryptophan Electrotherapy Elavil & Nardil	Elavil Elavil & Marplan Elavil & Parnate Lithium Electrotherapy
Electrotherapy treatments.	113	52	38
Hospital Admissions	7	4	5
Total Hosp. Days	228	87	145
Date of Surgery	7/1/75	9/24/76	12/13/76
Postoperative treatment	Elavil 150 mg.	Elavil Lithium L-tryptophan Cafergot Nardil Thyroid	Elavil Parnate (discontinued Jan., 1977)
Treatment July, 1978.	Elavil 125 mg.	Elavil 150 mg.h.s. Lithium 1200 mg. Nardil 45 mg. Thyroid 2½ gr.	---
Present condition	Symptom free (new job, promotion, husband, baby)	Some symptoms	Symptom free
Treatment category	3	7	1

TABLE "C" (contd.)
SUMMARY OF TREATMENT HISTORIES OF PATIENTS
REFERRED FOR ANTERIOR CINGULOTOMY

AGE & SEX	4. 22.F.	5. 61.F.
Duration of treatment prior to surgery.	26 mths	12 mths.
Previous treatment	Electrotherapy Prolixin Tofranil Psychotherapy	(Previous depression 1963 - 1966 - 166 Electrotherapies.
First seen	Mar., 1976.	Aug., 1976. (seen previously 1963-1966)
Diagnosis	Manic depressive disease (bipolar)	Manic depressive disease (unipolar)
Treatment	Elavil & Parnate Electrotherapy Narcosynthesis Demerol & Dexedrine Tofranil & Reserpine Prolixin Moban L-tryptophan	Elavil & Marplan L-tryptophan Elavil & Parnate
Electrotherapy treatments	31	30
Hospital Admissions	5	----
Total Hosp. Days	326	----
Date of Surgery	1/5/77	7/21/77
Postoperative treatment	Lithium following hypomanic attack	----
Treatment July, 1978.	----	----
Present condition	Depressed, less severely	Symptom free
Treatment Category	?	1.

TABLE "C"(contd.)

SUMMARY OF TREATMENT HISTORIES OF PATIENTS
REFERRED FOR ANTERIOR CINGULOTOMY

	6.	7.
AGE & SEX	67.F.	36.F.
Duration of treatment prior to surgery	4 yrs. 4 mths.	9 yrs. 7 mths.
Previous treatment	----	Psychotherapy Elavil Elavil & Marplan Electrotherapy
First seen	Aug., 1973.	July, 1977.
Diagnosis	Manic depressive disease(unipolar)	Manic depressive disease(unipolar)
Treatment	Elavil Lithium (1 yr.) L-tryptophan	Elavil 300 mg. daily Elavil & Marplan Elavil & Parnate L-tryptophan
Electrotherapy	38	7+
Hospital Admissions	6	----
Total Hosp. Days	113	----
Date of Surgery	12/16/77	2/24/78
Postoperative treatment	Elavil & Parnate L-tryptophan 13 Electrotherapies 3 Hosp. Admissions	Elavil & Parnate L-tryptophan Lithium Meds. discontinued after overdose 5 Electrotherapies
Treatment July, 1978.	Elavil 100 mg. Maintenance Electrotherapy	----
Present condition	Requires frequent Electrotherapy	Severely depressed Refuses Electrotherapy Willing to be re-referred for surgery.
Treatment category	8	8

References

1. Kiloh L.G. Psychosurgery for Depressive Illness in "Handbook of Studies on Depression (ed. Burrows, G.D.) p.p. 253-268. Excerpta Medica 1977. Elsevier/North-Holland Biomedical Press.

2. Ballantine, H.T., Jr., Levy, B.S., Dagi, T.F. and Giriunas, I.B. Cingulotomy for Psychiatric Illness.in Neurosurgical Treatment in Psychiatry, Pain and Epilepsy (Ed. Sweet, W.H. et al) 333-353. University Park Press, Baltimore, 1977.

3. Van Praag, H.M. Amine Hypotheses of Affective Disorders. In "Handbook of Psychopharmacology" (Ed. Iverson, L. et al) Vol. 13, pp. 187-297. Plenum Press, New York, 1978.

4. Coppen, A., Shaw, D.M., Herzberg, B. and Maggs, R. (1967): Tryptophan in Treatment of Depression. Lancet II: 1178-1180 (1978).

5. Grahame-Smith, D.G., Green, A.R. and Costain, D.W.: Mechanism of the Antidepressant Action of Electroconvulsive Therapy. Lancet I 254-256 (1971).

6. Winston, F. Combined Antidepressant Therapy:British Journal of Psychiatry 118:301-304.

7. Carroll, B.J., Mowbray, R.M., and Davies, B.M. (1970): Sequential Comparison of L-tryptophan with E.C.T. in Severe Depression. Lancet, I: 967-969.

8. Carroll, B.J. (1971): Monoamine Precursors in the Treatment of Depression. Clinical Pharmacology and Therapeutics 12: 743-761.

9. Bridges, P.K. (1972): Psychosurgery Today: Psychiatric Aspects. Proceedings of the Royal Soc. Med. Vol.65. 1104-1108.

10. Kelly, D. (1976): Neurosurgical Treatment of Psychiatric Disorders. In "Recent Advances in Clinical Psychiatry (Ed. Granville-Grossman) 227-261. Churchill Livingstone, New York.

11. Sargent, W., Slater, E.(1972): an Introduction to Physical Methods of Treatment in Psychiatry 129 Science House, New York.

© 1979 Elsevier/North-Holland Biomedical Press
Modern Concepts in Psychiatric Surgery
E.R. Hitchcock, H.T. Ballantine, Jr. and B.A. Meyerson, eds.

NEUROPATHOLOGICAL STUDY OF
BILATERAL CINGULOTOMY FOR MOOD DISTURBANCE

Peter G. Bernad[*], H. Thomas Ballantine, Jr.[**]
and Ida E. Giriunas[**]
Massachusetts General Hospital
Boston, Massachusetts

INTRODUCTION

Since the beginning of a systematic approach to the use of psychiatric illness in 1935, many reports concerning techniques, side-effects, indications and clinical experiences have been published (1, 2, 3, 4, 5, 6, 7, 8, 9, 10). Nevertheless, theoretical grounds for such operations are still controversial and thus further studies concerning anatomical and neuropathological changes in post-operative brains are important. There is unfortunately a paucity of such material available which, while disappointing to the neuroscientist, is a tribute to the relative safety of those operative procedures.

In the past 50 years, animal studies by neuroanatomists and neurophysiologists have shown an intimate working relationship between the frontal lobes and the limbic system, particularly in such states as fear, rage, sexual responses, passivity, aggression and pleasure (11, 12, 13). Corticocingulate and thalamo-frontal connections have been studied in apes and chimpanzees (14, 15). Researchers have shown that lesions of the prefrontal cortex induce retrograde degeneration of the dorsomedial thalamic nucleus (16, 17).

James Papez published his landmark contribution to neuroscience entitled "A Proposed Mechanism of Emotion" in 1937 (18). He was among the first to stress that the cingulum region was essential for the expression of emotion and that the experience of emotion depended on cortical function. He stressed the role of the afferent systems leading to the diencephalon and from there to structures of the forebrain. The stream of afferents to the corpus striatum he referred to as the "stream of thought" and the stream to the midline cortex (the cortex of the limbic lobe made up of

---

  * Department of Neurology
** Department of Neurosurgery

cingulate gyrus and hippocampal formation) he referred to as the "stream of feeling".

In expounding his proposed theory of emotion, Papez was at pains to point out connections whereby information from all sensory systems might be conveyed via the mammillary bodies to the cingulate gyrus. The cingulate cortex he noted "may be looked on as the receptive region for the experiencing of emotion, in the same way as the area striata is considered the receptive cortex for photic excitations coming from the retina". Thus Papez conceived of the cingulate gyrus as the central aspect of the limbic circuit and, further, that behavioristic manifestations of the variety of sensory imputs within the human brain is mediated through central viscero-emotive limbic-callosal connections. Both visceral and somatic receptors might relay appropriate stimuli to the brain stem from which they would pass into hypothalamus and its connections with the mammillary body, the anterior thalamic nuclei and via the anterior thalamic radiations in the cingulate region. From the cingulum, impulses could be transmitted to the hippocampus thence to the mammillary bodies via the fornix, the anterior thalamic nuclei via the tract of Vic D'Azyr, back to the cingulum and finally closing the circuit at the hippocampus.

As stated above, Papez's theory was that the cortex of the cingulate gyrus is the receptor site for these stimuli which set in operation inner emotional experiences. Propagation of this emotional process to the frontal cortex would, in his words, "add emotional coloring to the psychic process (18).

The frontal lobes undoubtably are closely connected to the limbic system. MacLean has stated, "The medial forebrain bundle and its continuation as the cingulum may be considered to be to the limbic system what the internal capsule is to the outer convexity of the brain" (13). This analogy is especially relevant since it has been demonstrated recently that the cytoarchitecture of the precentral gigantopyramidal field and the pyramidal cells of Betz within the cingulate gyrus is the same (19).

The connections between the limbic cortex and the brain stem have been delineated by Nauta (20). He considers the central gray and the paramedian reticulum which with the adjoining nucleus of Gudden constitute the "limbic midbrain area". From these areas ascending connections are made with the hypothalamus and through the medial forebrain bundle with the amygdala and septum from which fibers radiate to the limbic cortex of the temporal region.

Neurosurgeons, neurologists and psychiatrists have struggled with a variety of both medical and surgical treatments for those patients afflicted with chronic severe pain and devastating mood disorders. Bilateral surgical interruption of the sagitally positioned cingulate bundle of this so-called "limbic system", that is, bilateral cingulotomy, has benefitted sufficient numbers of patients suffering with intractable emotional disorders to validate recommendation of this procedure in selected patients (1, 3, 4, 5, 6, 21, 8, 9, 10).

The connections of the human cingulate gyrus constitute a problem in neurology. Discrete radio-frequency cingulotomy lesions offer an excellent opportunity for the neuroscientist to study the efferent pathways from it and we have studied the brains of three patients who died from various causes three months to 7 years after bilateral cingulotomy. (Fig. 1)

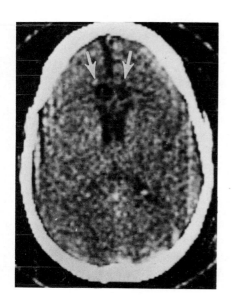

Figure 1: C.T. Scan Visualization of Radio Frequency (R.F.) Cingu- lotomy Lesions (Case #1)

The brains were fixed in formalin, and sectioned to demonstrate the cingulotomy lesion and the fiber tracts. The serial sections were stained with hematoxylin, eosin, Loyez, and cresyl violet.

The purpose of this communication is to depict some neuro-anatomic connections of the limbic system and to report on the neuropathologic correlations in these three cases of bilateral cingulotomies for intractable mood disorder and/or pain.

The findings in these cases will be compared to those of Yakovlev and others in reference to those afferent and efferent connections which travel via the cingulate white matter.

Case Summary 1:   N.H. was a right handed 65-year-old woman who was always thought by her family to be vivacious, healthy, active and devoted to her husband and relatives until the age of 32. At that time she began to have numerous somatic complaints such as burning pain, headaches, numerous ill defined dizzy spells and hoarseness.

At the age of forty-two, a staff psychiatrist at the Massachusetts General Hospital thought that she was "focusing a great deal of attention on her somatic symptoms which tended to represent screening, a tendency to depression". Between the age of 40 and 50 during the initial phase of treatment of her illness, she received one dozen electroconvulsive shock treatments with minimal improvement. After 4 years she was again noted to be depressed and followed in Psychiatric Clinic being on Amitriptyline. During her psychiatric follow-up she was noted to have frequent crying spells, poor appetite, and thought that people were against her, and that she should kill herself. After many consultations and admissions for mood disorder, she underwent bilateral stereotactic cingulotomy in 1970 by one of us (HTB, Jr.).

The burr holes were placed bilaterally 9.5 cm. from the nasion and on either side of the midline. Dura and cortex beneath the burr holes were lightly cauterized. There was some difficulty with bleeding from the right burr hole which was satisfactorily controlled during the procedure. The wound was then closed and stereotactic lesions at a distance of 2 cm. from the tip of the frontal horn of the lateral ventricles were placed in the cingulate gyrus bilaterally using 8 watts for 75 seconds. The procedure was well tolerated by the patient. (Fig. 2)

For three years after operation the patient did remarkably well on low doses of Amitriptyline. Subsequently, however, she became upset and depressed when her daughter's marriage was dissolved.   She experienced diurinal mood fluctuation, worse in the morning, with constipation and depression. She would complain "I can't do anything any more". There

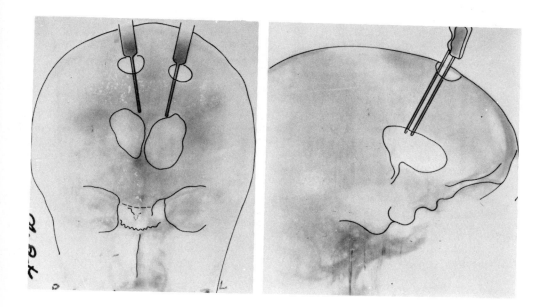

Figure 2:   Outlined A.P. and Lateral X-Ray Views
of Cingulotomy Procedure on N.H. (Case #1)

were no hallucinations or ideas of reference. At no time was she thought
to be psychotic. General medical and neurological evaluations were negative.
She was treated symptomatically and gradually improved in a period of a
few months.

In 1975 she fell and suffered a subcapital fracture in the right hip
which required surgical nailing. While in hospital she was noted to be
psychiatrically well and was not depressed and had been living happily

taking only aspirin, Propoxyphene and Flurazepam but was not taking any antidepressants.

She was admitted for the last time in June of 1976 for right hip pain, abdominal pain and symptomatic right pleural effusion. She was found to have metastatic carcinoma of the ovary. After exploratory laparotomy and right oophorectomy she had a stormy course and died with terminal bronchopneumonia.

General Post Mortem: The general autopsy revealed stage IV, grade IV widespread metastatic endometrial ovarian carcinoma, bronchopneumonia, pulmonary edema, pleural effusion and nephrosclerosis, most likely secondary to hypertension.

Neuropathological Post Mortem: Bilateral frontal burr holes were noted. The fresh brain weighed 1140 grams. The dura was normal. There was little atherosclerosis of the cerebral arteries. No occlusion was demonstrated. The external surface of the brain showed one 0.5 cm. cavity in the vertex of the cortex 1 cm. to the right from the midline. The rest of the external surface of the brain was normal without softening or asymmetry. The brain stem and cerebellum appeared normal. (Fig. 3)

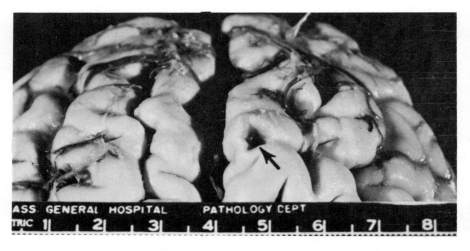

Figure 3: Site of needle insertion on right. Note cortical defect 0.5 cm. from mid-line (Case #1)

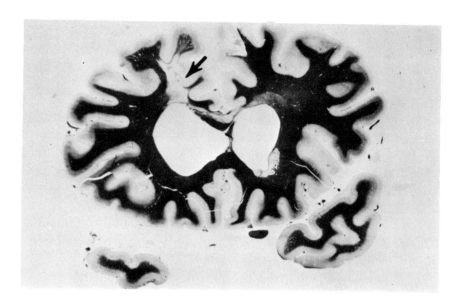

Figure 4: Cingulate lesion on left side

A block of tissue measuring 3 inches incorporating the cingulotomy sites was taken for serial section (35 microns each) for celoidin embedding. These sections were stained with Loyez and C.V. to study the post-cingulotomy lesions. Complete serial sections were performed; all sections were examined and every 20th section stained. Bilateral asymmetrical lesions are demonstrated in the coronal sections. The left sided lesion measures 7 mm. in transverse diameter and 9 mm. in the dorsal ventral plane, appearing as a quadrilateral defect. (Fig. 4) On the right side the lesion was more irregular, largely triangular and barely reached the alba of the cingulate gyrus. It measured 5 mm. at the widest diameter. (Fig. 5)

The left sided lesion was in a lateral position, 13 mm. to the left of the median plane. The right sided lesion was 5 mm. lateral to the median plane.

Detailed Descriptions: The microscopic study of the seven year old radio-frequency surgical lesion shows on the left side the lesion as it enters the crown of the superior frontal convolution at the level of the

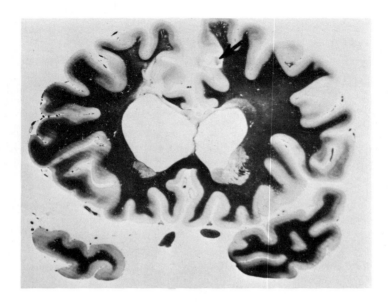

Figure 5: Cingulate lesion on right side

genu of the corpus callosum. It minimally involves the cortex over the
convexity, between two gyri in the tertiary sulcus and at progressively
more caudal levels it extensively destroys the white matter deep to the
interhemispheric part of the superior frontal convolution extending
ventrally to involve the corpus callosum, throughout its entire extent in
the coronal section. The cortex of the cingulate gyrus is involved minimally in the depth of the cingulate sulcus. The cingulate bundle appears
to be incompletely interrupted in the myelin stain. The corpus callosum
at the level of the lesion is virtually devoid of stainable myelin. The
subcallosal bundle appears severely atrophic and in all likelihood the
lesions had involved the major superficial part of the subcallosal fasciculus.
(Fig. 6) The white matter of the corona radiata is involved as well as the
centrum semiovale with marked pallor associated with marked dilatation of
the ipsilateral lateral ventricle suggesting widespread loss of myelin
fiber tracts on that side.

On the right side, the surgical lesion begins at the same level in the
crown of the superior frontal convolution involving the white matter of the

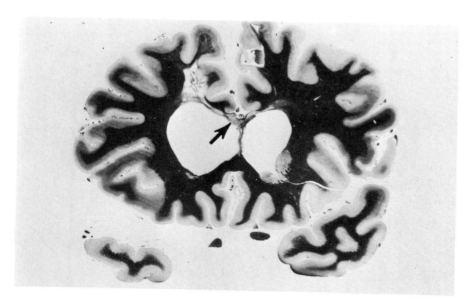

Figure 6: Atrophic Subcallosal Bundle

convolution and in part the interhemispheric cortex. At more caudal levels
it pierces the cingulate sulcus destroying a small frontal convolution in
this sulcus and adjacent cingulate sulcus and reaches its deepest penetration in the alba of the cingulate gyrus just dorsal to the cingulate bundle.
On this side there is also pallor of the corona radiata and to a lesser
extent centrum semiovale. The subcallosal bundle appears to be spared.
The lateral ventricle on the right side is only moderately enlarged as compared to the other side (no change from time of operation). C.V. and Nissl
staining reveals some gliosis on both sides in the cingulate fasciculus
area suggesting incomplete involvement from the surgical procedure. An
incidental finding is the occurrence of several lacunes in the corpus
striatum bilaterally but sparing the internal capsule.

 What seems clearly evident upon detailed examination of this neuropathologic material is that on neither the left or right side is the
cingulate fasciculus completely interrupted by the radiofrequency lesion.
On the right side the epicenter of the lesion was too dorsal and on the
left side approximately 1 cm. too far lateral. Further serial sections

are being prepared that include the corpora striata and thalami.

Case Summary 2:   A 20-year-old female from Finland had been diagnosed
as "schizophrenic" at age 16. She manifested severe self-mutilating behavior and depression. Her mother (who had committed suicide) and a brother
were also diagnosed as "schizophrenic". Bilateral subrostal cingulotomies
were performed on the patient at age 18 by Dr. L.V. Laitinen which produced
clinical improvement for many months but manic, aggressive and self-abusive
behavior recurred. A second surgical procedure aimed at the genu of the
corpus callosum was under consideration when the patient was found comatose
with evidence of self-induced head injury.

Neuropathological Post Mortem: Cerebral contusion and edema were noted
with minor subdural hematoma. The brain, which was received for whole-
section and histo-anatomical study by Dr. P.I. Yakovlev, demonstrated
grossly bilateral uncal and inferior anterolateral herniation. There was
recent hemorrhagic swelling of the left temporal lobe and focal traumatic
hemorrhages in the pontine tegmentum of the brainstem close to the midline.

Detailed Descriptions: Microscopic study of this nearly two-year-old
surgical lesion revealed two parallel needle tracks 1 mm. in diameter
through the alba of the right frontal lobe extending to the genu and rostrum
of the corpus callosum. At the end of each track, a single electro-
coagulative cyst, measuring 10-12 mm. across the mid-sagittal plane, had
destroyed subrostral sections of the cingulate gyri, completely inter-
rupting the subjacent cingulate bundles along with the rostrum of the
corpus callosum to the ventricles but without performation. The cyst on
the right side of the midplane was larger than its counterpart on the left.
From each electro-coagulative cyst a wide band of dense gliosis throughout
the cingulate bundle extended over the genu and anterior part of the
corpus callosum gradually fading out posteriorly. (Fig. 7)
    New bands of dense gliosis penetrated from the cyst through the genu of
corpus callosum branching off from the band of gliosis in the cingulate
bundle into the corpus callosum at right angles with the calloso-commissural
fiber tracts. The latter, however, were intact and showed gliosis only
within the knee where they had been disrupted by the surgical lesion.
    The stratum subcallosum between the caudatum and corpus callosum in the
dorso-lateral angle of the lateral ventricle was densely gliotic bilaterally.

degeneration in the caudata is not evident. Retrograde degeneration in the thalami, however, appears prominent and severe.

DISCUSSION

Analysis by Ballantine et al of an extensive clinical experience with frontal cingulotomy for mood disturbance indicated that about 80% of individuals disabled psychiatrically by severe depression or psychic pain could be improved following one or more cingulotomies (6). Achievement of a satisfactory status for a patient after a second operation when the first one had failed was explained on the basis of a need for a larger lesion or a lesion in a different site, or both.

Researchers have shown that the core of the corpus callosum is formed mostly of commissural fibers which unite the homotopic cortical areas of the two hemispheres. The superficial layers consist of the transcallosal cingulostriate fibers which have their origin in the cingulum. In Case 1, these superficial fibers were markedly atrophic and had lost their myelin in the myelin stain. Some fiber tracks run in the ventral lamina of the corpus callosum to the septum and to the contralateral stratum subcallosum and caudate nucleus. Others run in the dorsal lamina and perforate the commissural fibers in the contralateral hemisphere. (Fig. 12) Of these, some descend in the internal capsule and others are distributed in the putamen and according to Showers (22) even in the pallidum, subthalamic area and substantia nigra.

It may be argued that in anxiety, tension schizophrenia, chronic mood disorders and psychogenic painful states the interhemispheric cingulo-striate fibers are hyperactive. These pathways may constitute the link between an emotional integrative system and its motor output. Laitinen (5) had advocated bilateral stereotactic rostal cingulotomies in which he included the superficial fibers of the genu of the corpus callosum. Others have criticized that procedure and described it as a paramedian frontal lobotomy. Turner (4) had made lesions in the frontal paramedian structures 1 cm. in front of the genu of the corpus callosum and obtained good results in the treatment of anxiety and aggressiveness. He thought that mesoloviotomy interrupts the same anatomical pathways. However, Laitinen disagrees and claims that cingulotomies close to the callosal target but definitely in the cingulum do not give the excellent results observed when the superficial fibers of the corpus callosum are also

298

involved. These most dorsal fibers are thought to connect the cingulum
with the corpus striatum of the contralateral hemisphere or they may
simply connect the two cinguli across the corpus callosum.

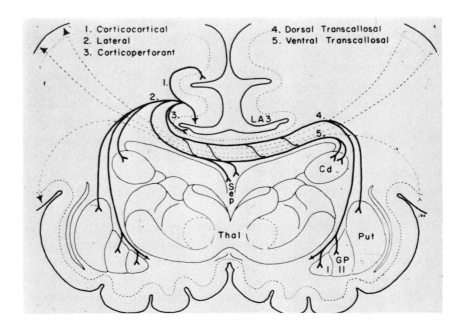

Figure 12: Major Branches of Cingulum in Coronal Plane.
(Yakovlev and Locke, 1961) Superior (corticocortical),
callosoperforant (lateral, dorsal, and ventral transcallosal), and corticoperforant branches are shown.
Contralateral projections to lenticular nucleus are
only tentative.

Thus, from an examination of the neuropathological material it seems
intriguing that clinically excellent results could be obtained by lesions
not significantly involving the cingulate fasciculus as in the first
patient. This striking observation correlates well with the early

cingulotomy experience of Ballantine (9). When the dorsal fibers of the corpus callosum or the most superficial fibers were not involved in the radio-frequency surgical lesion, a significant number of the patients failed to achieve a satisfactory post-operative state. It was only after a deeper lesion was performed that the patients improved. The initial lesions were above the cingulate fasciculus and were apparently related to misinterpretations of the lateral radiographic films during the early period of cingulotomy studies. There was no allowance made for the fact that the cingulum lies in a "depression" below the lateral ventricular shadow and that a lesion which would appear in the lateral projection to be placed in the corpus callosum or even within the ventricle itself was actually in the cingulum bundle. It is now advocated to place the tip of the electrode on the ventricular roof.

Another interpretation would seem to be related to the fiber tracts on the superficial surface of the corpus callosum and centrum semiovale or corona radiata which may subserve efferent and afferent projections of the cingulate gyrus. In the first case there is ample evidence for extensive destruction of white matter around both lateral ventricles and corpus callosum but not directly involving the cingulate fasciculus. In the other cases the cingulate fasciculi are involved as well as the fiber tracts of the corpus callosum. There is evidence that the cingulum projects to and receives impulses from the anterior nucleus of the thalamus. However, other fiber tracts as yet not identified may be involved in limbic circuits.

Our experience would favor the explanation that the most superficial fibers of the corpus callosum have to be involved in the surgical lesion if improvement in psychiatric status is to occur.

It is proposed that cingulotomy favorably affects patients with intractable disorders of affect because of demonstrated anatomic disruption and as yet to be documented neurochemical effects of such disruption. The delay in post-operative improvement documented by Ballantine argues for a major secondary neurochemical rather than a primary neuroanatomical effect of cingulotomy. The occasional regression in psychiatric status after an initial satisfactory result may also support that conclusion.

A succinct summary concerning the possible effects of cingulotomy has been put forth by Yakovlev who formulated the following: "The cingulum

is a bundle strategically situated to mediate activities of the limbic
cortex to the entire forebrain. On general grounds one might speculate
that these activities have something to do with the outward expression of
the visceral, that is, of the internal states or emotions. Its interruption in cingulotomy modifies in some way the behavioral expression of
the distraught internal states. The changes effected by cingulotomy
apparently are not different in kind from those effected by the classical
leucotomies. However, these effects appear to be more selective, less
damaging to the intellectual faculties and obviously much less damaging
to the brain". (7, 14, 21)

Further research should concentrate on cerebra obtained from long-term
survivals which have been donated by persons who had undergone psychosurgical procedures involving the limbic system. Indeed, an international
"brain bank" should be established, which would collect these brains and
would perform neuropathological studies in serial section. It seems
evident that only with thorough, detailed scientific investigations will
the unknown border areas between neurology, psychiatry and neuropharmacology
be paved so that these patients with tortured self-concern, severe
anguish and psychic pain could be helped.

ACKNOWLEDGMENTS

The authors wish to express their profound appreciation to
Drs. P. Yakovlev, W. Nauta, T. Kemper, E.P. Richardson, Jr., and
H. Hamlin for their invaluable contributions. We are deeply indebted
to Valerie Giorgione, Sheila O'Brien, and Nancy Davidson for their
editorial and secretarial assistance.

REFERENCES

1. Foltz, E.L. and White, L.E.: "Pain 'Relief' by Frontal Cingulumotomy."
   J. Neurosurg. 19: 89-100, 1962.

2. Pribram, K.H. and Fulton, J.F.: "An Experimental Critique of the
   Effects of Anterior Cingulate Ablation in Monkey." Brain 77: 34-44,
   1954.

3. Hurt, R.W. and Ballantine, H.T., Jr.: "Stereotactic Anterior Cingulate
   Lesions for Persistent Pain: A Report on 68 Cases." Clinical
   Neurosurgery 21: 334-351, R.H. Wilkins ed., Williams and Wilkins,
   Baltimore, 1974.

4. Turner, E.: "Stereotaxic Lesions in the Knee of the Corpus Callosum
   in the Treatment of Emotional Disorders." Lancet 1: 755, 1972.

5. Latinen, L.V. and Vilkki, J.: "Observations on the Transcallosal Emotional Connections." Surgical Approaches in Psychiatry, Proceedings of the Third International Congress of Psychosurgery, 74-80, L.V. Laitinen and K.E. Livingston eds., Univ. Park Press, Baltimore, 1973.

6. Ballantine, H.T., Jr., Levy, B.S., Dagi, T. and Giriunas, I.B.: "Cingulotomy for Psychiatric Illness: Report of 13 Years' Experience." In 'Neurosurgical Treatment in Psychiatry, Pain, and Epilepsy', Sweet, W.H., Obrador, S. and Martin-Rodgrguez, J.G. eds., 333-353, Proceedings of the Fourth World Congress of Psychiatric Surgery, 333-353, Univ. Park Press, Baltimore, 1977.

7. Yakovlev, P.I., Discussion of Cassidy, W.L., Ballantine, H.T., Jr., and Flanagan, N.B.: "Frontal Cingulotomy for Affective Disorders." Rec. Adv. Biol. Psychiat. 8: 269-275, 1965.

8. Ballantine, H.T., Jr., Cassidy, W.L., Flanagan, N.B. et al: "Stereotactic Anterior Cingulotomy for Neuropsychiatric Illness and Intractable Pain." J. Neurosurg. 26: 488-495, 1967.

9. Ballantine, H.T., Jr., Cassidy, W.L., Brodeur, J., et al: "Frontal Cingulotomy for Mood Disturbance." Hitchcock, E., Laitinen, L. and Vaernet, K. eds., Psychosurgery, 221-229, Charles C. Thomas, Springfield, Ill., 1972.

10. Long, C.J., Pueschel, K., and Hunter, S.E.: "Assessment of the Effects of Cingulate Gyrus Lesions by Neuropsychological Techniques." J. Neurosurg. 49: 264-271, 1978.

11. Cobb, S.: "Emotions and Clinical Medicine." New York, W.W. Norton and Company, 1950.

12. Bard, P.: "Neural Mechanisms in Emotional and Sexual Behavior." Psychosom. Med., 4: 171-172, 1942.

13. MacLean, P.D.: "Contrasting Functions of Limbic and Neocortical Systems of the Brain and their Relevance to Psychophysiological Aspects of Medicine." Am. J. Med. 25: 611-626, 1958.

14. Yakovlev, P.I., and Locke, S.: "Cortical Connections of the Anterior Cingulate Gyrus, the Cingulum and the Subcallosal Bundle in Monkey." Arch. Neurol. 5, 364, Chicago, 1961.

15. Mettler, F.A.: "Corticofugul Fiber Connections of the Macaca Mulatta." J. Comp. Neurol. 61, 509, 1935.

16. Meyer, A., Beck, E., and McLardy, T.: "Prefrontal Leucotomy: A Neuro Anatomical Report." Brain 70, 18, 1947.

17. McLardy, T.: "Thalamic Projection to Frontal Cortex in Man." J. Neurol., Neurosurg., Psychiat. 13: 198, 1950.

18. Papez, J.W.: "A Proposed Mechanism of Emotion." Arch. Neurol. Psychiat. 38: 725-743, Chicago, 1937.

19. Braak, H. and Braak, E.: "The Pyramidal Cells of Betz Within the Cingulate and Precentral Gigantopyramidal Field in the Human Brain." A Golgi and Pigmentarchitectonic Study, Cell Tiss. Res. 172, 103-119, 1976.

20. Nauta, W.J.H.: "Hippocampal Projections and Related Neural Pathways to the Midbrain in the Cat." Brain 81: 319-340, 1958.

302

21. Yakovlev, P.I., Locke, S., and Angevine, J.B., Jr.: "The Limbus of the Cerebral Hemisphere, Limbic Nuclei of the Thalamus and the Cingulum Bundle." In The Thalamus, Purpura and Yahr, M. eds., 77, New York, Columbia Univ. Press, 1966.

22. Showers, M.J.C.: "The Cingulate Gyrus: Additional Motor Area and Cortical Autonomic Regulator." J. Comp. Neurol. 112, 231, 1959.

© 1979 Elsevier/North-Holland Biomedical Press
Modern Concepts in Psychiatric Surgery
E.R. Hitchcock, H.T. Ballantine, Jr. and B.A. Meyerson, eds.

RESULTS OF PSYCHOLOGICAL TESTING OF COGNITIVE FUNCTIONS IN PATIENTS
UNDERGOING STEREOTACTIC PSYCHIATRIC SURGERY

TALIS VASKO AND GUNVOR KULLBERG
Departments of Psychiatry and Neurosurgery, University Hospital, Lund,
Sweden

All patients undergoing functional brain surgery in our unit are subjected
to routine testing of cognitive functions for the purpose of continuous
assessment of possible side effects of these operations. A review of the
test results in a series of patients who underwent psychiatric surgery is
presented.

MATERIAL AND METHODS

The series comprised 44 operations in 37 patients. Bilateral lesions
were placed with stereotactic technique in the anterior internal capsule
in 21 patients, in the anterior cingulate area above the frontal horn in
15 patients, and in the frontobasal subcaudate area in 8 patients (for
more detailed description of the lesions, see[1]). Seven of the patients
had operations in two of these sites with an interval of about one and a
half year. The second operations have been treated as independent cases
in the analysis of the test results.

The majority of the patients suffered from neurotic disturbances; a
few had a diagnosis of borderline psychosis or schizophrenia, with well
preserved personality. All had longstanding, "intractable" emotional
symptoms, which in most cases were ameliorated after the operation.

The age of the patients, which might be pertinent to the occurrence of
organic cognitive deficit, is shown in Fig. 1.

The patients were tested before the operation and again postoperatively,
when they had recovered from the operative trauma and seemed fit for testing. The interval from the operation varied from one to five weeks. If
test performance had declined compared to preoperatively, which actually
occurred in about half the patients, testing was usually repeated in connection with later follow-up examinations, some months to a year after
the operation. In the analysis of the results the data from these re-
-testings were combined with the data from the one postoperative testing

of the rest of the patients, in order to express the average outcome of
the total group.

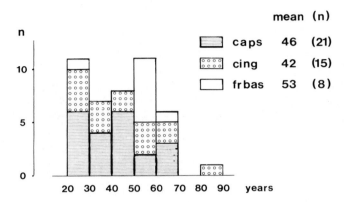

Fig. 1. Age distribution over 10-year periods in relation to type of
operation.

The test batteries administered varied somewhat, but the tests listed
below were given in most instances and provided data, which could be used
for statistical analysis and group comparisons.

Test	Function measured
Raven's Progressive Matrices and/or Koh's Block Design	Non-verbal intelligence
SRB Synonyms	Verbal intelligence
Kendall's Memory for Design Test and/or Benton's Visual Retention Test	Spatial perception and memory
Paired-Associates Test	Verbal memory

RESULTS

Intellectual level

There was little change in individual performance on the intelligence
tests after the operations. The mean value for the (first) postoperative
testing was slightly higher than the preoperative mean, but the difference was not statistically significant (Table 1).

TABLE 1

INTELLECTUAL LEVEL

Test	n	preop Mean $\pm$ S.D.	(first) postop Mean $\pm$ S.D.	signi- ficance
Non-verbal (IQ)	31	93.9 $\pm$ 14.0	95.6 $\pm$ 14.6	N.S.
Verbal (stanine score)	19	5.1 $\pm$ 1.9	5.3 $\pm$ 2.0	N.S.

Spatial perception and memory

As two different tests had been used, in combination or as alternatives, the raw data were not suitable for comparison. The results were therefore classified in four grades, 0 indicating no defect, 1 borderline performance, 2 clear but moderate defect, 3 marked defect.

The individual results at preoperative and early postoperative testing
are shown in Fig. 2, with each operative group represented separately. It
should be noted, that test performance indicating defect was seen already
before the operation in some patients. Postoperatively, a few had improved but a large proportion of the patients showed a decline in performance.
This tendency was most marked in the cingulotomy group. At later re-test-
ing, however, performance had improved towards the original level, as
demonstrated by the mean values in Table 2. The average final result of
the whole group was little different from the average preoperative performance.

TABLE 2

SPATIAL PERCEPTION AND MEMORY

Patient category	n	Mean defect (graded 0-3)		
		preop	postoperative	
Decline - retest	12	0.2	1.7	0.7
One postop testing	30	1.0		1.0
Total	42	0.8		0.9

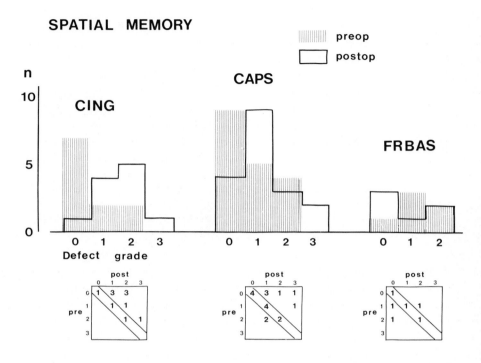

Fig. 2. Spatial perception and memory: Preoperative and early (< 5 weeks) postoperative results. Each operative group is represented by a histogram and a correlation table.

Verbal memory

Fig. 3 shows the preoperative and early postoperative performance on immediate recall of 30 word-pairs. There were large individual changes from pre- to postoperative, both in positive and in negative direction, especially in the capsulotomy group. Retesting of the patients with post-operative impairment (Fig. 4) showed return to or above the original level, with the exception of three capsulotomized patients, who remained considerably below their preoperative scores.

Table 3 summarizes the results expressed as mean values. The final mean score of the whole group was somewhat higher than the preoperative mean, but the difference was not statistically significant. The subgroup who showed decline at early postoperative testing, turned out to have significantly higher preoperative score than the rest of the patients.

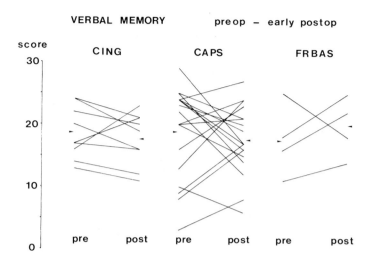

Fig. 3. Verbal memory: Preoperative and early (< 5 weeks) postoperative results. The mean values for each operative group is indicated by arrows.

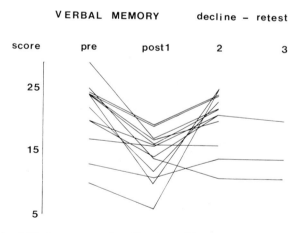

Fig. 4. Verbal memory: Results in patients who declined postoperatively and were retested later. By then performance level was stable as judged by the results in three patients who had a third postoperative test. Three patients from the capsulotomy group remained below their preoperative score.

TABLE 3

VERBAL MEMORY

Patient category	n	Mean score preop	postoperative
Decline - retest	13	21.2	14.5[a/] 20.6
One postop testing	22	16.9[b/]	20.1[a/]
Total	35	18.4	20.3[c/]

Statistics (t-test): a/ sign.different from preop. (as could be expected, due to the selection) b/ sign. different from "decline group" c/ not sign.different from preop. - Significance level p < 0.001.

Age

There was no obvious correlation between the patients' age and the various changes in test performance.

DISCUSSION

These tests did not disclose any significant lasting deterioration of cognitive functions in the group of patients studied, as judged by the mean values for preoperative and final postoperative performance (Tables 1-3). This result agrees with the findings of other authors who studied the effects of similar psychosurgical lesions with various cognitive tests and generally found no or little impairment, sometimes even improvement[2].

The temporary changes in the early postoperative period are of certain interest for the analysis of the effects of the operations. The transient impairment of spatial and verbal memory functions does not seem wholly explainable as an unspecific postoperative depression of performance, as the two functions sometimes changed in opposite directions in the same individual. Furthermore, decline in spatial memory tended to be most marked after cingulotomy, decline in verbal memory after capsulotomy, suggesting that the two operations may have differential effects on cognitive functions, although these effects are attenuated with time. Other differences between cingulotomy and capsulotomy, for example in the occurrence of postoperative confusion, have been described previously[1]. Deterioration on spatial tests following cingulotomy was reported also by Teuber et al[3].

Marked bi-directional changes from pre- to postoperative were found on the verbal memory test (Fig. 3), presumably due to two oppositely directed effects of the operation: an untoward effect of the operative lesion on brain functions subserving memory, and a positive effect related to the relief of emotional distress, which preoperatively prevented some patients from demonstrating their true cognitive capacity. The latter assumption is supported by the finding, that those patients whose performance improved,scored significantly lower on the preoperative test compared to the patients whose performance declined (Table 3). These observations serve as a reminder that emotional improvement might in some cases conceal a cognitive deficit caused by the operation; unchanged or even improved postoperative test performance, although satisfying from a practical point of view, does not exclude the possibility that damage has been inflicted to the cognitive function tested. Further elucidation of this problem would require methods which take the emotional and behavioural factors into account.

SUMMARY

A series of 44 psychosurgical interventions (capsulotomy 21, cingulotomy 15, frontobasal tracotomy 8) was reviewed with regard to the results obtained on psychological tests measuring intelligence level, spatial perception and memory, and verbal memory. The patients were tested before the operation and within 5 weeks after. If test performance had declined postoperatively, testing was repeated in connection with later follow-up examinations.

There was no significant change in intelligence level from pre- to postoperatively. About half the patients showed some decline on the spatial or the verbal memory test at the early postoperative examination, and there was some evidence of differential effects of the three types of operations: capsulotomy tended to interfere with verbal memory more than the other operations, cingulotomy with spatial functions. At later retesting, however, this initial impairment had disappeared in all but a few patients. Test performance above preoperative level was seen in many patients following the operation, presumably reflecting relief of emotional symptoms, which had previously prevented them from fully utilizing their true cognitive capacity. The mean values for preoperative and final post-operative performance, based on the whole group of patients, showed no significant difference. It was emphasized, that the effects of emotional improvement might in some cases conceal a cognitive impairment caused by the operation.

References

1. Kullberg, G. (1977): Differences in Effect of Capsulotomy and Cing-ulotomy. In 2, pp 301-308.

2. Several reports containing information on results of psychological testing,as well as further references, will be found in the Proceedings of the Fourth World Congress of Psychiatric Surgery: Neurosurgical Treat-ment in Psychiatry, Pain and Epilepsy. Eds Sweet, W.H., Obrador, S. and Martín-Rodríguez, J.G. University Park Press, Baltimore 1977.

3. Teuber, H.-L., Corkin, S.H. and Twitchell, T.E. (1977): Study of Cingulotomy in Man: A Summary. In 2, pp 355-362.

© 1979 Elsevier/North-Holland Biomedical Press
Modern Concepts in Psychiatric Surgery
E.R. Hitchcock, H.T. Ballantine, Jr. and B.A. Meyerson, eds.

Monitoring Psychosurgery:

Clinical and Research Observations

by

J. Bartlett, P. van Boxel

P.K. Bridges and P. Sepping

The Geoffrey Knight Psychosurgical Unit is independently organised within the South-East Thames Regional Neurosurgical Centre. which is responsible for emergency and routine neurosurgery for those living in the southeast of England from London to the coast. The Unit consists of eight beds specifically for patients admitted for assessment for operation, and for psychosurgery and subsequent rehabilitation. The operation employed is almost invariably Knight's stereotactic subcaudate tractotomy (Knight, 1965). About eighty patients are assessed for possible psychosurgery each year, about 30% are either not accepted as suitable or themselves decline. In all, over 850 operations have now been performed. Thus, there is a regular flow of patients through the Unit. with one operation being carried out per week and with patients in conditions that are quite well controlled. This enables systematic organisation of clinical monitoring with an associated comprehensive research programme. The aim of this chapter is to present an over-view of the work, giving examples of recent research effort.

Psychosurgical lesions will, of course, vary both by site and by size but both can be standardised using Knight's operation which produces a lesion of predetermined size in a standard operation site, both of which are therefore closely similar for all patients.

The patients are admitted two weeks before operation and stay at least two weeks afterwards, sometimes considerably longer, for purposes of rehabilitation. During admission all the patients are asked to accept a controlled diet avoiding foods containing large amounts of monoamines the diet being as that taken by patients receiving monoamine oxidase inhibitor drugs. For similar reasons, we exclude as far as possible foods such as bananas, nuts and orange juice which have a relatively high tryptophan content.

A primary purpose of monitoring is to try to establish a reliable diagnosis and also to attempt to record progress and decide on the outcome after operation. The problem of diagnosis is considerable because in psychiatry there will be little opportunity for objectivity, but reliable diagnosis is important as a means of assigning prognosis and also as a crucial parameter to which research findings can be related. There is, first, uncertainty as to what type of concept should be used. For example, a phobic anxiety state beginning for the first time in the second half of life, perhaps associated with early morning waking and suicidal ideas, would generally be regarded as quite clearly as a depressive illness essentially and would be more likely to respond decisively to antidepressant medication than to anxiolytic compounds. Should this case be labelled as one of anxiety or one of depression? In order to avoid clinical assumptions as to the basic cause of psychiatric illnesses. it seems better to give a diagnosis on the basis of the presenting symptom and other characteristics of the illness can be added.

Table 1

DIAGNOSTIC SCHEME

PRESENTING SYMPTOMS

Depression

Primary	Bipolar	Chronic	Agitated
Secondary	Unipolar	Recurrent	Retarded
		Uncertain	Uncertain

Anxiety or Tension

Primary	Chronic anxiety	Recurrent anxiety
Secondary	Chronic tension	Recurrent tension
	Chronic phobic	Recurrent phobic

Obsessional neurosis

Primary

Secondary

Other: specify . . . .

PRESENT STATE

Well. Unwell, not at worst. At worst. Anomalous.

specify . . . .

The chart places patients into three diagnostic categories, namely those with primary anxiety, primary depression and primary obsessional neurosis. This may verge on the simplistic but, in the present state of knowledge about aetiology in psychiatry. it may be as far as one should go. Additional information can be added and there is provision to note for example, bipolar or unipolar illnesses, agitation or retardation and

and chronic or episodic conditions. Another important aspect is that the patient is not necessarily ill when operated on. In the case of recurrent depression, for example, the patient may be entirely well at the time of operation but wishes to accept the treatment in order to avoid future attacks. It is therefore important for research purposes especially, to know whether patients are, at the time of admission when specimens may be collected, well or unwell. Finally, at the assessment for suitability for psychosurgery, if the patient is accepted for operation, a note is made of the anticipated outcome one year after operation, as follows:-

I   Recovered, no symptoms and no treatment required
II   Well; mild residual symptoms. little or no interference
        with daily life
III Improved, but significant symptoms remain which interfere
        with the patient's life
IV   Unchanged
V   Worse

Another attempt at an objective approach to diagnosis is by the use of the Present State Examination (PSE) (Wing, Cooper and Sartorius, 1974). This was carried out two weeks before the operation by an observer specially trained in the use of the method. Preliminary results are as follows in Table 2.

There is moderate agreement between the diagnostic groups assigned on clinical grounds.and the P.S.E. Catego classes established on the basis of symptomatology. Class B (obsessional) included nearly all the cases of obsessional neurosis, diagnosed on clinical grounds, however, Class B also included most cases of depression but an additional nine cases of depression came into Class R (retarded depression).

The lower part of the table relates P.S.E. syndromes obtained before operation with the outcome one year later. Classes B and N (neurotic depression) were associated with good outcome in about half the cases, while of the patients in Class R, only 25% responded. Study of the data continues but this would appear to be an objective and original approach to the problem of diagnosis and the possibility of separating individual symptoms may offer a new means of aiding suitability for psychosurgery and prognosis after.

Table 2
PRESENT STATE EXAMINATION

Clinical diagnostic group

P.S.E. Catego Class	Depression	Anxiety	Obsessional Neurosis	other	
B	13	3	6	3	25
R	9	1	-	2	12
N	8	4	1	2	15
	30	8	7	7	52

P.S.E. Catego Class

Outcome at 1 year	B	R	N	
Good (I & II)	12(48%)	3(25%)	8(53%)	23
Poor (III & IV)	13	9	7	29
	25	12	15	52

The clinical assessment of outcome (I - V) is carried out in the Unit by inviting the patient to attend one year after operation, and the outcome category is decided by a senior psychiatrist otherwise not associated with the Unit. We have felt that the definitions for outcome given above have proved useful in practice and it may be that other units could use the same or modify them in a way that a number of workers would agree to, hence aiding uniformity of research into psychosurgery. However, objective data is needed as far as possible to support the clinical assessment and this may be carried out in several ways. The use of self-completed psychological tests is an obvious method and some results are shown in Table 3(Göktepe et al., 1975). The clinical assessment of outcome at one year was compared with two psychological tests carried out at the same visit, The Wakefield Inventory for depression (Snaith, Ahmed, Mehta and Hamilton, 1971) and the Taylor Manifest Anxiety Scale (Taylor, 1955). The results for those of good outcome were significantly lower than for patients in Group III and in Group IV.

Table 6

Mean Plasma Cortisol (nmol/1) values by Outcome

I and II n = 8	Control	After dexamethasone	After tetracosactrin
Pre-operation	378	130	775
Post-operation			
3 weeks	416	119	595
1 year	392	91	704
III and IV n = 5			
Pre-operation	397	119	827
Post-operation			
3 weeks	409	185	902
1 year	570	147	832

Table 7

Mean Plasma Tryptophan values (μmol/1)

before and after operation

Diagnosis.	n	Total tryptophan pre- post-		Free tryptophan pre- post-		Free/Total % pre- post-	
Depression	26	63.8	60.5	5.9	5.6	9.2	9.2
Anxiety	5	68.1	69.0	5.8	6.2	8.6	8.9
Obsessional neurosis	4	62.2	69.0	5.7	5.6	9.2	8.2
Other	5	49.0	48.5	4.0	4.5	8.7	8.8
Controls	20	72.1		6.1		8.5	

Sandler, Bonham-Carter, Cuthbert and Pare (1975) found that a group of depressed patients. given a single dose of 100 mg of tyramine, subsequently, in the first three hour period showed significantly reduced conjugated tyramine output compared with controls. A further study including some of our psychosurgical patients has recently been reported (Bonham-Carter. Sandler, Goodwin. Sepping and Bridges, 1978). Again, there was a significant difference, and this time tyramine was also given to the same patients one year after operation. While it was found that six had virtually recovered and ten were only somewhat improved or else unchanged. nonetheless, the same reduced conjugated tyramine output was observed in both groups. This suggests that an abnormality associated with depressive illnesses is present continuously and becomes mani-

Table 8

Mean Noradrenaline and Adrenaline Excretion

(nmol/24 hr)

	n	Pre-operation Adren.	Noradren.	Post-operation Adren.	Noradren.	Differences Adren.	Noradren.
Depression							
I and II	8	152	873	259	314	+107	-559
III and IV	12	245	686	211	477	-34	-209
All other diagnosis	15	156	483	185	480	-29	-3
Controls	7	323	514	420	1124	+97	+610

T-tests	Post-operation Adren. Noradren
Controls v all other diagnoses	$p < 0.05$ < 0.001
Controls v depression	$p < 0.05$ < 0.01

T-tests of differences	Differences between pre- and post-operation
Depression	noradrenaline $p < 0.02$
Controls	noradrenaline $p < 0.02$

Table 9

Ventricular C.S.F.

Diagnoses	n	Age years	Tryptophan (μg/ml)	5-HIAA (μg/ml)
Depression	21	54	0.63[a]	0.066[d]
Other diagnoses	8	52	0.71	0.070
Agitation, anxiety, tension	5	49	1.05[b]	0.106[e]
Neurological probably normal CSF flow)	5	40	0.85[c]	0.087

a - b $p < 0.001$, a - c $p < 0.02$, d - e $p < 0.01$

only in certain circumstances. This study is being extended.

During the operation of stereotactic tractotomy air is routinely injected into the ventricles in order to facilitate stereotactic calculations. This offers an opportunity for the collection of ventricular C.S.F. and Table 9 summarizes the findings in the study by Bridges, Bartlett, Sepping, Kantamaneni and Curzon (1976). Suitable control values were very difficult to obtain for this study but it appears that reduced values for tryptophan and its metabolite 5-HIAA in C.S.F. reflects more the presentation of the case than the basic diagnosis, patients with anxiety and tension having significantly higher levels than those presenting with depression even although that last group had significantly lower concentration than the controls.

We are at present attempting to examine relationships between plasma tryptophan, lumbar C.S.F. tryptophan and ventricular C.S.F. tryptophan which will have importance for the research being done with depressed patients as a way of assessing the significance of plasma tryptophan in relation to central nervous system tryptophan metabolism. In this study blood was taken at 08.00 hrs., which is before the operation begins. Another specimen was taken after the start of the operation, about one hour later, at which time it is a convenient point in the operation to collect ventricular C.S.F. About one further hour later a third blood specimen was taken at the time when lumbar C.S.F. can be collected. All the significant correlations have been shown in Figure 1 by continuous lines and it can be seen that C.S.F. tryptophan, either lumbar or ventricular, relates significantly only to free plasma tryptophan taken one hour before. The ventricular and lumbar C.S.F. values did not significantly relate although they were taken only one hour apart. This is another study which requires considerable development.

Thus, investigations carried out partly to attempt to improve diagnostic and prognostic procedures in relation to psychosurgery show considerable promise as means by which psychiatric illnesses may be, in some ways, more effectively studied than hitherto. Psychosurgery now usefully involves biochemists, pathologists, and psychologists as well as psychiatrists and neurosurgeons, all of whom may co-operate to help the individual patient and improve our knowledge both of psychiatric illnesses and of some aspects of the function of the nervous system.

Figure 1

RELATIONSHIPS BETWEEN PLASMA, VENTRICULAR
CSF AND LUMBAR CSF TRYPTOPHAN AND 5HIAA

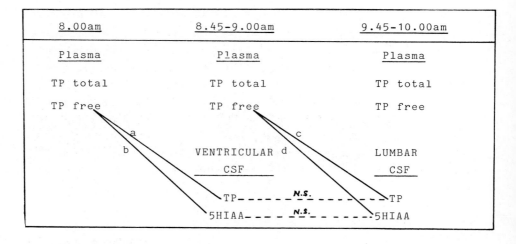

a   0.43   p<0.05   c   0.44   p<0.05
b   0.51   p<0.02   d   0.53   p<0.02

References

Beck, A.T., Ward, C.H., Mendelson, M., Mock, J. and Erbaugh, J. (1961) Arch. gen. Psychiat. 4, 561-571

Bonham-Carter, S., Sandler, M., Goodwin, B.L., Sepping P.and Bridges P.K. (1978) Brit. J. Psychiat. 132, 125-32

Bridges, P.K., Curzon, G, Newcombe, R.L. and Rosser R. (1975) Biol. Psychiat, 10, 211-217

Bridges, P.K., Bartlett, J.R., Sepping, P., Kantamaneni, B.D. and Curzon, G. (1976) Psychol. Med. 6. 399-405

Carroll, B.J. (1976) Psychosomatic Med. 38, No. 2 p.106-121

Carroll, B.J., Curtis, G.C., and Mendels, J. (1976) Arch. Gen. Psychiatry. 33. 1039-1044

Carroll, B.J., Curtis, G.C. and Mendels, J. (1976) Arch. Gen. Psychiatry. 33. 1051-1058

Coppen, A, Ecclestone, E.G. and Peet, M. (1973) Lancet ii, 59-63

Eysenck, H.J. and Eysenck, S.B.G. (1964) Manual of the Eysenck Personality Inventory, University of London Press, London

Göktepe, E.O., Young, L.B. and Bridges, P.K. (1975) Brit. J. Psychiat. 126, 270-80

Knight, G. (1965) J. Neurol. Neurosurg. Psychiat. 28. 304-310

Landon, J., James, V.H.T., Warton, J.J. and Friedman, M. (1967) Lancet ii, 697-700

Niskanen, P., Huttunen, M., Tamminen, T. and Jaasekelainen, X. (1976) Brit. J. Psychiat. 128, 67-73

Papeschi, R. and McClure, D. J. (1971) Arch Gen. Psychiat. 25, 354-358

Peet, M., Moody, J.P., Worrall, E.P., Walker, P. and Naylor, G.J. (1976) Brit. J. Psychiat. 128, 255-258

Salkind, M.R. (1972) Postgrad. med. J., Suppl. 48, 34-41

Sandler, M., Bonham-Carter, S., Cuthbert, M.F. and Pare, C.M.B. (1975) Lancet, i, 1045-1048

Schildkraut, J.J. (1965) Amer. J. Psychiat. 122, 509

Sepping, P., Wood, W., Bellamy, C., Bridges, P.K., O'Gorman, P. Bartlett, J.R. and Patel, V.K. (1977) Acta psychiat. scand. 56, 1-14

Snaith, R.P., Ahmed, S.N., Mehta, S. and Hamilton, M. (1971) Psychol. Med. 1, 143-149

Taylor, J.A. (1955) J. abnorm. soc. Psychol. 48, 285-290

Wing, J.K., Cooper, J.E. and Sartorius, N. (1974) Measurement and Classification of Psychiatric Symptoms. Cambridge University Press: Cambridge.

J. R. Bartlett, MA. FRCS.
Consultant Neurosurgeon
P. van Boxel, MRCPsych,
lately Research Fellow
P. K. Bridges, MD. PhD. MRCPsych
Consultant Psychiatrist
P. Sepping, MRCPsych.
lately Research Fellow

Geoffrey Knight Psychosurgical Unit, Brook General Hospital, Shooters Hill Road, London, S.E.18

SOCIETY AND PSYCHIATRIC SURGERY

© 1979 Elsevier/North-Holland Biomedical Press
Modern Concepts in Psychiatric Surgery
E.R. Hitchcock, H.T. Ballantine, Jr. and B.A. Meyerson, eds.

FURTHER EXPERIENCE OF LIMBIC LEUCOTOMY

NITA MITCHELL-HEGGS, DESMOND KELLY, ALAN RICHARDSON AND JOHN
McLEISH
St. George's Hospital Medical School at Atkinson Morley's Hospital
London, SW20, England

INTRODUCTION

At the fourth World Congress of Psychiatric Surgery in 1975 the
results of the first 66 consecutive patients to undergo stereotactic limbic leucotomy were reported[1]. The data of the first
100 patients, followed up for a mean interval of 20 months, are
now being analysed and this is a preliminary communication of the
ongoing assessment of limbic leucotomy.

THE PATIENTS

Thirty-two males and 68 females in the series had a mean age of
38 years (range 19-74 years) and were all suffering from severe
intractable psychiatric illness. They had failed to respond to,
or to maintain improvement from, alternative forms of treatment;
their mean duration of illness was 12 years, and they had spent on
average nearly two years in psychiatric hospitals. Forty-four
percent of the patients had made one or more suicidal attempts
prior to surgery. If there was any doubt about the adequacy of
previous treatment, they were admitted to the inpatient psychiatric unit of St. George's Hospital and re-treated before surgery
was seriously considered. The Consultant Behaviour Therapist on
the academic staff of the unit independently reviews and treats
all the patients with obsessional neurosis, or other conditions
which may respond to behaviour therapy, before surgery is contem-
plated.

The following criteria are used in assessing the patients'
suitability for psychosurgery:

1. The severity of illness, which in most cases results in total
incapacity and/or an intolerable life.

2. The chronicity of the condition.

3. Failure to respond to other appropriate forms of treatment:
such as ECT 90%, Psychotherapy 70%, or Modified Narcosis 50%.

328

4. Absence of contraindications such as psychopathy, alcoholism or drug addiction, uncontrollable violence or intracerebral pathology.

5. The patient's full agreement to the operation. Only patients who are NOT compulsorily detained in hospital under the Mental Health Act are deemed eligible.

THE OPERATION

The stereotactic technique used by Dr. Richardson has replaced the rostral leucotomy of Sir Wylie McKissock. Limbic leucotomy is designed to interrupt frontothalamic and hypothalamic connections in the <u>lower medial quadrant of the frontal lobe</u>, and the main limbic circuit, the Papez circuit in the <u>cingulate area</u>[2] (Fig.1).

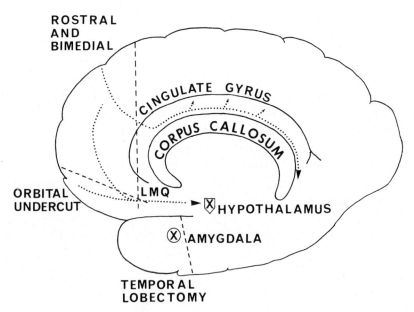

Fig.1. Frontolimbic pathways and sites of some free-hand psycho-surgical procedures. In stereotactic tractotomy lesions are made in the posterior 2 cm of the orbital undercutting incision, and in stereotactic limbic leucotomy small lesions are made in the lower medial quadrant (LMQ) of the frontal lobe and in the cingulum bundle (dotted) in the cingulate gyrus. The amygdala (A) and hypo-thalamus (H) are target sites for operations on the defence react-ion circuit for uncontrollable violence associated with epilepsy. (Reproduced with permission of Br.J.Hosp.Med.).

Both bony and ventricular landmarks are used for calculating
the target sites (indicated by a dot in a circle; Figs.2 and 3),
and electrical stimulation of these invariably results in physiological changes, especially in respiration. If adequate responses
are not obtained the target may be moved a few millimeters prior to
lesion-making by thermocoagulation or with a cryogenic probe.

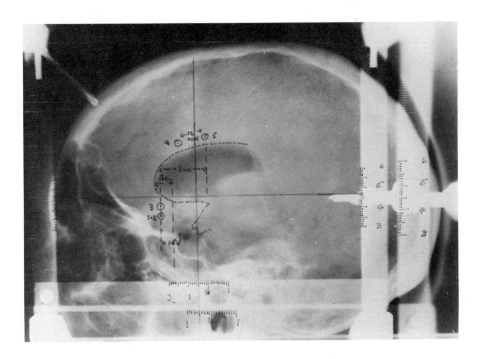

Fig.2. Lateral X-ray of the skull showing air in the ventricles and
the stereotactic frame in place. The lower medial quadrant target
sites (1, 2 and 3) and cingulate sites (4 and 5) are shown.
(Reproduced with permission of Postgrad.Med.J.)

The majority of patients had three small lesions in each frontal
lobe and four in the cingulum bundle as shown in Figs.2 and 3.
Some patients had frontal lobe lesions with others in the genu of
the corpus callosum instead of the cingulum, following Laitinen's
report at the Second World Congress where he advocated such placement for reducing chronic anxiety.

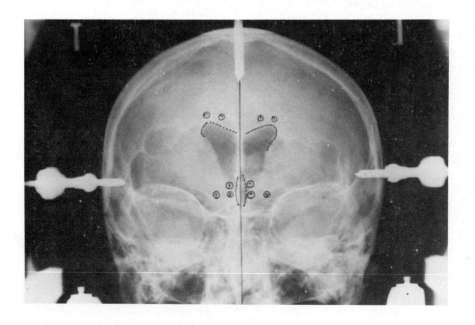

Fig.3. Anterior-posterior view of the skull with air in the lateral
ventricles. The 3 lower medial quadrant target sites form a triangle, while the cingulate sites are above the roof of the lateral
ventricles. (Reproduced with permission of Postgrad.Med.J.).

FOLLOW-UP

The patients were reviewed with rating-scales after a mean interval of 20 months post-operatively. Since the forms used were not
scored until some weeks later, the results were not
known at the time of the two independent psychiatric assessments
by Dr. Mitchell-Heggs and Dr. Kelly. The less favourable of
their two clinical ratings is used; I Symptom free; II Much
improved (minimal residual symptoms); III Improved (definite
improvement, but significant residual symptoms); IV Not improved;
V Worse: i.e. the clinical state is less satisfactory than preoperatively, although not necessarily because of the operation,
but because of continuing illness leading to further deterioration.

Categories I, II and III are placed together to give a percentage of overall improvement.

TABLE I

STEREOTACTIC LIMBIC LEUCOTOMY - IMPROVEMENT RATINGS AT FOLLOW-UP
(N = 100)

N	Diagnosis	Clinical ratings I,II,III	IV,V.	% Improved
32	Obsessional neurosis	28	4	88
21	Chronic anxiety/Phobic neurosis	12	9	57
18 +1	Depression	11	7+1	61
15	Schizophrenia/Schizo-affective disorder	11	4	73
3	Anorexia nervosa	1	2	
1	Personality disorder with anxiety	1	–	
4	Personality disorder with depression	2	2	
1	Depersonalization with depression	–	1	
1	Dementia with depression	–	1	
1	Intractable pain with depression	1	–	
1	Paranoid state with depression	–	1	
1	Palilalia with Parkinsonism	–	1	
100		67	32+1	67

Of the total sample, 32 patients were suffering from obsessional
neurosis of whom 88% improved. Twenty-one anxious patients had a
57% improvement rate, which was similar to the figure (61%) for

the 18 depressives.   One patient died from a pulmonary embolus 4
months post-operatively; she is indicated separately as one of the
depressives on the table.

An unexpected finding was that of 15 patients suffering from
schizophrenia or schizo-affective disorders: 73% improved.   There
was usually little change in the underlying schizophrenic process,
but the affective component, i.e. anxiety or depression, or the
obsessional component of the illness improved, and the patients
were appreciably less distressed by their symptoms.   Of the other
diagnostic categories listed, worthwhile improvement generally did
not occur.   The results in anorexia nervosa have not been encouraging.

The clinical ratings appear to be a valid measure of change.
When pre- and post-operative psychometric scores were retrospect-
ively determined for each clinical category at follow-up, it was
found that before surgery the mean scores were very similar (Table
2).   There was no significant difference between the mean preoperative scores of the categories for Neuroticism (Maudsley Personality Inventory) or Depression.

TABLE 2

CLINICAL RATINGS AT FOLLOW-UP WITH PRE- AND POST-OPERATIVE MEAN
NEUROTICISM AND DEPRESSION SCORES

Clinical ratings	I Symptom Free	II Much Improved	III Improved	IV Not Improved	V Worse	F
Pre-operative						
Neuroticism (M.P.I.)	30	35	32	33	36	NS
Beck Depression	22	27	26	29	32	NS
Hamilton "	17	25	23	25	26	NS
Middlesex "	9	10	10	10	11	NS
Self-rating "	5	6	5	6	7	NS
Observer-rating "	5	6	5	6	7	NS
Post-operative						
Neuroticism (M.P.I.)	10	24	26	34	40	.001
Beck Depression	4	13	20	27	44	.001
Hamilton "	3	11	16	24	33	.001
Middlesex "	3	7	7	9	10	.001
Self-rating "	1	3	5	6	8	.001
Observer-rating "	1	3	4	6	7	.001

Twenty months <u>post-operatively</u>, however, there were highly significant differences between the patients who were rated Symptom
Free and those rated as Worse. On the Neuroticism scale those rated as Symptom Free had a score of 10, i.e. a 20 point decrease in
N score; Much Improved had a score of 24, i.e.an 11 point decrease;
Improved had a score of 26, i.e. a 6 point decrease, while those
rated as Not Improved had a score of 34, an increase of one point,
and those who were Worse a score of 40, an increase of 4 points.

The findings for <u>Depression</u> were very similar, with post-operative values on the Beck Depression Scale (Table 2) as follows:
Symptom Free,18 point fall; Much Improved,14 point fall; Improved,
6 point fall; Not Improved,2 point fall; Worse,12 point increase.

When the total sample of patients was examined, it was found
that the pre and post-operative scores on the Middlesex Hospital
Questionnaire for <u>Anxiety</u>, <u>Obsessional</u>, <u>Depressive</u>, <u>Phobic</u>, and
<u>Somatic</u> symptoms were all significantly less at follow-up (Fig.4).

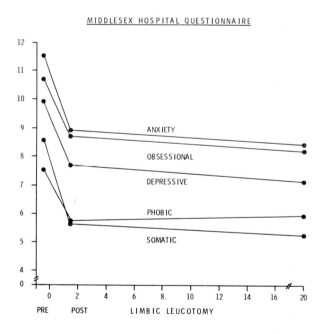

Fig.4. Mean pre and post-operative scores at 6 weeks and 20 months

334

The obsessional patients were also assessed pre and post-operatively on the Leyton Obsessional Inventory. Post-operatively, Obsessional Symptoms and Traits had fallen significantly, as well as Resistance (the distress caused by symptoms) and Interference (intrusion caused by symptoms) p<.OO1.

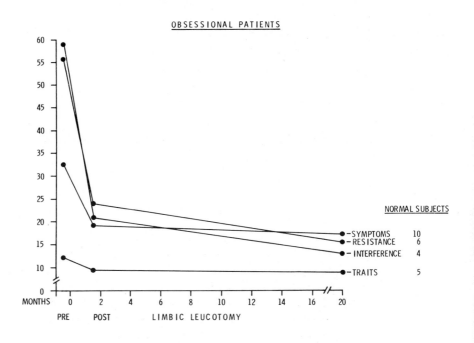

Fig.5. Mean pre and post-operative scores on the Leyton Obsessional Inventory at 6 weeks and 20 months

ASSESSMENT OF INTELLECTUAL FUNCTION PRE AND POST OPERATIVELY

There was no fall in IQ on the Wechsler Adult Intelligence Scale as a result of surgery. The mean values for Verbal and Performance as well as Full Scale IQ had in fact increased (see difference column on right of Table 3) 6 weeks post-operatively. Practice effects, generally observed when the WAIS is repeated are probably largely responsible for this. There was no fall-off in any of the sub-scales on the WAIS, indeed all the Performance sub-scales increased significantly,as did two of the Verbal sub-scales.

TABLE 3

THE MEAN SCORES ON THE WECHSLER ADULT INTELLIGENCE SCALE BEFORE
AND 6 WEEKS AFTER LIMBIC LEUCOTOMY (N = 88)

	Before	After	Difference	p
Verbal IQ	106.5	109.7	+ 3.2	.01
Performance IQ	96.7	101.1	+ 4.4	.001
Full scale IQ	102.3	105.8	+ 3.5	.001
Verbal sub-scales				
Information	10.4	10.9	+ 0.5	.001
Comprehension	12.6	13.0	+ 0.4	NS*
Arithmetic	9.8	10.4	+ 0.6	.01
Similarities	10.9	11.2	+ 0.3	NS
Digit span	9.5	9.8	+ 0.3	NS
Vocabulary	12.5	12.7	+ 0.2	NS
Performance sub-scales				
Digit symbol	7.4	7.8	+ 0.4	.05
Picture completion	9.2	9.8	+ 0.6	.001
Block design	9.3	9.7	+ 0.4	.05
Picture arrangement	8.5	9.2	+ 0.7	.01
Object assembly	8.6	9.6	+ 1.0	.001

*NS: Not significant
(Reproduced with permission of Br.J.Psychiatry)

CONCLUSION

1. Limbic Leucotomy produced a 67% overall improvement rate in a
very severely ill and suicidal group of patients who had failed
to achieve sustained improvement with any other method of
treatment.

2. One third of patients, however, received no appreciable
benefit from surgery, the risk of suicide remained, and further
deterioration in clinical state sometimes occurred.

3. The results in obsessional neurosis were particularly good,
while those of depression left something to be desired. In view
of this, patients with primary depressive illness now have
frontal lobe lesions in a very similar configuration to that
employed by Knight[3] without cingulate lesions.

4. The detailed methods of assessment reported here enable
different types of lesion placement to be compared. It was
encouraging to find that the psychiatrists' clinical ratings at

follow-up corresponded well with changes in psychometric scores.
5. Stereotactic methods allow for much smaller lesions to be
placed with a high degree of accuracy, hence the risk of mortality
is reduced to almost zero. Compared with 'free-hand operations',
an adverse personality change is much less likely to occur.
6. Although it was not possible to get the financial support of
the Medical Research Council for the Prospective Controlled Trial
of Stereotactic Surgery planned by the Royal College of
Psychiatrists[4], much valuable work can still be done to refine
methods of patient selection, surgical technique and psychiatric
and psychological evaluation.

ACKNOWLEDGMENTS

We are most grateful to the Wellcome Trust who financially
supported this research over a number of years. Dr. Tony
Coughlan, Tony Halil and Hilary Evans gave us invaluable
assistance.

REFERENCES

1. Mitchell-Heggs, N., Kelly, D. and Richardson, A.E. (1977)
   in Neurosurgical Treatment in Psychiatry, Pain and Epilepsy.
   ed. W.H. Sweet, S. Obrador, J.G. Martin-Rodriguez. University
   Park Press, Baltimore, P.367.
2. Richardson, A.E., Kelly, D. and Mitchell-Heggs, N. (1977) in
   Neurosurgical Treatment in Psychiatry, Pain and Epilepsy.
   eds. W.H. Sweet, S. Obrador, J.G. Martin-Rodriguez. University
   Park Press, Baltimore, p.363.
3. Knight, G.C. (1969) Bi-frontal stereotactic tractotomy.
   Br.J.Psychiat. 115, 257.
4. Royal College of Psychiatrists (1977) in Neurosurgical
   Treatment in Psychiatry, Pain and Epilepsy. eds. W.H. Sweet,
   S. Obrador, J.G. Martin-Rodriguez. University Park Press,
   Baltimore, P.175.

© 1979 Elsevier/North-Holland Biomedical Press
Modern Concepts in Psychiatric Surgery
E.R. Hitchcock, H.T. Ballantine, Jr. and B.A. Meyerson, eds.   337

A PARADOX OF PSYCHOSURGICAL EVALUATION

JOHN SCOTT PRICE

Northwick Park Hospital and Clinical Research Centre, Watford Road, Harrow,

Middlesex. HA1 3UJ, United Kingdom.

PREAMBLE

Many branches of medicine and surgery are going through difficulties, if not
actual crises, in relation to the evaluation of therapy. A new generation
trained in the principles of clinical science is refusing to accept the
"bedside" evidence which is given to justify many of our established treatments;
they have been taught in medical school of the biases which can distort the
results of uncontrolled trials; they are demanding, as they have been taught to
demand, evidence from one or preferably several randomised prospective
controlled trials before they make up their minds about the effectiveness of a
new (or even an old) treatment. Those in senior positions in our professional
organisations are sympathetic to this demand for well-controlled evaluation;
indeed, they themselves have largely stimulated it. In actual practice,
however, it is proving unexpectedly difficult to carry out these trials. There
is no shortage of research units or personnel with the necessary skills or of
motivation; but for some reason the trials just do not get done. The reason
for this difficulty in responding to a logical, widespread and persistent
demand is obscure.

The problem as it affects surgery in general has been stated very lucidly
by David H. Spodick of the University of Massachusetts Medical School and
twelve colleagues from all over the U.S.A.[1] On the day that Dr. Spodick's
letter appeared in the Lancet, there was editorial comment in the British
Medical Journal[2] regretting the lack of controlled trials of palliative surgery.
In psychiatry, we have had extensive recent agonising over the evaluation of
ECT, and an extremely well-mounted trial of psychotherapy[3] ended in dismal
failure with the general conclusion that psychotherapy is barely amenable to
evaluation. In general it appears to be the "important" treatments which are
difficult to evaluate – important in terms of time, money, skill of the
therapist and significance to the patient. Less "important" treatments such as
drug therapy have had their problems of evaluation[4] but in more recent years
very large numbers of well-controlled studies have been carried out; for example,
the long term trials of maintenance therapy in schizophrenia and affective
disorders reviewed by John M. Davis.[5]

The important question arises, is the evaluation of "important" therapies just running a bit behind the evaluation of drugs, or is there some fundamental impediment about the "important" therapies which makes them in some way not susceptible to the techniques of clinical science?

I hope that a discussion of the particular case of the psychiatric surgeon may throw some light on this difficult problem. I make no excuse for offering the contribution of a general psychiatrist with no special knowledge or experience of psychiatric surgery; from a distance one may see the wood rather than the trees; and from this vantage point it does appear, as I hope I shall be able to demonstrate, that one possible difficulty in our attempts at evaluation is the relative contribution we expect of the generalist and the specialist in the common task. I do ask pardon, however, for stating my case rather baldly and brashly, for overstating it in places, and for contradicting myself at one stage in the main thesis of the argument.

THE PARADOX

Brain operations for mental disease are too important to evaluate, too important not to evaluate.

INTRODUCTION

Of all the therapies available to the psychiatrist, brain surgery deserves the most rigorous evaluation. The most rigorous method we have of evaluating a new treatment is to compare it is a randomised trial with the best available conventional treatment. After 43 years of psychosurgical practice, there is no reported instance in the literature of a patient being randomised between psychiatric surgery and non-surgical treatment.

The three preceding statements underlie the paradox of psychosurgical evaluation.

I will not argue the case for the first statement; suffice it to say that the decision to advise referral for evaluation by a psychosurgical team is one of the most important a psychiatrist is likely to make. There are not only the usual hopes and anxieties about a grave procedure; there are also specific anxieties about the effect of damage to that part of the brain which deals with feeling and higher mental function; and there is the ever-present awareness of hostility to psychosurgery both within the profession and outside it. In these circumstances the psychiatrist should have exceptionally fool-proof evidence on which to base his decision and by which he can justify it to the patient, the relatives, the general practitioner, his junior medical staff

and the other members of his multi-disciplinary team – all of whom are likely
to have strong and usually negative feelings about psychosurgery.

Nor will I argue the case for the randomised trial; this has been given a
recent exposition[6] and those who do not accept it now are not likely to be
influenced by anything that can be said here.

Rather I will devote this paper to an exploration for the reasons for the
third statement. The lack of randomised trials has been documented and deplored
in the literature with reference-clogging regularity[7] and strong pleas for such
trials have been made in the editorial columns of medical journals at least
since 1962.[9,10] It has been assumed that the situation they deplore is due to
inertia. This may not be true, and we should consider the possibility that
there is some real impediment to a randomised trial of psychosurgery, which if
discovered might be overcome; but if left covert might block our research for
many years. Anticipating the results of my own thinking, it seems likely that
there is a serious impediment which derives from that very importance of
psychosurgery which makes evaluation so necessary. But first I will consider
some other possible impediments which may seem fanciful or even cynical.

POSSIBLE IMPEDIMENTS

Resources. The pharmaceutical companies dispense large sums for the
evaluation of drugs, but they are not interested in surgical treatment. This
might account for some of the hundreds of controlled trials of psychotropic
drugs, but it cannot account for the complete absence of trials of surgery
because other sources of funds are available. Moreover, the element of
randomisation in drug trials has been introduced not so much on the initiative
of the drug companies but because of adverse editorial and other commentary on
uncontrolled trials. Considerable resources of time and money have been devoted
to uncontrolled evaluation of psychosurgery. Randomisation is cheap; it is the
pre- and post- operative evaluation that is expensive.

Administration. The very small proportion of patients who might be suitable
for surgery raises a problem. However, now that psychosurgery is largely
confined to specialist units which carry out something in the region of 50 to
100 operations a year, this should no longer apply. Patients are considered
carefully for surgery by a multi-disciplinary panel consisting of at least a
surgeon and a psychiatrist. There is no administrative reason why a
randomisation element should not be introduced at this stage.

In the proceedings of the Fourth World Congress, the research committee of
the Royal College of Psychiatrists presented a protocol of a trial[10] in which it

was planned that the college would co-operate with two well known psychosurgical teams. This trial has unfortunately been abandoned, but not for lack of potentially competent administration.

Politics. There is a certain amount of public feeling hostile to psychosurgery, and it may be that grant-giving bodies close to the government do not wish to appear to be supporting "experiments" on the human brain. Such considerations do not appear to have influenced the fate of the Royal College trial. Our Department of Health is already perceived to be supporting psychosurgery, and a controlled trial would give it evidence on the basis of which it could either justify its support or withdraw it.

In recent years the West has been rightly critical of the abuse of psychiatry for political purposes in the Soviet Union. There are several aspects of our own psychiatry which could be critisised in return, and psychosurgery is one of them. Stalin banned psychosurgery in the Soviet Union in 1944; his successors could claim that we are using it to silence those members of our society whose depression, anxiety or aggression is a manifestation of their inability to cope with our competitive capitalist culture. In the face of such potential critisism it would be useful to have the most rigorous evidence that operated patients, when compared to non-operated controls, showed not only a reduction of complaints but an actual improvement in the quality of their lives.

Unethical to do dummy operations. Some dummy operations have been performed, but unfortunately the results have only been reported anecdotally.[11] There are arguments for and against such procedures, and my own personal preference,[12] in the unfortunate event of being a patient in a randomised trial of psychosurgery, would be to have a dummy operation and not to know I was in a trial. However, the weight of opinion is against dummy operations,[13] and it is unlikely that a protocol which included them would be accepted by ethical committees or funding organisations.

The lack of dummy operations in the control group creates two difficulties; a placebo effect cannot be ruled out, and the rating of outcome cannot be completely double-blind. Although a placebo effect may seem unlikely with follow-up at one or two years, it cannot be ruled out. The lack of double-blind ratings should not be so much of a problem with relatively objective measures applied by independent and impartial raters. However, scientists tend to be pernickety people and it may be that, to some extent, the evaluation of psychosurgery has been impeded by the feeling that "if a thing can't be done properly, it is not worth doing at all".

Of course, from the point of view of the patient, it does not really matter whether the improvement is due to operation or placebo and what the referring psychiatrist wants to know is whether his referral will increase his patient's chance of recovery; it would be interesting, to it clinically irrelevant, to know which component of the treatment programme was effective. If a placebo effect cannot be obtained in any other way, then let it be obtained by operation.

Possibly the introduction of a new technique might help to overcome this problem? Lesions have been successfully induced on both simian and human brain by induction heating.[14] In this technique a piece of electro-magnetically sensitive metal is placed at the target site in the brain, and at a later date the lesion is created by placing the patient's head in an electro-megnetic field — the metal becomes hot and destroys the surrounding tissue. A very felicitous property of some metals is that they have specific temperatures above which they cease to take up electro-magnetic energy, so that by varying the components of an alloy it is possible to create an implant which on induction reaches a constant temperature just above that required to destroy brain tissue — the size of the lesion can then be carefully controlled by varying the duration of the inducing current. The efficacy of the treatment could be estimated by comparing the effects of randomly allocated lesion sizes, or possibly it might be considered ethical to permit, in the control group, a delay of several months between insertion of the implant and the application of the inducing current.

Reluctance to submit skill to evaluation. Not only psychosurgery but also psychotherapy has been found very difficult to evaluate, and one thing that psychotherapy and psychosurgery have in common is the need for considerable skill, acquired over a long period of training, on the part of the practitioner. To administer a relatively new psychotropic drug, on the other hand, requires relatively little skill specific to that drug. It is one thing to carry out a trial which may show that a drug is without therapeutic value — it is quite another thing to take part in a trial which may show that one's surgical technique is ineffective. Nevertheless, this was not a problem in the case of the Royal College trial, where the co-operation of two surgical teams was freely offered.

The problems of evaluating psychosurgery and psychotherapy are different, and this suggests that their common element of skill may not be relevant. The main problem encountered in a psychotherapy trial[3] was an insistence on the part of the therapists to include only "eminently suitable" cases in the trial, making it virtually impossible to achieve the requisite numbers. One objection to the Royal College psychosurgery trial was the insistance of the psychosurgical teams

on excluding very suitable cases so that they could receive surgery without risk
of allocation to the control group; they were confident that their skill could
be amply demonstrated on less than "ideal" patients.   It is this firm belief of
psychosurgical teams in the effectiveness of their treatment which gives rise
to the next impediment, which I suspect is the most important of all.

   Ethical Conflict between present and future patients.   The profession as a
whole has a general ethical duty to evaluate new treatments so that the
advantages and disadvantages may be known for the benefit of future patients.
This general ethical duty leads to the carrying out of randomised controlled
trials.   It conflicts with the individual ethical duty to the patient who
presents for treatment, to whom one's duty is to advise on the best treatment
available.   Most doctors would interpret this rather ambiguous word "best" to
mean, not what appears best from a statistical review of the literature, but
what the doctor concerned really believes is best for the patient, after taking
the statistical review of the literature into consideration along with a lot of
other factors.

   If a treatment is perceived as very important it is likely to be invested
with strong belief either for or against, even in the absence of evidence on
which to base the belief − this is a property of belief which is not only
evident from everyday experience but is predicted from cognitive dissonance
theory.[15]   In the case of an important treatment, it is therefore difficult to
maintain that attitude of doubt which is necessary for a randomised trial.
Furthermore, the more important the treatment, the more exactly must be balanced
the possible advantages and disadvantages for randomisation to be acceptable.
Finally, the more concerned a person is with the treatment the more likely he
is to have strong beliefs about it.

   In view of these considerations, it would be unrealistic to expect the
members of a psychosurgical team not to believe in the effectiveness of their
treatment.   And if they have such a belief, how can they participate in a
decision to randomise a patient in such a way that he has to accept a 50−50
chance (or any chance, for that matter) of being denied the only treatment which
can help him?

   According to this view of ethics, psychosurgical teams cannot take part in
randomised trials, and randomised trials of psychosurgery cannot be done without
psychosurgical teams.   If our profession is ethical, randomised trials of psychosurgery are impossible.   Therefore, the absence of reports of randomised trials
in the literature is not so much a disgrace to our general ethics as a tribute
to the individual professional ethics of those who have practised psychosurgery

in the past – a considerable tribute, in view of the pressures to which they have
been subjected.

IMPORTANCE OF THE FLOW DIAGRAM

Who, if anyone, is in a position to advise a patient to enter a randomised
trial of psychosurgery, knowing that he would give the same advice to his sister
or his mother-in-law, and feel confident afterwards that he had done the very
best for his patient? Certainly, as I have argued above, no member of a
psychosurgical team – even if any were undecided at the beginning of the trial
it is almost certain that they would have formed a view either for or against
before the trial was far advanced. Randomisation therefore cannot take place
after referral to the psychosurgical unit, at which time the members of that
unit take over clinical charge of the patient. The Royal College trial was
doomed either to stagnate or to place intolerable ethical strains on the staff
because it had the following flow diagram:

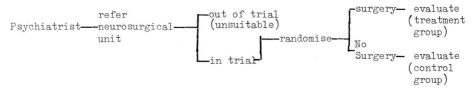

For some reason we have become obsessed in the design of our trials with the
idea that the specialist should be closely concerned with the randomisation
procedure, in spite of the impossible situation to which this method of
organisation gives rise. Let us consider the experience of an attempt to
evaluate psychotherapy,[3] which might well have appeared in the final report of
the Royal College trial of psychosurgery if that had ever been mounted:

"The investigating team itself must, of necessity, contain members who are
experienced in the therapy under examination; they are much more troubled by
ethical problems than other members of the team, who see the study simply as
an attempt to evaluate a treatment the effectiveness of which has not yet been
established". One hundred and thirteen patient were referred to this trial, of
whom 8 were accepted by the evaluating panel. What we must question is the
necessity for the investigating team to contain members who are experienced in
the therapy under examination, for this clearly does not work either in theory
or in practice. For a trial of psychosurgery we might propose the following
flow diagram:

344

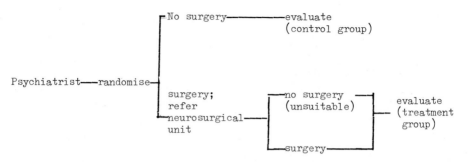

There are disadvantages in this flow diagram, but they are not insuperable.
A proportion of the treatment group would be found unsuitable by the psychosurgical team and would not have the treatment. This does not matter provided
it is a relatively small proportion. In any trial some of the treatment group
do not get treatment. In a drug trial they may fail to take their drugs, or
they may be fast metabolisers of drugs and not achieve a therapeutic blood
level on the schedule permitted in the trial. Even when surgery is given,
there may be a proportion of patients in whom the lesion is not made in the
right place. Such untreated patients in the treatment group merely reduce the
mean treatment effect; they do not negate the trial, they just increase the
sample size required to detect a treatment effect of any given size.

Pre-trial ratings could not be made under controlled conditions in the
psychosurgical unit. Even if pre-trial ratings were considered necessary, and
many would argue that they are not, all patients could be visited at home or
in hospital after randomisation and before referral of the treatment group.

The most serious objection is that even general psychiatrists with no
particular experience of psychosurgery are likely to have beliefs about its
efficacy, even though they may be irrational. And certainly after one referral
belief is likely to develop depending on the outcome of that one case.
Therefore if a small group of referring psychiatrists is selected and trained
in the indications for surgery, the supply of patients to the trial is likely
to dry up. It would be realistic to expect one referral from each psychiatrist;
in fact there are good reasons for asking each psychiatrist to refer 2 well-
matched patients at the same time, one of whom would be allocated to the
treatment group and one to the control group. It is possible that there are
enough psychiatrists with an interest in psychosurgery and a very genuine doubt
about its efficacy to make a randomised trial possible without any compromising
of ethical standards.

THE ETHICS OF DOUBT OR DOUBTFUL ETHICS

Let us imagine, in the distant past, two general practitioners meeting in their club and discussing the claim of Arbuthnot Lane that neurasthenia is due to toxins entering the system from the large bowel and that he can cure it by means of total colectomy. We can sympathise with their interest, as they each have a patient with a long-standing neurasthenia which has proved unresponsive to all known remedies. We can also sympathise if they show scepticism and are worried about the possible adverse effects of total colectomy. Each might be in a state of genuine doubt about whether to refer his patient. It would be quite reasonable for them to decide to refer one patient and see what happened to him or her before sending the second. But which patient to refer? Which of the two should make the referral? In this situation I do not think it would be unethical for them to toss a coin to make the decision for them. And thus an element of randomisation can be introduced into a grave treatment decision without the ethical standards of either being brought into doubt.

Let us now turn our imagination to the consulting room of Arbuthnot Lane, who has spent several years perfecting the technique of total colectomy and advising patients to undergo the procedure. How will he feel if he has finally been persuaded by professional opinion to subject his operation to controlled evaluation? Can we envisage the mental process by which he advises a patient that it is in her best interest if he tosses a coin to decide whether to operate on her or not? Can we imagine the great surgeon telling his patient that his operation is of such doubtful value that she would be just as well off without it? And, if she is allocated to the control group, what will she say to her general practitioner who has spent several months persuading her to accept referral to the surgeon and representing colectomy as her only remaining chance of leading a normal life? This hypothetical situation jars on my sense of ethics and also on my sense of what is correct professional behaviour between the general practitioner and the specialist.

Before the days of clinical trials evaluation (such as it was) took the form of evaluation of the claims of the specialist by the generalist who referred him patients. Only the generalist could afford to have doubt, and to express his doubt to the patient. For some reason, with the introduction of modern clinical science, we have abandoned this form of procedure and have had the expectation that the specialist should evaluate his own treatment, or at least be clinically involved with its evaluation. This only works with relatively unimportant treatments in which it is possible to fudge the ethical issue, and in which the thought of benefit to patients in the future can distract the mind from the fact that the advice being given to the patient on the other side of the table is not the very best that one could give. I have had this experience personally and I imagine it must be not uncommon in specialist centres.

Every level of specialisation should be evaluated by the level below. In the case of psychosurgery, psychosurgical teams should be evaluated by general psychiatrists, who should be evaluated by general practitioners, who should be evaluated by non-medical representatives of the general public. This is the only ethical flow-diagram of evaluation, and even then it may be impossible to find sufficient genuine doubt on the part of the referring doctors to justify randomisation unless the doubt is augmented by shortage of the treatment concerned.

SHORTAGE OF CLINICAL FACILITY

If a treatment is not only of doubtful efficacy but is also in short supply, its evaluation becomes very much easier. Thus because of shortage of drug supplies the Medical Research Council was able to mount an excellent randomised trial of streptomycine in the treatment of pulmonary tuberculosis in 1947. If the demand for psychosurgery in an area was more than twice the capacity of the local psychosurgical unit, that unit could quite ethically accept patients only from the randomising agency of the trial. In fact it would be more ethical to do this than to favour any other method of selection, since each patient who required surgery would have an equal chance of getting it. Such a method of selection might be more humane than attrition on a long waiting list, and since all patients would be severely ill a selection procedure according to severity would not be appropriate.

If all referrals for psychosurgery went through a randomisation procedure, the ethical problem for the referring psychiatrist would disappear. He could refer all patients whom he felt might benefit from surgery, knowing that half of them would be evaluated by the psychosurgical team and knowing that the other half could not have surgery anyway. He could advise his patients to their best advantage without any shadow of an ethical doubt — in fact, with an assurance which I personally do not believe it would be possible to obtain in any other way.

Naturally, one deplores shortage of opportunities for treatment. But they do occur, and I cannot see any ethical or other reason why they should not be exploited in the interest of controlled evaluation. Psychosurgery is now very unpopular in many areas; due to many factors not the least of which is the influence of the delegates to this conference, it is likely to become much more popular in the future. No doubt the setting up of new psychosurgical teams is likely to lag behind the increasing demand for treatment. One hopes that these new teams would take advantage of their inability to supply demand and begin their practice on a randomised sample of their potential patients, for the imbalance between supply and demand might not last for long.

SUMMARY

There is an ethical conflict between the need to evaluate treatment with randomised trials and the process of advising an individual patient to accept randomisation. The latter requires a genuine doubt about the efficacy of the treatment. Doubt is less likely in the case of important treatments such as psychosurgical operations; it is also less likely in those who are closely concerned in the administration of the treatment. Randomised evaluation is therefore not likely to be successful unless the randomisation occurs before referral to the specialist team; and it will be easier if the specialist team has facilities to treat only a proportion of the potential referrals. The best opportunity for effective evaluation would be the establishment of a psychosurgical team in a country which had previously been unfavourable to psychosurgery, where the local psychiatrists were interested in but doubtful about psychosurgery and possessed the organisation to randomise potential referrals, and where the new psychosurgical team agreed to accept referrals only from the randomising organisation.

REFERENCES

1. Spodick, D.H., Aronow, W., Barber, B., Blackburn, H., Boyd, D., Conti, C.R., Loberfo, J.P., Lown, B., Mathus, V.S., McIntosh, H.D., Preston, J.A., Selzer, A. and Takaro, T. (1978) Lancet 1, 1213–1214.
2. Editorial (1978) Brit. Med. Journal 2, 1438–1439
3. Candy, J., Balfour, F.H., Cawley, R.H., Hildebrand, H.P., Malan, P.H., Marks, I.M. and Wilson, J. (1972) Psychol. Med. 2, 345–362
4. Blackwell, B. and Shepherd, M. (1967) Lancet 2, 819–822.
5. Davis, J.M. (1976) Am. J. Psychiat. 133, 1–13.
6. Byar, D.P., Simon, R.M., Friedwald, W.T., Schlesselman, J.J., DeMets, D.L. Ellenburg, J.H., Gail, M.H. and Ware, J.H. (1976) New Eng. J. Med. 295, 78–80
7. Templer, D.I., (1974) Biol. Psychiat. 9, 205–209
8. Editorial (1962) Lancet 2, 1037–1038.
9. Editorial (1971) Brit. Med. J. 3, 595–596
10. Research Committee of the Royal College of Psychiatrists (1977) in Neurosurgical Treatment in Psychiatry, Pain and Epilepsy, Sweet, W.H., Obrador, S.,and Martin-Rodriguez, J.G., ed., Univ. Park Press, Baltimore, pp. 175–188
11. Livingston, K.E., (1953) Assoc. Res. Nerv. Ment. Dis, 31, 374–378
12. Price J.S. (1978) Brit. Med. J. 2, 1200–1201

13. Laitinen, L.V. (1977) in Neurosurgical Treatment in Psychiatry, Pain and Epilepsy, Sweet, W.H., Obrador, S. and Martin-Rodriguez, J.G. ed., Univ. Park Press, Baltimore, pp. 483-488
14. Merry, G.A., Hale, R. and Zervas, N.T. (1973) IEEE Transactions on Biomedical Engineering 20, 302-303.
15. Chapanis N.P. and Chapanis A. (1964) Psychol. Bull. 61, 1-22.
16. Paul, N.L., Fitzgerald, E. and Greenblatt, M. (1956) J. am. med. Ass. 161, 815-820

AFTERTHOUGHT

If it had been possible for me to give this paper in Boston as I would dearly have liked, I would have spoken about Henry Cabot Lodge and the Cambridge-Somerville youth study. It is tantalising to think that such an excellent randomised trial could have been designed and implemented in the nineteen thirties, before the introduction of psychiatric surgery to Massachusetts. Even in psychiatric surgery the Bostonians were ahead of their time and produced the only randomised trial of different psychosurgical operations ever to be reported[16] if the influence of Lodge had been greater the Boston Psychopathic Hospital trial might have had larger numbers, independent evaluation and a non-operated control group. In that case, I suspect that either we would now be attending the Twentieth International Congress of Psychiatric Surgery, or we would not be here at all.

ACKNOWLEDGEMENT

I should like to thank my fellow members of the erstwhile Psychosurgery Subcommittee of the Research Committee of the Royal College of Psychiatrists, and particularly its chairman Dr. Brian Barraclough, who stimulated my interest in the field of psychiatric surgery and who taught me most of what little I know of it.

© 1979 Elsevier/North-Holland Biomedical Press
Modern Concepts in Psychiatric Surgery
E.R. Hitchcock, H.T. Ballantine, Jr. and B.A. Meyerson, eds.

PAST AND PRESENT TRENDS OF PSYCHIATRIC SURGERY IN JAPAN

SADAO HIROSE

Department of Neuropsychiatry, Nippon Medical School, Sendagi, Bunkyo-ku,
Tokyo (Japan)

Before starting this short report, I wish to pay tribute to the late great
Professor Antonio Egas Moniz as a pioneer of psychosurgery and a Nobel Prize
winner.

I had the privilege of communicating with Professor Egas Moniz only once.
I received a cordial letter with a picture of himself of March 28th, 1955,
also one with his monograph on psychosurgery and some other reprints of his
work. I can't forget the memory of that occasion.

In Japan the first brain operation for mental disorder was performed in
November 1938 by Mizuho Nakata (1893-1975) of Niigata Medical College, who
was a pioneer of neurosurgery in our country, using prefrontal lobectomy for
disturbed schizophrenia, epilepsy, and hyperkinetic idiocy, and had been used
in 52 cases by 1941. In January 1942, Nakata applied Freeman and Watts'
prefrontal lobotomy procedure for mental disorder inspired by an epoch-making
monograph written by Egas Moniz, "Tentatives Opératoires dans le Traitment
de Certaines Psychoses", and Freeman and Watts' papers on prefrontal lobotomy.
He reported the results of his operations during the World War in 1942 at
the annual meeting of the Japanese Society of Psychiatry and Neurology, but
most of the psychiatrists did not have an interest in such a neurosurgical
treatment for psychiatric patients and some psychiatrists were rather sceptical
of the operative results. Moreover, owing to the cultural isolation during
the wartime, very few psychosurgical operations were performed in Japan until
1945.

Immediately after the World War released Japan from such an international
isolation, the American Medical Sciences were introduced into Japan with
a rush.

In 1946, Paul Schrader, who was working for the U.S. Armed Forces retained
in Osaka as a medical officer, introduced the surgical approach to the treatment of mental disorders in the United States of America. In 1947, the 12th
General Assembly of the Japan Medical Congress was held in Osaka and some
of the papers on psychosurgery were adopted at the meeting, especially
Schrader's special lecture on "Indications and After-Treatment of Prefrontal
Lobotomy", which was a hilight in the Surgical Section. From that point on

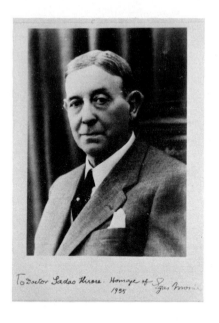

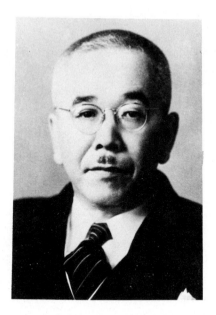

Fig. 1.   Egas Moniz (1874-1955)   Fig. 2.   Mizuho Nakata (1893-1975)

prefrontal lobotomy became acceptable, and many Japanese psychiatrists and
surgeons were employed in the work. Several thousands psychosurgical operations have been performed in Japan since that time. In those days, I was
a young psychiatrist at Matsuzawa Mental Hospital of Metropolitan Tokyo,
and I was very much impressed by a lot of articles concerning frontal lobes
and psychosurgical problems in the American Journal of Psychiatry, Archives
of Neurology and Psychiatry, the Journal of Nervous and Mental Disease, and
so on.

   During the wartime most of the young doctors underwent military service
as medical officers of the Japanese Army or Navy. Some of them were trained
in surgery, including brain surgery. During the period 1942 to 1945 I was
mostly engaged in surgery and neuropsychiatry in the Japanese Navy as a medical
officer. When I returned to the Department of Neuropsychiatry at the University of Tokyo and then began to work at Matsuzawa Mental Hospital, I saw

many disturbed patients who unfortunately remained in the hospital in spite
of any somatic treatment such as ECT, Insulin coma treatment, and continuous
sleep treatment. And I planned to treat them via prefrontal lobotomy. So,
I frequently visited a national hospital in Tokyo and learned from the neurosurgical operations. After that I performed my first operation of prefrontal
lobotomy on a 34-year-old female schizophrenic patient, who had suffered for
more than ten years.

On May 4th, 1948 the first meeting of the Japanese Society for the Study
of Brain Surgery was held in Niigata Medical College in collaboration with
Professor Nakata and Professor Makoto Saito (1889-1951) of Nagoya. I attended
this meeting twenty five years ago with excitement immediately after the annual
meeting of the Japanese Society of Psychiatry and Neurology in Kanazawa, where
I read my paper, "Prefrontal Leucotomy in 37 Cases". It was a nostalgic and
memorable event. At the meeting, Nakata presented an important paper, "On
the Limit of Effectiveness of the Frontal Lobotomy" and we had a lot of heated
discussion between psychiatrists and surgeons. By the way, neurosurgery in
Japan had not separated from general surgery by 1951.

On September 1st, 1948 Professor Percival Bailey came to Japan as a consultant physician to the Far East General Headquarters and gave a special lecture
on "Recent Developments in Neurology" at the University of Tokyo. He strongly
criticized the prefrontal lobotomy, transorbital lobotomy, and topectomy
procedures. Since then, psychosurgery in Japan entered a critical period.
In September 1949, a special issue on "Criticism on Prefrontal Lobotomy" by
some psychiatrists, including myself, appeared in a Japanese Journal, "Brain
and Nerve".

In April 1950, at the 47th annual meeting of the Japanese Society of Psychiatry and Neurology in Kyoto, two special reports on prefrontal lobotomy
were presented. One of them was "Psychosurgical Treatment in Psychiatry"
by Hidezo Nakagawa of Sapporo, a psychiatrist and another one was "Functional
Brain Surgery for Extrapyramidal Hyperkinesia" by Hiroshi Takebayashi of Osaka,
a surgeon. Nakagawa reviewed statistical data of 2,000 cases from 28 hospitals
in Japan and the operative results were good in 33.9 per cent, fair in 24.3
per cent, poor in 28.1 per cent, worse in 1.6 per cent, and operative deaths
in 3.1 per cent. Also at the meeting, various types of selective lobotomies
were reported. I reported on my experience in orbital leucotomy (sections
of the orbital areas only by Hofstatter et al.) and Narabayashi et al. reported on "Stereotaxic Instrument for Operation on Basal Ganglia".

In the same year, a heated discussion on indications, postoperative personality changes, and working mechanisms of psychosurgery between Hirose and Nakagawa came out in the Japanese Medical Journal. These articles caused a great sensation among psychiatrists and surgeons.

In January 1951, I published a monograph on "Prefrontal Lobotomy" for the first time in Japan and afterwards in that year Nakagawa also published a monograph on "Surgical Treatment for Mental Disorder".

Between March and July, 1956 Professor Gösta Rylander of Stockholm, who is here today, stayed in Pusan, Korea as a Commanding Officer of the Swedish Red Cross Field Hospital and often came to Tokyo. He told me that the better way to perform Scoville's cortical undercutting method by suction. So I wrote to Dr. Scoville and I received his very kind letter with some reprints of his paper on cortical undercutting and its congeners. Immediately, I adopted selective cortical undercutting method and performemed this type of operation on 16 cases. Then I initiated an improved method of orbito-ventromedial undercutting, which is characterized by focusing upon much more restricted areas of operative lesions compared with Scoville's orbital undercutting, and I performed this method on 123 cases between July 1957 and June 1972. Following the development of psychotropic drugs since the middle part of the 1950's, a marked world-wide decline in the number of psychosurgical operations has been observed in Japan. But, I have continued my operations for very carefully selected cases until 1972.

On a terribly hot summer day, namely on July 28th 1956, Rylander gave a guest-lecture, "Mental Symptoms and Therapeutic Results after Different Types of Frontal Lobe Operations in Mental Disorder", at the University of Tokyo, Medical School. His lecture awoke the great interest of a large audience, at a time when psychosurgery had declined.

In April 1959, the 15th General Assembly of the Japan Medical Congress was held in Tokyo and the subject "Functional Brain Surgery" was taken up at one of the plenery sessions. The titles of the session and the panelists were as follows: 'Psychosurgery - Evaluation of 406 Cases' by Hirose,'Stereotaxic Pallidotomy and Ventrolateral Thalamotomy for the Extrapyramidal Disorders' by Narabayashi, 'Cerebral Hemispherectomy' by Ueki, 'Surgery of Epilepsy' by Shimizu, and 'Experience of Epilepsy Operation' by Araki.

Since January 1960, I have been a professor of Neuropsychiatry at Nippon Medical School. Through June 1972 I had operated on 83 cases by orbito-ventromedial undercutting after strict case selection in good cooperation with our neuropsychiatric staff.

At the same time, Sano carried out the stereotaxic posteromedial hypothala-

motomy for severe aggressive or violent behavior in 1962 and stereotaxic
amygdalotomy was first introduced by Narabayashi for control of abnormal
behavior such as aggressiveness, violence, and erethistic feeble-mindedness
in children in 1963.

From the beginning of the introduction of psychosurgery in Japan, some
psychiatrists have maintained a sceptical and contradictory attitude toward
the psychosurgical operation. Recently, radical psychiatrists oppose the
use of psychosurgery just as in the United States. Actually, three lobotomized
patients supported by some anti-psychosurgery groups of radical psychiatrists
are still in litigation to demand compensation from the Japanese Government
or doctors, who were concerned in the operation.

Moreover, since 1969 the Japanese Society of Psychiatry and Neurology
and some psychiatric departments of national universities have been continuously in the vortex of controversy. The radical psychiatrist and student radicals
have continuously been proposing prohibition on the use of psychosurgical
operations including brain stimulation and cerebral biopsy. They fear that
the operations might be misused to supress the political activists with undesirable ideas. Owing to such unavoidable circumstances I have not done
my operation since 1973. Recently the Japanese Society of Psychiatry and
Neurology introduced a resolution opposing the use of psychosurgery for any
types of psychiatric patients, because the majority of the members of the
board of directors were dominated by the radical psychiatrists. I think
they are alarmist and hold extreme, onesided, dogmatic views. I hope that
"after rain comes fair weather", but I feel very pessimistic. Anyway, we
are awaiting sound developments.

Concerning my operative series of 523 cases since 1947 I have already
reported at the World Congress of Psychiatry and the World Congress of
Psychiatric Surgery every time[1-6]. New Year's Day and midsummer in Japan
is a good time for general remembrances. I have continued to send out my
greeting cards in both season to my patients who underwent my operation as
much as possible, and often patients spontaneously write notes to give me
news of their progress. I know even now by personal communication with my
patients that more than one hundred among them are still working or keeping
house adequately. They have shown the long duration of the improvement.
There are professors and scholars, business and professional men, a female
medical practioner, and housewives. They have mostly made progressively
better social adjustment in the later years following the psychosurgical
operation. Once in a while, some of them visit my home or our clinic in

354

order to renew their old friendship with me.

Finally, I would like to relate a most dramatic example of superior social adjustment following my orbito-ventromedial undercutting. This case was reported at the Copenhagen meeting[4] in 1970.

A 37-year-old male statistician had suffered from a periodic schizophrenic disorder with an atypical clinical picture at the age of 23, when he was a university student, and showed varying clinical features often associated with exhausted depressive state, stupor, perplexity, delusions of reference and persecution, emotional turmoil, insomnia, anxiety, and excessive worry. His father's personality was syntonic and harmonious. His mother showed viscous personality. His maternal aunt died in a psychotic state in a mental hospital. The patient had been a sensitive, serious, intellectual, conscientious, hardworking, good-natured, and attractive premorbid personality. He had highest intellectual power. He graduated from the University of Tokyo School of Physical Science and was employed in the Japanese Prime Minister's Office as a statistical officer of great ability, but soon after this employment he had his second nervous breakdown. Thereafter he had numerous attacks of an acute schizophrenic nature, appearing always under the strain of the hard work required. He had been hospitalized five times during thirteen years before the operation. He made a complete recovery under ECT, insulin coma treatment, and various neuroleptics or antidepressants, but relapsed each time. He underwent my orbito-ventromedial undercutting on June 28, 1967. Within a month after the operation he became hypomanic with loss of inhibition. Two months after the operation he returned to his job. On March 31, 1969 he married a girl friend who worked in the same office. In April 1970 he took an official trip to Okinawa and also in June of the year he represented Japan at the ECAFE (the Economic Commission for Asia and the Far East) meeting in Bangkok, Thailand. Thereafter he wrote some papers on stochastics or mathematical statistics. In April 1973, six years after the operation, he was appointed a professor of statistics at a national university of commerce and works full time. In 1975 he published a monograph, "An Introduction to Statistics" from a famous publishing company in Tokyo. At present, over eleven years after the operation, he works teaching, studying, attending the congress, and so on. He visits my home or our clinic once or twice a year and does not show any personality deficit. He is sensitive even now, but he is controlling himself adequately.

Figure 3 shows the lateral extent of my operation by use of tantalum powder as a marking substance.

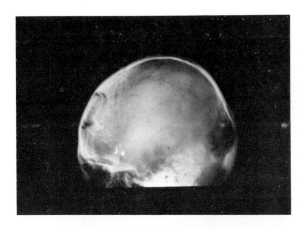

Fig. 3. Case 100, 37-year-old male, who operated upon June 28, 1967. Tantalum powder demonstrating the lateral extent of orbito-ventromedial undercutting, extending approximately 4 cm posteriorly from the frontal tips.

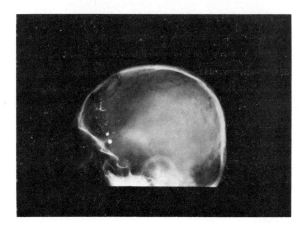

Fig. 4. Tantalum powder demonstrating the lateral extent tenyears and four months following the operation. The position of tantalum powder is still the same.

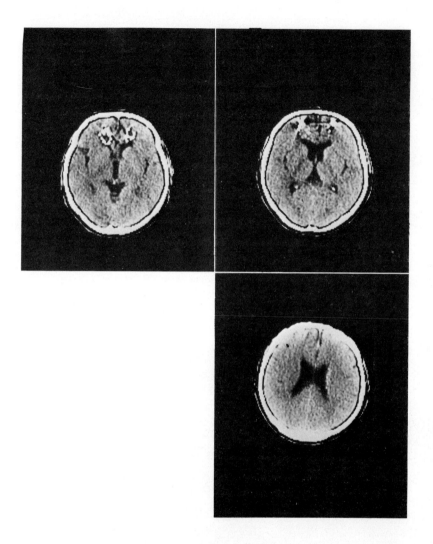

Fig. 5. Computed tomography performed by EMI scanner CT 1010 ten years and four months after the operation. There are sliced in parallel with OM line. There is a ring like high density due to tantalum powder in bilateral orbito-medial frontal regions, however no ventricular dilatation, cortical atrophy, or cystic change can be observed.

Figure 4 shows the same lateral roentgenogram ten years and four months after the operation. The position of tantalum powder is still the same.

Figures 5, 6, and 7 show computed tomography performed by EMI scanner CT 1010 ten years and four months after the operation. There are sliced in parallel with OM line. There is a ring like high density due to tantalum powder in bilateral orbitomedial frontal regions, however no ventricular dilatation, cortical atrophy or cystic change can be observed.

In concluding my speech, I would like to say again, the prejudice that all psychosurgical operations are followed by undesirable deficit of personality and damage to human dignity ought to be dispelled. I expect the operation will be resumed for most tortured patients in the near future.

ACKNOWLEDGEMENTS

My thanks are due to Professor Shozo Nakazawa in the Department of Neurosurgery and Dr. Kazuyoshi Honda in the Department of Radiology at Nippon Medical School, for helping criticism on the findings of computed tomography.

REFERENCES

1. Hirose, S. (1962) Psychosurgery 1947-1960. Evaluation of 450 Patients Treated by Prefrontal Lobotomy and a New Method of Orbito-Ventromedial Undercutting. Proceedings of the Third World Congress of Psychiatry, Vol. 1 (Montreal), pp. 138-141.

2. Hirose, S. (1965) Orbito-Ventromedial Undercutting 1957-1963. Follow-up of 77 Cases. Amer. J. Psychiat. 121, 1194-1202.

3. Hirose, S, (1966) Present Trends in Psychosurgery. Folia Psychiat. Neuro. Japon. 20, 361-379.

4. Hirose, S. (1972) The Case Selection of Mental Disorder for Orbito-Ventromedial Undercutting. IN: Psychosurgery (Eds. Hitchcock, Laitinen, & Vaernet) pp. 291-303. Charles C. Thomas, Springfield, Ill.

5. Hirose, S. (1973) Long-Term Evaluation of Orbito-Ventromedial Undercutting in "Atypical" Schizophrenic Patients. In: Surgical Approaches in Psychiatry (Eds. Laitinen & Livingston), pp. 196-205. University Park Press, Baltimore.

6. Hirose, S. (1977) Psychiatric Evaluation of Psychosurgery. In: Neurosurgical Treatment in Psychiatry, Pain, and Epilepsy (Eds. Sweet, Obrador, & Martín-Rodrígues), pp. 203-209. University Park Press, Baltimore.

© 1979 Elsevier/North-Holland Biomedical Press
Modern Concepts in Psychiatric Surgery
E.R. Hitchcock, H.T. Ballantine, Jr. and B.A. Meyerson, eds.

SOME THOUGHTS ON THE ANTI-PSYCHOSURGERY ATTITUDE IN SWEDEN

PER MINDUS MD

Psychiatric unit, Department of Neurosurgery, The Karolinska Hospital,
S-104 01 Stockholm, Sweden

Communication at the V World Congress of Psychiatric Surgery, Boston 1978.

ABSTRACT. In his editorial (the Bulletin 8, 9, 1978), Meyerson challenges
psychiatrists for their biased and ignorant attitude to psychiatric surgery. He expresses the hope that more research and information would promote
a dialogue between neurosurgeons and general psychiatrists, but fails to
indicate anything that would render such information efficacious. Being a
psychiatrist myself, I should like to discuss some of the psychological
mechanisms which may be thought to underlie the sometimes unduly critical
attitude to psychiatric surgery taken by many psychiatrists and laymen, at
least in Sweden. I believe that an insight in these mechanisms would improve the way in which researchers in the field of psychiatric surgery inform their colleagues and patients, thereby promoting the dialogue. Some
mechanisms may be denoted 1.anxiety reactions, 2.defensive reactions and
3.transference reactions. Some consequences of anxiety-provoking features
of psychiatric surgery will be discussed, focussing on the patient, his
relatives, members of the general psychiatric team, the neurosurgeon himself, and the general public. Some defensive reactions will be described
such as rationalization or denial of the "side-effects" of no treatment at
all. It is illustrated how classical lobotomy is projecting its shadow on
modern psychiatric surgery by means of a transference reaction influencing
peoples' attitudes and actions. Some measures to counteract the non-objective anti-psychosurgery attitude will be discussed and hints will be given
on how to improve the way in which advocates of psychiatric surgery may
reply to their critics.

INTRODUCTION

   Meyerson probably speaks for many neurosurgeons interested in psychiatric surgery when he states that: "I had the impression that among some
of the psychiatrists the attitude towards psychiatric surgery is a result
of ideology, rather than of an unbiased evaluation of the method as a
treatment of mental disease". (The Bulletin of the International Society
of Psyciatric Surgery, 8, 9, 1978). He expresses the hope that more research and information would promote a dialogue on psychiatric surgery

between neurosurgeons and general psychiatrists. But Meyerson fails to indicate anything that would render such information efficacious. I believe that the current information problem has (at least) two aspects. First, one must have something to inform about. As Meyerson points out, very few original publications on psychiatric surgery have appeared lately. It may be added that those which appeared are generally published in proceedings from international meetings and not in psychiatric journals of high repute. Therefore, reports do not get adequate publicity. Secondly, one must know how to inform. Being a psychiatrist myself, I should like to discuss some mechanisms which may be thought to underlie the sometimes unduly critical attitudes to psychiatric surgery taken by most general psychiatrists, clinical psychologists, social workers and laymen, at least in Sweden. I believe that an insight in these aspects may perhaps improve the way in which advocates of psychiatric surgery reply to their critics. Since negative attitudes to psychiatric surgery is by no means limited to Sweden, I hope that the viewpoints below are relevant to the situation also in some other countries.

Before going into detail I hasten to state here that my own experience with psychiatric surgery is very limited. Since 1976 I am working at the Department of Neurosurgery at the Karolinska Hospital, Stockholm, where a neuropsychiatric unit has existed for many years. Patients referred to us by general psychiatrists are independently evaluated by us and closely followed throughout the procedure. We perform anterior capsulotomies with thermolesions or with radiosurgery, so called gamma-capsulotomies on patients with anxiety, phobic or obsessive-compulsive neurosis. I have thus no personal experience of other types or indications of psychiatric surgery. During my psychiatric training, (which included personal analysis and analytic training), I saw patients who were evaluated for psychiatric surgery. The education on psychiatric surgery that I have had was poor and biased and, I believe, representative of the training of most university clinics in my country. (No wonder then, that I experienced myself many of the emotional reactions described below). Scientifically, I have been interested in various aspects of ECT (electro-convulsive treatment). ECT has since long been subject to intensive anti-propaganda in many countries. The psychological roots of these negative feelings have attracted my interest. I have noticed so many similarities between probable mechanisms behind the anti-ECT and the anti-psychosurgery reactions that I feel that a comparison is of relevance when it comes to understanding and counteracting the non-objective anti-psychosurgery attitude.

Classical lobotomy.

The advent to Sweden of classical lobotomy in the late 40-ies implied a considerable improvement in the therapy of mental disorders. Not surprisingly,surgery was tried with enthusiasm as a universal remedy in several mental disorders. It must be remembered that good therapeutic alternatives were nonexistent. As was the case with ECT, the enthusiasm lead to an overuse of the treatment. During the following years undesired side-effects were recorded (in Sweden by Rylander 1948 and by Bingley 1949) and a counter-reaction ensued, which was reinforced when first ECT and later psychotropic drugs became available. Today, most neurosurgeons and psychiatrists would agree that the initial enthusiasm for classical lobotomy was inappropriate but understandable. To my mind, the present negative attitude to psychiatric surgery taken by most workers in the field of psychiatry in Sweden, also seems inappropriate but understandable. As appears to be the case with ECT, some of the possible psychological mechanisms involved may be denoted 1. anxiety reactions 2. defence reactions and 3. transference reactions.

Anxiety reactions.

To the present audience, it may seem redundant to elaborate on the anxiety-provoking features of psychiatric surgical procedures. On the other hand, the neurosurgeon who is repeatedly and extensively exposed to these features may well have become "de-sensitized" and may minimize (or even overlook?) that some aspects of the procedures seem very frightening to the patients. For instance, when informing patients pre-operatively, I have repeatedly noticed that, in particular, the idea of drilling burr holes under local anaesthesia seems frightening. Many individuals have expressed the fear that the burr might perhaps "run into my very brain". Also, thoughts on the insertion of electrodes elicit anxiety reactions. The gamma-capsulotomy, although closed and appealingly "clean", also induces particular anxiety reactions. As one patient put it: "Just the thought of being locked up into that 'igloo' (referring to the shielding) for hours exposed to irradiation freightens me". Obviously, it must take considerable ego strength, motivation, and suffering by the patient to submit himself to psychosurgical treatment.

Anxiety reactions in others than the patient.

Whenever psychiatric surgery is discussed with regard to a particular

patient, anxiety seems to be provoked also in members of the general psychiatric team. As regards the general psychiatrist, that has various consequences. One is that he becomes (actively of passively) disinterested
in a treatment which he believes is harmful, obsolete and un-scientific.
Since he wants to be helpful, modern and scientific, the whole concept of
psychiatric surgery disturbs him and he discourages patients who are candidates. Other psychiatric colleagues simply disregard the very existence of psychiatric surgery an do not care to read and learn anything about
it. Therefore they are not competent to provide patients and their relatives with adequate information. Apparently, anxiety reactions induce a
vicious circle which tends to preserve an ignorant and emotional attitude.
Defensive reactions.

In order to cope with anxiety, we may use various defensive reactions
such as rationalization and denial. In the Swedish debate it is often argued that the mode of action of psychiatric surgery is "unknown". (This
holds true also for ECT). I think that the contributors to this congress
have shown that they now know a great deal about the mode of action of
psychiatric surgery. And knowledge in this field is not less than that
of, say, ECT or psychopharmacology. Another argument is that psychiatric
surgery is "only symptomatic". If this is so, it would certainly not be
unique for psychiatric surgery, since it applies to many forms of therapy
in medicine. Both remarks may be characterized as rationalizations. Another example is the following: When psychiatric surgery is discussed
among general psychiatrists or with the patient, its possible adverse side-effects are often emphasized. But the "side-effects" of no treatment
at all, or the prolongation of ineffective treatment (and suffering), is
not always taken into account. This may perhaps be referred to as denial.
Transference reactions.

As an example of transference reactions I should like to point at the
following: Like ECT, psychiatric surgery has been used now for several
decades. The fact that a modified (!) therapeutic procedure, which is
still in use, is old, would scarcely seem to be a disadvantage. On the
contrary, this would be an indication that it is of value. But when psychiatry is concerned, it probably appears as a disadvantage, because the
modality will easily be associated with therapies used in the past. One
must, of course, condemn the dark sides of old psychiatry and psychosurgery, but it seems that modern psychiatric surgical procedures have to
bear the brunt of criticism more properly aimed at classical lobotomy.

Moreover, it seems that nonpsychiatric interventions in the brain appear
to the general public as "more modern" than psychiatric surgery. Therefore such operations seem less prone to transference reactions, despite
the fact that they contain many technical features that are equally or
more frightening to the patients. (Even some neurosurgeons disapprove of
psychiatric surgery, perhaps on similar grounds). Some senior psychiatrists have recollections of patients who have undergone lobotomy with undesired side-effects. These experiences will of course influence the attitudes of younger colleagues, who, in addition, often prefer non-biolo-
gical therapies, such as psychotherapy. In brief, classical lobotomy is
still projecting its shadow on modern psychiatric surgery. It influences,
by way of a transference reaction, consciously and unconsciously, peoples'
thoughts, attitudes and behaviour. We may disapprove of this - but we
cannot disregard it. Doctor G. Kullberg has called my attention to the
fact that the psychological mechanisms behind the emotional reactions outlined here are eloquently illustrated by Shakespeare in Julius Caesar
(Act 2, scene 2):

> "The evil that men do lives long after them;
> The good is oft interred with their bones."

Some measures to counteract the anti-psychosurgery attitudes.

Given this background, what can be done and what may be said in order
to promote a dialogue on psychiatric surgery between neurosurgeons and
general psychiatrists? Again with reference to the ECT debate, some measures are listed below:

1. High level of competence in the neuropsychiatric team.
2. Limited and well-defined indications.
3. Careful pre- and post-operative evaluations.
4. Careful follow-ups.
5. More basic research.
6. Better clinical research.
7. Adequate information to general psychiatrists.
8. Adequate information to medical students.
9. Adequate information to the general public.

Comments.

I believe that some workers with self-esteem now sit back confortably,

thinking that they, at least, have always taken the above, self-evident
steps. Also, some of them may perhaps think that they know of one or two
colleagues who do not quite live up to these standards. According to the
National Commission Report and other sources researchers in the field of
psychiatric surgery do meet with many but not with all of the above criteria.

Ad 1. This is essential for the creation of a trustful atmosphere within the team and particularly between the team and the patient. Also, I
believe that the psychosurgical team should contain representatives of
different clinical disciplines.

Ad 2. Cases with uncertain or ill-defined diagnosis or so called "hopeless" cases should not be considered for operation. Apart from obvious
ethical contraindications it should be kept in mind that bad results will
compromize the method, and more suitable patients will not be referred.

Ad 3. The neuropsychiatrist should make his evaluation independently
of that of the referring general psychiatrist.

Ad 4. Follow-up evaluations should be made under standardized conditions and with regular intervals and include informations from relatives
or other informants. Independent evaluations by the team's and the referring psychiatrist should be made. Personality inventories, rating
scales and psychometric tests should be given pre- and post-operatively.

Ad 5. More basic experimental research is needed for a better understanding of the effects (and side-effects) of various psychosurgical procedures.

Ad 6. The literature on psychiatric surgery is difficult to evaluate.
Some authors report on small samples with heterogenous diagnoses, targets
(varying in numbers, size and localization) aimed at with differing techniques, results evaluated with un-standardized methods and described in
terms of value judgements ("excellent"), and follow-ups performed with
varying methods at varying (sometimes short) intervals after operation,
all of which underline the need for better clinical research.

Some hints on how to inform.

Ad. 7. 8. 9. When it comes to information, I have noticed that many
senior advocates for psychiatric surgery take a defense position in the
dialogue with general psychiatrists and laymen. They often start by
pointing at positive results, beneficial effects, etc and may wrongly
seem to try to evade the question of side-effects. In the audience, on

the other hand, some may be anxious to hear about the "horrible side-effects" that they think they know of. Therefore they may feel that the speaker tries to hide something and will contemplate what. As a consequence, the audience does not listen to what is said, but to what is not said and the message does not get through. I believe that one way to avoid this lies in using a reverse order of information, as sometimes is done when a serious diagnosis is to be told to an apprehensive patient. The information should perhaps start with the possible drawbacks of the method. Perhaps one should establish frankly, that the mode of action of psychiatric surgery is (relatively) "unknown", that the therapy is "empirical" and "only symptomatic" etc. Perhaps one should admit in a straightforward way that some features of psychiatric surgery are anxiety provoking to the persons concerned. One should perhaps emphasize that, of course, this treatment also has adverse side-effects – most if not all effective therapies have – but that they may not be easily detected with modern psychometric methods. Further, any side-effects of a treatment must be weighed against the effects and side-effects of other treatments for that disorder and with the "side-effect" of no treatment at all. Now that the advocate of psychiatric surgery has himself "admitted" a few things, tension may perhaps decrease in the audience which, hopefully, will sit back and listen. Now time has come to inform on beneficial effects etc.

If no adequate action is taken soon, psychiatric surgery may continue to be as underused today as it was probably overused during its past period. It is a difficult task to inform well on something that so easily evokes strong emotions. But our patients need it – and psychiatric surgery deserves it.

AUTHOR INDEX